Health spaces

Hospital Outdoor Environment

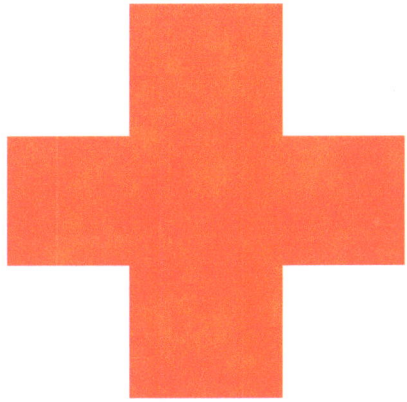

Edited by Francesca Giofrè and Zoran Đukanović

Copyright 2015 Health space. Hospital Outdoor Environment / Edited by Francesca Giofrè and Zoran Đukanović.
Copyright of individual chapters is retained by copyright holders as detailed for each chapter.

All rights reserved for the publisher *Inter-University Research Centre TESIS "Systems and Technologies for Healthcare Buildings"* Univerity of Florece, Street San Niccolò 93, 50125 Florence; Sapienza, University of Rome, Department Planning Design Technology of Architecture, Street Flaminia 72, 00196 Rome.
No part of this publication may be reproduced, stored in a retrieval system or transmitted in any form or by any means electronic, mechanical, photocopying, recording or otherwise without the prior written permission of the publisher. For more information on all TESIS publications visit *http://www.tesis.unifi.it*

Authors: Rosalba Belibani, Nađa Beretić, Ružica Božović-Stamenović, Martina Cardi, Rosalba D'Onofrio, Zoran Đukanović, Anna Maria Giovenale, Francesca Giofrè, Vesna Mandić, Ivana Miletić, Valentina Napoli, Giuseppe Primiceri, Fabio Quici, Tamara Stanisavljević, Ferdinando Terranova, Elio Trusiani
Foreword: Romano Del Nord and Vladan Đokić
Design credits: Nađa Beretić

ISBN: 978-88-907872-9-4

First edition, 2015

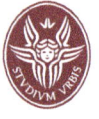

Sapienza University of Rome, Department Planning Design Technology of Architecture, Italy

Faculty of Architecture, University of Belgrade, Serbia

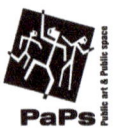

Public Art & Public Space program, Faculty of Architecture, University of Belgrade, Serbia

Health spaces

Hospital Outdoor Environment

Content

Foreword
Romano Del Nord vi-vii
Vladan Đokić viii-ix

Introduction
Francesca Giofrè and Zoran Đukanović x-xv

01_ Hospital open spaces and urban open spaces
Zoran Đukanović_ 16-57

02_ Regeneration and restoration of the hospital spaces
Ferdinando Terranova_ 58-95

03_ Healing environments design
Nađa Beretić_ 96-125

04_ Observation as a way of knowing and measuring open hospital spaces
Fabio Quici_ 126-147

05_ Exploring the relationship between outdoor and indoor environments in the hospital design process
Francesca Giofrè_ 148-169

06_ Hospital outdoor environments on dualities and contradiction
Ružica Božović Stamenović_ 170-199

07_ Health facilities and open spaces: integrated policies at the landscape and territorial level
Rosalba D'Onofrio and Elio Trusiani_ 200-219

08_ A Master Plan for regeneration: Piacenza Hospital complex, Italy
Anna Maria Giovenale_ 220-237

09_ Barriers between hospital and city: seven Italian case studies
Francesca Giofrè_ 238-261

10_ Image of a hospital city: clinical center of Serbia
Ivana Miletić _ 262-287

11_ The role of outdoor public space in a pavilion university hospital. Case study: Policlinico Umberto I of Rome, Italy
Valentina Napoli and Giuseppe Primiceri_ 288-311

12_ Hospital open spaces. Healing or threatening environments. Case study: Clinical centre of Niš and Clinical centre of Vojvodina in Novi Sad, Serbia
Vesna Mandić and Tamara Stanisavljević_ 312-343

13_ Analysis of some renovation projects indoor and outdoor. Case study: Policlinico Umberto I of Rome, Italy
Rosalba Belibani and Martina Cardi_ 344-369

Foreword by Romano Del Nord

Director of Tesis, Inter-University Research Centre "Systems and Technologies for Healthcare Buildings", University of Florence, Italy

The important growth attributed to sensory perceptual stimulations on the path to healing of hospitalized patients is increasingly pushing designers of social and health care facilities to enhance the physical and environmental elements of 'nature' until they are considered fundamental inputs in order to optimize the quality not only of the care spaces but of all the spaces that help in the process of regenerating the physical and emotional conditions of people who are sick. It is no coincidence that, since the earliest antiquity, the fundamental principles of design in the *Asclepia* in ancient Greece included the "insertion of structures to be used for care in areas highly integrated with nature (in connection with the sacred forest)", equipped with open spaces for leisure and physical activities and geared towards creating visual relationships with the dwelling places of the deities, for the psychological effect that this performance could have in patients.

Spaces "without walls" increasingly tend to assume a strategic value in the spatial and physical configuration of the hospital complex and require particular attention from the initial preparation of masterplans for social and health care facilities, going on to influence, where possible, the territorial planning of urban voids in all their multiform manifestations.

There are a variety of ways in which expressions of nature, plants, flowers, colours, scents, water, noise, and birds can have a positive effect on the senses of those who are physically and psychologically debilitated, and expertise is required to understand how individuals react to the stimuli perceived in relation to their state of wellbeing/malaise. However, we cannot forget that, together with patients who spend limited periods of time in healthcare facilities, the medical and care staff due to their continued presence are subject to fatigue and burn-out that would justify – even in terms of efficiency, productivity and risk reduction – design solutions that consider the design of suitable open spaces to be a valid and recognized contribution to the containment of this critical issue.

All this leads us to make some reflections that are difficult to dispute:
- the design of the spaces outside the functional units of hospitals should be

approached so it is fully integrated with the design of the interior spaces;

- as there are many types of outdoor spaces and they are highly differentiated in terms of their potential to support the restoration of wellness (internal courtyards, gardens, parks, footpaths), it is not easy to define design rules or guidelines that are generally applicable;

- certain solutions can only be deemed effective if supported by post-occupancy checks that help to classify as "evidence-based" the design solutions that turned out to be of actual therapeutic benefit and where wellbeing was perceived by the users;

- the close correlation that exists between the different user categories and their different ways of reacting to psycho-sensory stimulations make it clearly apparent that the performances of an outdoor space for sick children cannot be considered similar to those intended, for example, for those suffering from Alzheimer's disease or for cancer patients: the type of building configures the different specificities.

Being mindful of the above, the aim of this book is not to compile a set of guidelines with systematic discipline, nor to act as a manual to be added to the already numerous publications on the design of Healing Gardens, rather it has attempted to extract – from experiences, projects and research – some principles aimed at highlighting the contribution offered by designers in treating, with equal dignity and equal purpose, the outdoor spaces as interior spaces in healthcare facilities.

The inclusion of case studies that refer to contexts with different social-cultural as well as geographical-territorial connotations offers the reader the opportunity to reflect on how the diversity of different contexts makes it difficult to generalize about design approaches to the problem and how important it is to derive solutions from knowledge of the culture of those places.

The range of case studies examined tends to construct a sort of database – and not necessarily best practices – that can continuously be enriched by new contributions to stimulate the sensitivity of designers and clients on the topic addressed and to create a widespread culture of human-centred design for spaces of health and wellness rather than spaces for treatment alone aimed at recovery.

Romano Del Nord

Foreword by Vladan Đokić

Dean of the Faculty of Architecture, University of Belgrade, Serbia

Having in mind that present considerations regarding good public health to be highly prioritized resource for the sustainable development, the 'ambiance' of a space generally must be reconsidered. In recent years design for public spaces especially begun to include designing enhancements in an attempt to reduce stress and anxiety, increase users' satisfaction, and promote health throughout the urban territory. Lately was established a process for designing and applying several techniques based on pro-health architectural and urban improvements of hospital outdoor environment. Thus this book presents some of the existing research on this subject as the information base in order to widen aspects considered in planning and designing built and natural environment, and to enlist opportunities that already exist and to predict new in order to make meaningful contributions in this area that are likely to make a significant impact to achieve both individual health (at micro level) and public and environment health outcomes (at macro level). The book includes the views of educationalists and practitioners and raises considerations of an added social value to be asked for as an important dimension in people's well-being and recovery from ill health or social exclusion. Such outcomes emerge from the idea of public spaces becoming a 'product' delivered to the community, and contributing and being healing or promoting health in public space generally.

The high demographic shift towards urbanization and a rise of people living in urban areas pose environmental problems among others and a need to promote health effects in urban design and planning. The space has an effect on people using the space, therefore current tendencies are aimed at creation and design of spaces "providing a positive context" and being actively salutogenic. Recent researches have been concentrated on a limited number of settings and design guidelines for the physical elements of an optimal healing environment, also the description, development and reflection of relations between experience of health and access to open and public spaces in cities.

Public urban space is used as a comprehensive term for all urban areas in the city: parks and green spaces, nature areas near population centers, gardens, residential and school courtyards, etc. With this in regard, public urban spaces are viewed as a health-promoting element of city planning. Open spaces provide benefits linked to physical activity and reported stress and quality of life, as well as social and natural capital outcomes related to general wellbeing.

Finally, the book provides a narrative summary for urban planners and designers and, especially, health policy-makers and demonstration that consideration of health becomes an element of high importance in city planning. Presented findings of the relationship between physical and social dimensions of urban spaces and their association with health protection sought to pull together clear relevance public outdoor spaces have for public health and to encompass the wider social and economic determinants of public health.

Vladan Đokić

Introduction

Francesca Giofrè and Zoran Đukanović, Editors

It was February 2012 at the Faculty of Architecture, University of Belgrade during the course "Health Urban Design" when we have developed the topic of Healthy spaces around the hospital complex. Thanks to the Basileus Erasmus Mundus programme, we had the chance to work together for one month and then we have received the funds by Sapienza International Office, on the basis of the mutual agreement between our Institutions, to go on with our research and teaching activities.

The Serbian students, during the Course, worked on the regeneration of the outdoor environments at the Clinical Center of Serbia in Belgrade. To let them fully understand the topic, the students together with us, met the board of management of the Clinical Center and they interviewed, through a questionnaire given by us, 108 users amongst which there were patients, hospital staff, students and visitors. The interviews' results were really interesting. On the one hand the results highlight the bad feelings of users towards outdoor environments, on the other hand the great importance of outdoor environments for the users as an integral part of surroundings city and the importance of the relation with the indoor activities of the hospital.

We discussed the topic in deep, concluding that there are a lot of places around the world where the outdoor environments around the big hospitals are not properly taken into account by the designers. Even if the hospitals occupy a big portion of the city, the outdoor spaces are not integrated into the city, nor used as an extension of the healthcare activities.

It can be argued that the 'outdoor spaces' are not 'places characterized' but only physically 'open spaces'.

The book "Health spaces. Hospital Outdoor Environments" comes from that teaching experience and from the studies made during these years.

We decided to write this book involving different experts in the healthcare design and landscape, aware of the need for interdisciplinary approaches and of the significant importance that landscape design gains in these last years. The book discusses and shows design solutions aimed at creating the right balance as much between the city and the hospital's outdoors, that much between hospital open spaces and indoor environments, in accordance with users' needs and behaviors.

The book develops the topic of "Health spaces: Hospital Outdoor Environments" starting from a general approach to go on in the real case study's analysis. According to that, the book is divided in two parts: the first part collects essays on planning and design approach and the second part shows significant case studies located in Serbia and in Italy.

The first part of the book collected six papers. They explore theoretically the main topic from different points of view, from different disciplines.

The paper "Hospital open spaces and urban open spaces" (by Z. Đukanovic), which is opening the book, presents a brief review of the relation between urban open space as a wider, complex system of contemporary cities and the hospital open spaces as its, not less complex, sub-element. There are several different types of approaches to researching and defining the 'openness' of the open spaces and the author discusses the main five approaches: landscape, formal, functional, cultural and economic.

The paper "Regeneration and restoration of the hospital spaces" (by F. Terranova) proposes a critical path that a designer should follow in designing a meta-project of a hospital, starting from the analysis of the importance of the social determinants. The paper also argues that the goal of a good design is to find solutions aimed at mitigating environmental pressures and the increasing gaining importance of the landscape design. At the end the author closes the paper with some recommendations to address the designers.

The paper "Healing environments design" (by N. Beretić) researches a gap between urban open spaces and health care facilities and it symbolically presents green spaces as health promoters, but considered balance between notions and presents theories dealing with the research of urban open spaces within healthcare facilities. It researches those notions trough two lenses: the first is a review of existing literature about defining the main theories in the field of healthcare outdoors, and the second one observes historical and cultural conception of outdoor spaces within healthcare facilities.

The paper "Observation as a way of knowing and measuring open hospital spaces" (by F. Quici), discusses two main questions: "Can open hospital spaces be considered 'places'? Can it be said that the open spaces of today's hospital structures present characteristics sufficient to qualify them as public spaces?". The paper argues that the first step towards understanding the nature and the function of such spaces is to investigate the behavior and the expectations of the users. It discusses some methods that can be useful to address the designers.

The paper "Exploring the relationship between outdoor and indoor environments in the hospital design process" (by F. Giofrè) discusses the relationship between the city, the hospital and its indoor and outdoor environments. It contends that the outdoor spaces need to be integrated as part of the design process through a multidimensional design approach that involves the user groups. The paper introduces new categories in relation to the different levels of usability – public, semi-public, private. The design of these spaces is of great importance insofar as it potentially influences and alters the behavior of the people that use it, even more so if those same people are involved in its design.

The paper "Hospital outdoor environments on dualities and contradiction" (by R. Božović-Stamenović) closes the first part of the book. It discusses a number of dichotomies and paradoxes intrinsic to the nature of the hospital outdoor spaces. The outdoor realm is put in perspective with the urban, social and personal domains. The paper argues that the healthfulness of the outdoor hospital environment is deeply imbedded in design's qualitative substance rather than in its formal appearance. In that sense narrative strategies and exploration of indeterminacy and multifaceted character of outdoor spaces seem more opportune for achieving the lasting positive effects on users.

The second part of the book is opened by the paper "Health facilities and open spaces: integrated policies at the landscape and territorial level" (by R. D'Onofrio, E. Trusiani). It examines the relationship between health facilities and open spaces from a landscape and the territorial point of view, considering not just the hospital closest surroundings, but also more distant areas. It argues that the open spaces' network is a connection system of different green areas and natural amenities, inside and outside the city, and comprises a variety of functions at very different levels. The paper discusses some national and international examples in order to show how a different use of natural parks and other protected areas could represent a precious opportunity, still unexplored, for human health and social wellbeing.

The paper written by A.M. Giovenale illustrates an Italian case study" A Master Plan for regeneration: Piacenza Hospital complex, Italy" as the result of the synergy of different skills and different specializations. It examines the design of a hospital building, in particular the prevalence of functionality rather than architecture, highlighting how the Master Plan represents a possible solution which is 'outside the box'. The paper discusses as the master plan reinterpreted the hospital in Piacenza as a place where citizens should be able to meet, in order to recover the sense of the hospital being an 'urban site'.

What are the types of barriers between hospitals and city in Italy? The paper "Barriers between hospital and city: seven Italian case studies" (by F. Giofrè) analyses six university hospital complexes with more than 950 beds. The study applies a quantitative research method and its aim is to offer a reading, also photographic, of the current situation of those hospital complexes and their relationships with the city and also to analyze the data collected in order to understand the redevelopment potential of the external spaces of the hospital complexes.

The paper "Image of a hospital city: clinical center of Serbia" (by I. Miletić), discusses the open spaces within the Clinical Center in terms of the urban environment. The analysis shows a very varied and confusing conglomeration of buildings that passed through different social systems and therefore constantly changes its organization, methods of management and urban planning with significant repercussions on the physical layout.

Another interesting case study is analyzed in the paper "The role of outdoor public space in a pavilion university hospital. Case study: Policlinico Umberto I of Rome, Italy" (by V. Napoli, G. Primiceri). The paper investigates the outdoor space of the Policlinico Umberto I of Rome, through the analysis of its phases of evolution from the original project to current day proposals. The analysis of the external space in its current state is based on considerations and also on the basis of understanding the relationship with its urban surroundings. Along with the study, a questionnaire on the use and perception of the space was submitted by different categories of users. Through the process the possibilities that could be linked to the use of outdoor space are highlighted, especially in large university pavilion hospital situations.

The paper "Hospital open spaces. Healing or threatening environments. Case study: Clinical Centre of Niš and Clinical Centre of Vojvodina in Novi Sad, Serbia" (by V.

Mandić and T. Stanisavljević), analyses the existing open space in the two Clinical Centers. Methodology of research process includes desk and internet research, field research, site surveys and interviews with patients, local inhabitants and employees of the Clinical Centers. The goals of the study are to present the emerging need for developing integrated healthcare systems focused on overall well-being of patients and other users.

The last paper "Analysis of some renovation projects indoor and outdoor. Case study: Policlinico Umberto I of Rome, Italy" (by R.Belibani and M. Cardi), shows some of the several renovation projects of the hospital, particularly focusing on the one regarding the re- functionalization of Pediatrics and Obstetrics Clinics. The paper investigates also the tools for the design of green spaces pertaining to a hospital, in order to satisfy a high quality of the hospital landscape.

Matching and putting in order the key words written by each author, it's possible to give to the readers a word map of the book (see Figure 1).

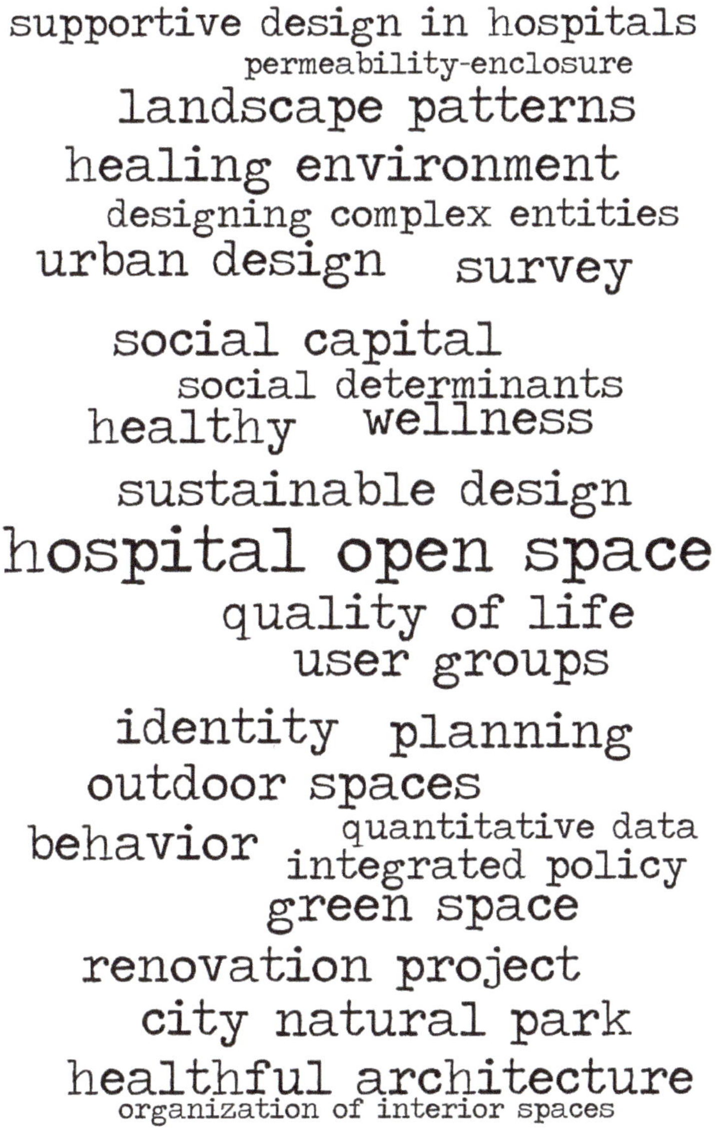

supportive design in hospitals
permeability-enclosure
landscape patterns
healing environment
designing complex entities
urban design   survey

social capital
social determinants
healthy   wellness

sustainable design
hospital open space
quality of life
user groups

identity   planning
outdoor spaces
behavior   quantitative data
integrated policy
green space
renovation project
city natural park
healthful architecture
organization of interior spaces

Figure 1: Word map of the book keywords

01

Hospital Open Spaces and Urban Open Spaces

Zoran Đukanović

Abstract: This paper discusses matters with the hospital's outdoors, respectively hospital open spaces, in the context of a wider field of the urban open spaces of contemporary cities. This kind of research approach wasn't used so much in the recent studies. While, the field of urban open spaces has been always, in the core focus of the experts from a wide range of the various disciplines (politics, planners, environmentalists, architects, developers, sociologists, anthropologists, economists, even the artists and philosophers, etc.), quite oppositely, interests of, anyway a few, experts who are researching, planning, design and managing the matters of the health spaces are mostly avoided the matter of the health open spaces. Additionally, even that there are many studies evaluating the success of housing schemes, there are many fewer of healthcare facilities, and only about the 1000 related to the hospital outdoors. Because of all of that, we decided to offer a brief review of the relation between urban open space as a wider, complex system and the hospital open spaces as its, not less complex, sub-element. The paper explores, defines, and explains the main characteristics of both the urban phenomena, using a simple comparative methodology, across the different typologies disciplinary approaches. As one of the important part of the research, at the end of the paper, we offer a very large, wide and comprehensive bibliography aimed to collect and review most of important recent works related to our core approach.

Keywords: urban open spaces, hospital open spaces, hospitals, nature, greenery.

Preface

The global rise of cities has been unprecedented. "In 1800, 2% of the world's population lived in cities. Now it is 50%. Every week, some 1.5 million people join the urban population, through a combination of migration and childbirth" (Powell, 2015). According to the UN Task Force (11/03/2015) counting of the 'world city population', every single day 187.066 new city dwellers are added to the world's urban population - 2 per second. Nowadays, more than half of the human population lives in the cities. Contemporary cities are growing faster, more than ever in history. Spatial needs of a growing urban population, are growing even faster, because the human needs (1) are not only rapidly increasing, but also widely diversifying, as well. Satisfying each of these human needs requires more space than ever before. On the other hand, the rapid growth of space requirements - for housing, working, transport, food production, energy, but also for health care, education, tourism, fun, sport, entertainments, etc. - lead us to an obvious crisis of available space. This spatial crisis is visible not only as a lack of available artificial space in the cities, but also as an extensive cultivation of huge wild-land areas which serving increased needs of the modern cities. Today, "cities occupy 0.5% of the world's surface, but consume 75% of its resources" (Powell, 2015). The future will be even more challenging. "The global urban population is expected to grow approximately 1.84% per year between 2015 and 2020, 1.63% per year between 2020 and 2025, and 1.44% per year between 2025 and 2030" (WHO, 2015).

This spatial crisis is already recognized as a critical matter. Sustainability, mobility, compact cities, mixed-use, energy efficiency, smart growth, etc. are only a few concepts of urban development which already linked to this problem - among the other problems they try to solve. Therefore, at the beginning of the twenty-first century, urban theory and policy throughout the world is returning to the issue of open spaces, particularly to public open spaces. The fact that open spaces do benefit daily urban living, and play a vital role in creating healthier, more sociable communities, is changing the attitudes, policies and actions (Wooly, 2003). It "alerted politicians of all political shades in developed countries to the cultural importance which good-quality public environments play in restoring popular confidence in urban living" (Worpole in Wooly, 2003, p.viii).

Introduction

This paper aims to discuss matters of the hospital's outdoors, respectively hospital open spaces, in the context of a wider field of the urban open spaces of contemporary cities. This kind of research approach wasn't used so much in the recent studies. There are many reasons for this kind of situation. "Though there are many studies evaluating the success of housing schemes, there are many fewer of healthcare facilities, and almost none of the hospitals' outdoors" (Cooper Marcus and Barnes, 1995, p.2). While, the field of urban open spaces has been always, especially last decades, in the core focus of the experts from a wide range of the various disciplines (politics, planners, environmentalists, architects, developers, sociologists, anthropologists, economists, even the artists and philosophers, etc.) (2), quite oppositely, interests of anyway the few experts experts who are researching, planning, design and managing the matters of the health spaces are mostly avoided the matters of the health open spaces. They are still predominantly focused mostly on the indoor hospital building spaces, their typologies, effective functionality, improving the organization of working process, efficient technologies and technical equipment, 'user friendly' interior design, rationalization of expenses, and so on. Esther M. Sternberg (2009, p.4) describes this situation in the way that "often, the hospital's physical space seemed meant to optimize care of the equipment rather than the care of the patients". Even if hospitals have some ground outdoor areas, they mostly don't use it as well as it is possible to do (Woolley, 2003, p.126). Cooper Marcus and Barnes, (1995) argue that land costs and pressure from insurance companies to minimize hospital stays have largely worked against the provision of gardens in these new or refurbished medical complexes. "Landscaping" is often seen as a cosmetic extra. (Cooper Marcus and Barnes, 1995, p.9). Money, being constrained, is not considered to be well spent on the external environment. Thus, traditional layouts and formal gardens have been lost (Hosking and Haggard, 1999 in Woolley, 2003 p.126). This sort of the bad maintaining of the hospitals outdoors started to give a bad impact in patient experiences. Simultaneously, some authoritative researches, realized in period from late 70's 'till today, indicate that the presence of the nature and well-designed natural greenery in the hospital's outdoor environment, have a various positive correlations with the process of rehabilitation of the patient and recognizable impact to reduction of time they spend in the hospital (3).

In the meantime, especially after 2000, health matter, have been expanded far from the hospitals and their belonging outdoors. Related to the 'WHO Health city project' (WHO/Europe, 1997) and 'Healthy urban planning - a WHO guide to planning for people' (Barton and Tsourou, 2000), which pronounce that human health and well-being are at the heart of sustainable development, our entire environment and public life are starting to be considered as the matter of health.

In accordance with these WHO documents, which generate an ideology of 'Health city movement', a number of states and cities from all around the world, especially in the EU, have been adapted their urban planning and urban management practice, policy and legislation. Proposed Health city principles have been promoted as priorities and the guidelines have been used as conductive to the health, wellbeing and a high quality of life.

All of that triggered fundamental changes into the contemporary urban planning and urban management practices, which results with big changes primarily in the field of urban open spaces and particularly in public open spaces.

Open spaces and public spaces

The terms: 'open spaces' and 'public open spaces', are not synonyms. These terms are related in many ways, but does not mean the same thing.

The term 'open' could be understood in different ways. To be properly understood, 'openness' of open spaces has to be related to, and explained by some of very specific sort of definition (this problem will be explained in the following text).

On the other hand, the term 'public' mainly relates to public or communal ownership, or mode of public use of the open spaces. Moreover, there are a many of the open spaces which are private. Although, there are many examples of private open spaces in public use (such as P.O.P.S. - Privately owned public spaces), there are uncountable examples of private open spaces without any kind of public use, nor any public activities, nor even public presence. On the other hand, the term 'public space' is mainly related to public open spaces, such as squares and piazzas, streets, parks, coastal areas and so on, but in the same time, the same term is addressing enclosed, indoor spaces of civic institutions such as: governmental buildings, schools, hospitals, police stations, fire stations, museums, etc., or religious buildings, for example. Exceptionally, there are some particular relations, with which is possible to synchronize meanings of 'open space' and 'public space', but this paper will avoid to use this "synchronization".

Health open spaces almost always relate to the 'public space', even if it is in private ownership, there are some obvious factors which limit this unlimited openness for public: concentration of illness, threat of possibilities of infections, higher density of worried and unhappy people, required specific behavior of users (e.g. silence) etc. These factors are more psychological than rational, but in any case it has some discouraging effect of unlimited openness of health open spaces for any kind of public. Although, these spaces are never 'closed' or forbidden for anyone, some people will avoid it persistently, until it was unavoidable to visit it, because of their own particular needs or interests related to the illness or business.

Defining the open spaces

For the purpose of this paper, it will be used the very general and very formal definition which was previously inspired by the definition of Benjamin W. Stanley and his team (2012, p.1089), who has been defined an open space as "any urban ground space, regardless of public accessibility, that are not roofed by an architectural structure". This definition would be applicable for our approach if it has not fixed the open spaces so much to the ground, and if it has not limited so much the 'openness' only to the sky. We decide to offer an approach which is slightly different, a bit more 'open' for systematization and classification of a bit wider range of appropriate urban phenomena which is possible to correlate with the term of the 'open space'. We define the urban open space as: *any urban space, which is permanently open to the open air with at least one of its sides* - no matter if it is a land or water, if it is built structure or undeveloped areas, regardless of the ownership status or mode of use (public or private), despite the type of the surface (green, gray or blue; porous or nonporous), or people access.

Although we are fully aware that this definition probably too much simplifies a complex matter of the field of open spaces, we decided to use it in this way just because of its obvious ability to accepting a various urban phenomena, from all levels of urban life. Whatever, comparing our definition with all other definitions which is possible to find in literature, we believe that this one, that we propose, is quite suffice and comprehensive enough for our research approach.

In this way, the definition includes the widest spectrum of various types of urban spaces which containing any, even the smallest possibility for users to experience the most immediate and the most direct contact with the open air, surrounding environment and the nature. Our main aim of such definition is to try to include into the systematization of open spaces, not only the prestigious 'Mona Lisas' of open spaces such as: squares, streets, parks, coastal areas, agricultural land, gardens and so on, but also to include an uncountable number of forgotten 'micro' open spaces, such as: roofs, roof terraces, balconies, passages, gaps between buildings and other 'junk spaces', even building facades. Potentials of these 'micro' open spaces are obviously visible at all levels of urban life. At the micro level (XXS), these 'micro' open spaces already have a peculiar impact in the ordinary life of every single user who own them, or who use them (arcades, balconies, terraces, passages, green roof terraces, porches, atriums and other different "openings" and "fractures" on the building etc.), but, on the other hand, numerous of other of them, are still waiting to be discovered, to be used and to be plugged in a daily city life in a better way than nowadays (unused roof terraces, roofs, facades, gaps between buildings, etc.). At the macro level (XXL) all of these 'micro' open spaces, related to their enormous total amount and almost incalculable total area of their "unfolded envelope", have a tremendous potential for improving the quality of the city life in numerous way, especially in the wider frame of the environmental and aesthetic matter.

It is obvious that all those 'levels' and types of open spaces are functioning mutually. Not just because they're exposed to each other. Basic calculation shown that the mutual impact of all notable levels of open spaces could exponentially arising environmental impacts. Therefore, it would be advisable to count immediately on these simultaneous effects, because of better predictions of the final results of urban planning and urban design.

There already are some of excellent examples which illustrate that way of using this kind of open spaces. Beside of the flowered balconies (among which some are real urban jewel), let's to name just a few: green roofs (extensive or intensive) (4), urban farming on roof terraces and balconies (with real 'zero distance' effect and respectable effects in reducing urban heat islands) (5), vertical greenery (with visible energy saving impact) (6), urban pockets (7), mural programs (8), etc.

The examples which could shed light on this kind of approach are as follows?

Research conducted in Manchester (UK), has shown that the ground level temperature in the forests around the city, is 12.8°C lower than the ground level temperature in the city core residential areas, which is such a drastic temperature difference (Cvejić, 2015). Regarding to this, they calculated that increasing of green space areas in rate of 10% in the residential complexes, could retain the temperature extremes at the current level until the end of the century, or might even be lower, despite climate changes. But, it is a huge problem to increase the ground space for green areas inside of city area which is already built. But, some of those percent can be earned with the serial, massive greening of the roofs. Such as it was done in the City of Toronto (CA). Research that has been conducted in Toronto has shown that if the 30% of 100% of all possibilities to make a green roof in the city would be realized, it would reduce the temperature in the city for about 0.5°C up to 2°C degrees. According to that, it was issued, a local-city-law, which encourages investors and architects to design and realize the roof greenery on all residential and commercial buildings (Cvejić, 2015).

It does not mean that Toronto authority was officially recognized the private building roofs as a type of urban open space, but it obviously means that the government of the city of Toronto has been recognized a huge potentials of the green roofs and their remarkable impact in the quality of life in their own city as a main public interest. Just because of that, they decide to include, by the law, the green roofs into the comprehensive system of the city greenery. In this way, officially or not, green roofs are recognized as an integral part of the network of urban open spaces.

On the other hand, there are more excellent examples, related to the urban open spaces, which are coming from quite different practices. One of the most interesting comes from the field of public art. Public awareness on this matter is particularly well developed in the US. There are numerous public, private and NGO institutions who care about public art in many cities all around the states. Among all of them, one of the best known is the Mural Program, which works in many of US cities and states a long time ago. Such programs were created "to make city neighborhoods more attractive, instill a sense of pride, provide employment for local artists in their own field, combat graffiti in neighborhoods, and engage young people in the beautification of their own communities, through participatory works with the city authorities, artists, neighborhoods, groups/associations and funding sources"

(Baltimore Arts, undated). Murals Programs are using different, artistic media (vertical greenery, as well) to realize artworks in various types of open spaces, but not only in open public spaces; moreover, very often, mural artworks are realizing on the facades of the private buildings, private fences, etc.

Over the several years, the authority of the City of Belgrade (RS) is participating, with public money, in investments of reconstruction of some of the important facades of the private buildings in the city core, with the aim "to improve the image of the neighborhoods, to reinforce identity of the specific quartiers and major city prospects, but also to preserve the capital examples of historical, cultural and architectural heritage and finally, in the cases where it is possible, to improve the energy efficiency of the building envelope" (City of Belgrade, 2014).

For a long time, many cities and municipalities all around Serbia, traditionally reward annually the 'most beautiful street side balcony' aiming to educate and motivate citizens to a balcony gardening with the main aim to improve their awareness and contribution to a "healthier, greener and more beautiful open public spaces in the city" (City of Belgrade, 2015).

This does not mean that facades and balconies of the private buildings are recognized officially as a type of urban open space, but it obviously means that it was recognized their remarkable impact on the aesthetic, environmental, health and cultural value of the urban open spaces and wider, on the quality of the city life at all. In this way again, officially or not, facades and balconies have been recognized as an integral part of the complex network of urban open spaces.

All of those, and many more similar or different examples, from all around the world, were the main reasons that we decide to define the urban open spaces such as we have proposed before.

Health open spaces / Hospital outdoors

The definition we propose could have a specific importance for the health spaces, particularly for the hospitals without belonging open spaces. This is a typical urban type. It appears inside of the "high density" central city areas. This type is characterized by a relatively small lot which is, more or less, completely fulfilled with a hospital building. Nothing, or negligible of belonging ground space remain to be used as an open space. On the other hand, often, these kinds of the hospitals is situated directly on the front lot line. That means the building is directly leaned to the public area, which means that adjacent public space undertakes some of functions of the hospital nonexistent-open-spaces (welcoming, basic information, direction, etc.), and vice versa, the hospital undertakes some of the functions of the public space (place-making, marking the place, representation, orientation etc.). Therefore, hospital and surrounding public city space have to share some of their functions between them, in this case. This is the most direct connection between the hospital and the city. Seemingly promising, but it isn't always desirable. There are some unsolved problems: direct merging of healthy and unhealthy people in sanitary uncontrolled space, uncomfortable vehicle access (car, ambulance, delivery, etc.), city noise, pedestrian crowd, traffic jam, etc., which could be very stressful for both for patients and for the staff, too. Lack of open spaces, for all of the users means to be mandatory "prisoned" inside of the hospital. On the other hand, even in the hospitals, which have some open spaces, there is many undesirable situations when it is not possible for the patients nor for the staff to leave out of the hospital building (infection risks, immobility, small kids, mental illness, the specificity of the therapeutic process, necessity of permanent supervising, etc.). Nowadays, hospitals indoors are strongly air-conditioned, fully disconnected with the fresh air and have a very specific smell which usually evokes not only bad memories and provokes doubtful moods, but also upsets the senses. "Healthcare facilities are high-stress environments for staff and patients alike" (Cooper Marcus and Barnes, 1995, p.59). Cumulatively, all of those characteristics, could have deeper, a claustrophobic impacts to the users, during their long staying inside of the building, without any contact with open areas.

Some researches (9) indicated several important beneficiary impact of the open-space-greenery to the patients' recovery and employees working routines. One of these studies, after the very comprehensive research find out that: "ninety five percent of the people, the users of the hospital's outdoors, reported a therapeutic benefit: employees said they were more productive, patients spoke of feeling better and having more tolerance for their medical procedures, and friends and relatives felt relief from the stress of the hospital visit" (Cooper Marcus and Barnes, 1995, p.65). According to these results, it is possible to assert that the any possibility to access and breath the fresh open air, for any of hospital users, would be more desirable than to spend the time in permanently closed, air-conditioned, artificial environment. Thus, all of the types of the open spaces which hospital can offer, even the smallest, provide various possibility for the hospital users to reach the sense of "getting away" from the interior hospital space (Cooper Marcus and Barnes, 1995, p.35), to breath immediate the open fresh air, to taking a warm touch of the sun, watching the birds while they flies over the top of the sky, hearing murmurs from the street - to be "plugged in" immediately in a daily city life and to be part of it again, to eat, to smoke and moreover to experience the nature in as much direct way that much it is possible to have. All of that should be more than desirable for all of the hospital users. Because all of that, Cooper Marcus and Barnes (1995) have been proposed the typology of the hospital's outdoor, which contents not only the "ground" types of the health open spaces, but also the types which are obviously belonging to the hospital building, such as: roof terraces, roof gardens, balconies, patios of daily room and cafeteria, even inaccessible atriums inside of the building structures. This typology is obviously fully related to the general definition of urban open spaces which was proposed in the previous text.

Openness of open spaces

Urban open spaces' are highly multidisciplinary matter. Different disciplines have different point of view on this multidisciplinary field. Although, the professional background of the authors, who write about the 'open spaces', is always known and visible, their approaches are meandering among various disciplines in various combinations. In different resources, which came from different disciplinary backgrounds, it is possible to notify several different types of approaches to researching and defining the 'openness' of the open spaces. Among all of them, we will pay attention at the main five:

1. Landscape / *green / environmental / horticulture*
2. Formal / *morphological / physical / shape / size*
3. Functional / *functions / type of activity / mode of use*
4. Cultural / *public life / community / politic / identity / proud / human rights*
5. Economic / *investments / money value.*

This list could look like a rigid systematization, because, in the matter of fact, there is no 'clean' - mono-disciplinary definition. Usually, all definitions of open spaces are hybrids. But, if we analyze them carefully, it would be possible to recognize each of the particular disciplinary background which is related to each of particular definition. Some of those definitions will be quoted in following text and correlated to the content of this work.

The 'landscape' approach

The 'landscape' approach addresses various 'openness' of the green open spaces. The most obvious is the matter of physical/formal openness, but it will be explained a bit later in following text. Even more important is sort of openness which addressing to wide openness to the natural and environmental impacts in all kinds of open spaces, particularly the green open spaces. Those 'natural' impacts are desirable, as much as it is possible to have it into the urban areas (wild life, biodiversity and such). 'Landscape' approach is more prominent in different academic resources compared to the other sort of approach. The term of "open spaces", is almost always strongly related to the green, environmental, and horticulture matter. Academics from these scientific fields are insisting that "ecological arguments are likely to play an even more important role in urban investment in our future, as it becomes clear that trees, plants, green corridors, pocket parks and urban natural settings can create much healthier micro-climates in the city, humanizing it and reclaiming it for the walker and the child at play, as much as for the motorist or shopper" (Worpole, 2003 in Wooly, 2003, p.ix). This approach is usually pretty influenced in the first phase of researching and in the last phase of design. For the authors who promote this approach, horticulture gives mostly all important "materials" for the design of the open spaces. Everything else is a bit ephemeral - shadowed by the trees. This specific sort of "good quality urban design moral" is basically focused on kinds of landscapes and gardens. They believed that this way brings us "recovering from illness or forms of mental distress - reminding us that our physical environment is as important a determinant of our mental well-being as our physical health" (Worpole, 2003 in Wooly, 2003, p.viii). Finally, their ecological arguments are not less healthy-oriented. Oppositely. Thanks to the huge power of "green" political strengths of today and its influence in public life (especially in developed countries), the ecological arguments are proclaimed in sort of ideology, such as it is in the matter of health (if it is possible to divide them totally apart, at all).

In the matter of 'health open spaces' the situation is quite similar. Among all recent research (10) which we have been already pointed out, all of them are related to the outdoor natural surroundings, green environment, greenery, gardening and so on, but also on their impacts to the health of patients and to the satisfaction and working abilities of the hospital staff. One of the first, and most important, was research of Roger Ulrich (1984, pp.420-421), a real pioneer in this matter, who have observed, during a long period of time, two groups of the patients after some of surgical intervention. He discovered and proved that the patients who were in rooms with a view on the outdoor nature, have been recovered less complicated, shorter in time, and with less pharmaceutical treatments than the patients who were in rooms with a view of the brick wall. Ulrich concludes that 'these findings strongly suggest that the view of the trees had comparatively therapeutic influences on the patients' (Ulrich, 1984, pp.420-421). This study was a real threshold in researching the field of health spaces, particularly in the matter of the health open spaces. But it was more studies around this central approach. Researches of Kaplan and Talbot (1983), Kimball (1983), Ewert (1990) indicates that significant psychological benefits arise from being in a natural environment. Greenway (1990, 1993) finds out that psychological changes caused by a natural environment are reflected as much in the short-term, ac in the long-term changes in functioning and behavior of the observed actors. Francis and Cooper Marcus (1991, 1992) research has revealed that people choose predominantly the natural settings as a preferable place where they would spend the time, when they feeling troubled, upset, or in grief. Some of the further studies have been related to the process of emotional change to specific qualities of the outdoor environment (Barnes, 1994), the use of hospital gardens and the therapeutic benefits of these outdoor spaces alike (Cooper Marcus and Barnes, 1995) as well as the impact that surroundings can have on patients, through the peculiar analysing of current conditions and possibilities of improving health the open spaces capacity for better use, design, management and maintenance (Hosking and Haggard, 1999). After these pioneering works, and after the promoting of WHO 'Health city' movement (2000), the interests in the hospitals' as well as for their outdoors have been suddenly expanded, and until today is possible to find about 1000 works related to this specific topic. Considering the notable importance of this topic, we believe that this number still is not respectable (11). This expansion of interests has been spread all over the widest range of disciplines and scientific fields, not only in landscape, horticulture and greenery, but also in architecture and planning, ecology, medicine and psychology, sociology, anthropology, behavioristic, culture, philosophy, wellbeing and quality of life, ecology, geography, resiliency, place making, art, design, economy, evidence-based management, healthy city ect. Although, the main pylon of researches is still based deeply in the incandescent core of the landscape approach, in the mean time, some of new topics appear. These new approaches, slowly but surely, started to generate the 'fine tuning' of existing types of the hospitals' outdoors and gardens, redirected slightly their definitions and meanings to the other various disciplines.

The 'formal' approach

The 'formal' approach addresses to the 'formal/physical' openness of the open spaces. This approach offers powerful tools for for researching a various morphological typologies. Research of the 'open spaces' from this kind of approaches is based on formal-spatial matter. Several authors discuss this problem through several criteria, among which more generalized is that one which starts from essential natural 'elements': land, water, air and even the light. From those 'basic elements' point of view, most simple definition of the open spaces is the one which explains it as any urban ground space, regardless of public accessibility, that is not roofed by an architectural structure (Stanley, 2012, p.1089). On the other hand, Gold (1980) has enlarged overview at this phenomena and define it as land and water in an urban area that is not covered by cars or buildings, or as any undeveloped land in an urban area. Both of those definitions are anticipated not only the land and water - they also speak about 'not roofed spaces' and 'uncovered spaces', both of them has anticipated crucial characteristic of 'openness'. On this way, they have been suggested that open space is not only the land, or the water surface or any undeveloped land in urban areas, which is not covered, nor by buildings, nor by cars, nor roofed, but is also the space and the light above the land (Tankel, 1963).

Along with basic 'formal' approaches, the other authors have been recognized some other characteristic of open spaces to research them: size, shape, patterns, proportion, but the types of the surface also, as well, etc. Those characteristic have been shown great potential to be a powerful tool for research of different morphological, formal classifications and typologies of open spaces. Camillo Sitte (1889) has offered his famous classification and design proposals of urban squares in his unique book. After him, many of the authors have been exploring his ideas. For example, Zucker (1959) has expanded Sitte's model and delineated five types: closed, dominated, nuclear, grouped, and amorphous. On the other hand, Krier (1979) has condensed the typology of all urban open space to two types only: the street and the square (and cross-referenced them with basic geometric shapes).

There are some more of 'this kind' of approaches. E.g. some of the authors are offering their own 'formally-physical' classification of open spaces based on the sort of surface: 'green spaces' - porous-permeable surface, fulfilled with vegetation; and 'gray spaces' - nonporous-impermeable surface covered by hard surface (Al-Hagla, 2008). Even that this kind of classification has deep impact on the 'landscape-ecological' matter, and it is very popular among landscape architects and environmental engineers and managers today, we have decided to classify it into the 'formal' approach. There is no any kind of urban plan today, which doesn't researched this aspect of landscape and environmental point of view. It is one of the most important 'control' criteria for evaluation of the vulnerability of ecological and natural environment in the cities. E.g. it has a deep impact at the matter of 'urban heating islands', management of ground rainwater in the city, etc. On the other hand, this kind of characteristic showed very directly, a 'formal' character of open spaces. Also, concerning that nowadays using of any kind of 'green spaces' are under the strong control and protection, it immediately and very obviously showed its potential for the further planning and design.

Finally, from this 'formal' point of view, it is very important briefly mention buildings which framed the open spaces. Related to Stanley (2012) and Gold (1980), these structures should be outside of the inner content of open spaces. But, on the other hand Tankel (1963) mentioned about "the space and light above the land". His assertion is directing far up to the ground level, exactly where the buildings are settled. Thus, these buildings are integral part of the open space. Buildings are the fundamental part of the public space. Both are the main reason of existence of each other. They are indivisible. Open spaces always relate to the surrounding buildings not only in 'formal' point of view, but also functionally, culturally, ecologically and economically, as well. Moreover, we believe that envelopes of the buildings, which fences the open spaces, are the distinctive part of the 'form' of the open space shape as well. We had already explained why the exposition to the open air of some parts of the envelope of the buildings posses obvious possibilities for defining it as the open spaces. This logic is deeply inserted in the definition of open spaces which we proposed at the beginning of this text.

The prevailing number of studies which research field of the hospital open spaces, mostly doesn't recognize the formal characteristics of them. Mainly, authors satisfy their ambitions about the 'formal' aspect with the dimensional analysis related to well-sized space for some of particular functions or equipment, or for some of specific group of users who demand variability of prevailing standards (people with disabilities, elder people, kids and so on). In a very few studies there are some 'formal spices' mainly related to perception or semantic character of some of landscape elements, e.g. "In wholeness, the sum of the landscape forms and elements is greater than the parts" (Dee, 2001, p.20).

The 'functional' approach

The 'functional' approach addresses the 'functional' openness of the open spaces relating to their ability to accept the widest range of the various activities. Open space provides and serve a variety of functions simultaneously, that satisfy human needs (Fausold and Lilieholm 1996, p.2). This functional flexibility and adaptability of an open space, usually called 'mix use', represent one of the most desirable, but also and most demanding conditions for every contemporary city, at all.

The 'functional' approach seems to be the most obvious. Many of the open spaces are named related to their main current function, or related to the memory of the main previous function, or more often, related to the function of the buildings which framed it, e.g. Piazza del Duomo, Place de l'Opéra, Town Hall Square, Harbor Square Park, Green Market street, even Riviera dell'Ospedale and so on. On this way, such as the 'formal approach' which was previously explained, this 'functional approach' is also proving how much the open spaces are unbreakable linked with its immediate built environment and how deeply they belongs each other.

In the traditional point of view, the function of the open spaces was mostly defined regarding to the basic communal matter: traffic and infrastructure, greenery and agriculture, market, social events, defense, etc. These matters are researched well, because it is pretty easy to measure it and calculate it. Accordingly, there is numerous of instructive "manuals" and "guidelines" - how to plan, design, and manage open spaces. Also, these basic functions of open spaces are researching from ordinary relational standpoints: 'how it works internally related to inner activities', 'how it works externally related to immediate surrounding activities ' and 'how it works related to the wider city matrix'.

On the other hand, contemporary approaches offer a bit more complex view. Beside of the basic functions which was noted before, nowadays we understand our open spaces also related to its cultural function, political and human rights function, economical function, environmental and ecological function, structural and aesthetic function etc., but moreover regarding to function of improving the quality of life.

Howover, in the practice, all of those systematization and categorization of functions of open spaces strongly depend on scientific discipline which lay in the background of the expert who define them. E.g.: Richard Stiles (2009), the landscape architect, starting from the lanscape point of view, in his study classified the functions of urban open spaces into the following three categories: 1) Environmental and ecological functions (which includes: Climatic amelioration; Noise screening; Influencing the hydrological cycle - storm water management; Providing habitats for wild plants and animals); 2) Social and societal functions (which includes: Providing space and facilities for leisure and recreation; Facilitating social contact and communication; Access to and experience of nature; Influencing human physical and psychological health and well-being) and 3) Structural and aesthetic functions (which includes: Articulating, dividing and linking areas of the urban fabric; Improving the legibility of the city; Establishing a sense of place; Acting as a carrier of identity, meanings and values). On the other hand, Boris Johnson, the Mayor of London, politician (2009) in the book "Open space strategies - Best practice guidance", has a quite different approach, which is more benefit oriented. As he defines, the benefit is the protection and creation of a network of the high-quality of open spaces which have a function to: reinforce local identity and civic pride; enhance the physical character of an area, shaping existing and future development; improve physical and social inclusion, including accessibility; provide connected routes between places for wildlife, recreation, walking and cycling, and safer routes to schools; protect and enhance biodiversity and ecological habitats; provide green infrastructure and ecosystem services; provide for children and young people's play and recreation; raise property values and aid urban regeneration; boost the economic potential of tourism, leisure and cultural activities; provide cultural, social, recreational, sporting and community facilities; protect and promote understanding of the historical, cultural and archaeological value of places; contribute to the creation of healthy places, including quiet areas; provide popular outdoor educational facilities; promote the opportunities for local food production; help mitigate and adapt to the climate changes; improve opportunities to enjoy contact with the natural world. Jan Gehl (1987), urban planner with strong orientation to the public-life-based-planning, starting from people behavior, understand that a function of open space has also been described from a user's point of view as being an arena that allows for different types of activities encompassing: a) necessary activities - 'almost compulsory' activities: transport, traffic, shopping etc., b) optional activities - 'if there is a wish and time': taking fresh air, jogging, sunbathing ect., c) and social activities - considered to be an social evolution from necessary or optional activities.

According to research on hospital outdoor spaces, there are many of very particular functions which are shown as desirable for hospital open spaces. In general, most often is possible to find sort of 'functional' typology of the hospital open spaces, which is derectly related to the main function of the hospital building, such as: healing, curing, therapeutic, restorative, positive, etc. Clare Cooper Marcus and Marni Barnes in their research published in the book 'Gardens in Healthcare Facilities: Uses, Therapeutic Benefits, And Design Recommendations' underlined as the most desirable: horticultural therapy, experience of a natural wilderness, stress-reducing and positive mood shifting, (Cooper Marcus and Barnes, 1995). Churchman and Fieldhouse (1990) underlined functional needs of solving problems of car parking, access to public transport, and access points into the buildings themselves and, but also access for services, not only ambulances but deliveries of goods and food too. Because all of that, they concluded that hospital site must surely be one of the busiest places in an urban center. People do not just fall ill or need medical attention and care between the hours of nine and five. In order to cover nursing provision for twenty-four hours in the day nursing, medical and support staff, working shifts, arrive and leave a hospital at different times of the day.

The 'cultural' approach

The 'cultural' approach addresses the most important sort of openness of the urban open spaces, the unlimited variety of 'openness to the people'. Just because of that, in various resources, this approach is mainly related only to the public open space. However, one would define the term public space, the definition has to take into account both the right of public access to it, and the right of participation in its use, on the individual, and on the collective level (as groups and communities). In the very ideal sense, a public space would be the one where everyone has a right to come in without being excluded because of economic or social conditions, and use it freely for any activity that does not conflict with the rights of other groups and individuals that may be using it as well (Vuković, 2011 in Đukanović 2011, p.172). Than, public open space is an arena of the social life, which should provide appropriate conditions for enjoying, expressing and protecting several important statements with particular importance for the contemporary urban community: human rights, access for all, cultural diversity, inclusion, participatory making decision, community responsible place-making, openness for creativity, freely expression of all varieties of lifestyles, preserving the memories and so on. In this respect, in general, we can say that open spaces which are widely open to the public are fundamental to social inclusion, community cohesion, health and well-being (Johnson, 2009, p.4). This way, we are approaching to the most valuable characteristic of the public open space: public open space is the core of the public interests / public sphere / public realm. Public open space is an urban arena where everyday life is guarding its right to the city (Lefebvre, 1968). "The right to the city is far more than the individual liberty to access urban resources: it is a right to change ourselves by changing the city. The freedom to make and remake our cities and ourselves is one of the most precious yet most neglected of our human rights" (Harvey 2008, p.23).

Public open space is attracting and connecting people. It is a stage where the ordinary daily routines of the people playing a unique 'sidewalk ballet' (Jacobs 1961) which have a power to convert the city to the magnificent 'oeuvre' (Lefebvre) (12). Some of the cities, but small towns and villages as well, from all around the world are very known just because of that kind of unique artistic sense which their ordinary daily life affect.

From the cultural point of view we can notice that local communities are always very tied to their own open spaces. There are many cases that urban open spaces, especially public open spaces, which are deeply rooted in the local tradition, provoke a particularly strong sense of local community. In these cases, open spaces are highly reinforcing the local identity and civic pride, improving physical and social inclusion, protecting and celebrating the memories and offer to people unique experience of enjoying their own everyday life.

To relate the cultural dimension of open spaces only to their 'public' content is limiting. Individuals, are spending most of their lives in their own private open spaces, warmly embraced by their families into the deep silence of their shaded gardens. This case, obviously also relates to the people. The cultural life of the city is flourishing there as well as in the public open spaces. Moreover, quite right on the thin edge between the public and private space is settled one of the most crucial cultural tension where culture defines itself basically. Around this line, public and private open spaces are merging each other, very often. There are a couple of categories which are somewhere in between, where Newman (1972) has been recognized a semi-public and semi-private open space. Those spaces are defined with sort of limited access to the people (semi private spaces) or to the public (semi public spaces). From this point of view, Helen Woolley (2003, pp.74-149) defines the scale of three groupings of urban open spaces - domestic, neighborhood and civic - based upon the concept of home range, which suggest three social levels of familiarity, sociability and anonymity. "Although any of these three social experiences might take place in any of the three types of urban open space, in general, there is likely to be a transition of experiences between them", she wrote (ibid. p.75).

Cultures and cities belong each other. Every specific culture is tailoring the city by its own specific shape and measure. Cities and culture are always fitted perfectly. They mirrored each other. These relations are primarily subscribed and visible in the open spaces.

There are countless of studies about relations between a culture, the city and their open spaces, especially in XX century. Also, there are many of comprehensive reviews which summarize those studies and explain them. Among all, related to our research's approach we underline one which is published as an important part of the book 'How to Study Public Life', Jan Gehl and Birgitte Svarre (2013). This book, reviewed all important resources, in relation to the public life research, whose impact is still visible in the contemporary urban planning practice. The review is very concise but comprehensive, cross-referenced and time-lined, and we warmly recommend it for further reading and better understanding of this important field.

However, no matter how we would define the 'cultural' dimension of the open spaces, regardless to our starting point of view, scientific field or cultural background, always in the central core of all of our researches will be a man and his life. This characteristic is particularly important and visible in researches related to the health open spaces (13).

Despite that, we argued before about the unsatisfying number of research of hospital's open spaces, everyone of them are carefully investigated and explain the relations between the open space and their users (14). Honestly, those researches are more psychological, behavioral and statistical then cultural. But, considering that, the matter of the researching of hospital's open spaces is still 'under construction', we believe that it is a very promising first step. Without cultural and architectonic studies, it is not possible so much to do, related to real improving of conditions of hospital open spaces. Simply, mathematical and statistical tools are not sufficient in this matter. Back in 1999, Hosking and Haggard was requiring of hospital's management boards to organize a serious team of top experts (architect, interior designer, landscape architect, arts coordinator and so on) with the main aim to provide highly professional, permanent care and support to design, built and maintaining of the hospital's outdoors. For example, many of datas, from the recent studies (15), which was kept by research on the users' behavior, is possible to translate in place-making design using the architectural methodologies and tools (e.g. Gehl's methodology should be quite adequate and sufficient). It means that, at the same time with collecting the statistical data, it is necessary to observe behavior of the users systematically and continuously, tracing their movements and the prevailing pathways, mapping activities and describe their character, evaluate it (but not only with statistical and mathematical tools) with the aim to understand "what happen" (but not only "how much") and finally, through immediate participatory work with the users, invent specific design guidelines and design solutions for any specific location. It is not useful wasting the time to inventing a "general guidelines" (although it can help sometime), because it is not possible to use it in every particular case, which basically means that it is not possible to use it at all. Every hospital is a case by itself. People are different and particularly specific, space is different and particularly specific, environment is different and particularly specific, places are different with particularly different meanings, illness is quite different but the grief is the same (16).

The 'economical' approach

The 'economical' approach addresses the openness in both: 'getting value' (which is not necessary to be only a 'value for money') as well as for various openness for the 'investments' (which is also not necessary to be only a 'money investments'). Those two kind of opennesses correlate each other, because both are obviously expecting to increase some new value comparing the existing one, and very often they work together. Beside, there is another kind of value which is possible to investigate: 'the current value' of the open space; but it is already included in previous two as a starting point for both of them. According to the huge impact that open spaces have in the city life, in economic matter as well, it is necessary to understand and estimate their value as precisely as it possible because of its impacts in the planning, management, governing and decision-making practice in the cities, at all (17).

However, as the matter of fact, open spaces still successfully avoid to be comprehensively calculated in the matter of the 'monetary value', although it has been much written about their 'economic value' (18). Moreover, as much as there are different disciplinary and methodological approaches to research and defining the matter of open space, that mush there are various ways of thinking about measuring the 'economic value' of it. To be more complicated, some of the values of open space cannot be valued in monetary terms, at all (Fausold and Lilieholm 1996a, p.2). Because of that this paper will try to refer, in general, to both of the open space value: measurable and non-measurable.

An open space is very challenging to be evaluated precisely from its value point of view, because of its complex matter. Consider that open space has an extremely wide spectrum of valuable characteristics, which are mostly very difficult to calculate only by 'monetary value', economists are using different kind of systematization, methods and tools, and there is no one which is prevailing and accepted by all.

Usually, beside of the 'real estate market value' which is the most direct measure of the economic value of open space, many of the other 'economic value' of the open spaces are associated with the 'open space activities' (i.e. uses: consumptive uses, non-consumptive uses and indirect uses). These activities generate the two main types of the value: 'use value' and 'non-use value'. Additionally, in relation to the market availability, the values are classified into the two groups: 'market value' and 'non-market value'.

However, it doesn't make the calculation much easier. Oppositely. There are more difficulties to assign the 'monetary value' to all visible value-parameters of the open spaces, such as Fausold and Lilieholm indicated (1996b, p.1): a) open space typically provides several functions simultaneously, b) different types of value are measured by different methodologies and expressed in different units, c) values are often not-additive and double-counting. On the other hand, there are also a wide variety of intangible values (e.g. cultural, aesthetic, historical, even spiritual) whose value most often is impossible to calculate. "Finally, some would argue that it is morally wrong to try to value something that is by definition invaluable. At a minimum, open space will always possess intangible values that are above and beyond any calculation of monetary values" (Fausold and Lilieholm 1996b, p.1).

It seems sometimes, that calculation of those values, looks like a calculation of 'apples and oranges' even for the economists who calculate them. But mostly, all of the authors invest respectable efforts to solve, seemingly, an impossible problem: to attempt a successful solution for finding the best way to estimate the real value of the open space.

Despite that methodologies which are used for estimation of the value of open spaces being mostly weak and non precise enough, the 'economical value' of open space is one of the most valuable and predominantly used tools and authoritative criteria for decision-making processes, as much for the public authority, that much for the private investors and external contractors.

The calculation of economic value in the particular matter of the hospital's outdoors is not much simplified. Such as in the wider field of the open spaces in general, there are all kinds of value but, concerning the importance of the healing processes of the weak people, some of the intangible values (e.g. cultural, emotive, human) are most visible and notable. Fortunately, these values are not possible to transfer in value for money (not just because it isn't moral or polite). Generally speaking, regarding to the economical befits of hospitals' outdoors, it is possible to say that: Well-designed outdoor spaces are an integral part of the healing environment, and provide benefits for everyone - patients, staff and visitors (Shackell, A. and Walter, R., 2012, p.iii).

'Designing outdoor spaces to have a therapeutic function represents a cost-effective approach. Such spaces can improve patient outcomes and lead to a range of other cost savings. Studies show that patients who are happier with their healthcare environments are easier to care for, and return home sooner. Evidence also indicates that, where the environment is improved, better staff retention results in cost savings in recruitment and training, with recruitment being enhanced in the first place.' (Shackell, A. and Walter, R., 2012, p.1).

Current value of the open spaces

'Current value' of the open space is the base point for any further researches and calculations. It is related, not only to value of the land (built or undeveloped), streets and infrastructure, but also to presence of the other valuable goods, product and attractions and moreover to specific value it has related to people: activities, behavior, believes and so on.

Different studies of the matter of 'open spaces' values, usually starts from, more or less, same or similar classifications, but they differ mostly concerning different approaches to definitions of appropriate methodologies of statistical analyses and various choices of optimal tools for mathematical estimations and calculations. These varieties are especially visible in the field of intangible or hidden values. For the purpose of this work we will not discuss the last two, statistical methodologies and mathematical tools, because they are irrelevant for systematization and classification of the open space values. Accordingly, we will focus our discussions to reviewing prevailing typologies which classify the wide spectrum of the values of open spaces.

Our approach to this matter is based on the research of Fausold and Lilieholm (1996a). They addressed a several possibilities for systematizations of open space's values related to their abilities to be estimated by 'fiscal impact analyses'. In the broadest sense of such approach was to provide a relevant, usable and sustainable method of estimation of values of open spaces aiming to facilitate the community decision-making processes. Among all, we decided to point-out a short list, sort of typology, of the 'open space' (OS) values and to investigate briefly some of possible relations with the particular field of the 'hospital open spaces' (HOS).

The Value of Open Space as a Natural System (OS): "Open space often supports natural systems that provide direct benefits to human society such as ground water recharge, climate moderation, flood control and storm damage prevention, and air and water pollution abatement (ibid. p.8)." (HOS): Relating to the hospital's open spaces, as we noted before, the presence of the qualitative nature provide a direct benefits, such as: presence of natural greenery in a scene have a high correlation with stress reduction (Ulrich, 1979, 1984, 1986; Honeyman, 1987; Hartig et al., 1990) which allowed that patients are recovering more quickly, i.e. needed shorter lengths of stay, with lower incidence of minor post-surgical complications, made fewer demands on nurses, including reduction of pharmaceuticals (Ulrich, 1984). Also, well planned and designed nature into the hospital's open spaces can have remarkable impacts to a micro-climate moderation, and so on. All of these characteristics could respectably reduce the costs, not only in the hospital, but also for the patients and staff as well.

Use and Nonuse Values of Open Space: (OS): "a)'consumptive uses' such as hunting, fishing, and trapping; b) 'non-consumptive uses' such as hiking, camping, boating, enjoying scenery, viewing and photographing wildlife, etc.; c) 'indirect uses' such as reading books or watching programs on open space-related resources or activities such as wildlife and travel (Fausold and Lilieholm, pp.9-10)." (HOS): In hospital's outdoors, in relation with our recent discussions: a)'consumptive uses' such as therapy, healing, curing, etc.; b) 'non-consumptive uses' such as socializing, eating, smoking, enjoying scenery, viewing a wild life, sunbathing, etc.; c) 'indirect uses' such as window scenic view, indoor presence of the natural sounds (birds, wind, rain) or rumors of the surrounding city life, even the consciousness, that the qualitative outdoor is allowed to be used, can provide some benefits to the users of the hospital.

Production Value of Open Space: (OS): "Lands valued for open space are seldom idle, but rather are part of a working landscape vital to the production of goods and services valued and exchanged in markets (ibid. p.12)." (HOS): In the hospital's outdoors, gardening and farming are on the top of the list of the most desirable therapeutic activity for some categories of the patients. These activities can be productive (flowers, fruits, vegetables etc.) and additionally, those products could cover some expenses which hospital usually have (decoration, food, replanting).

Revenues Generated by Open Space-Related Activities: (OS): "Activities directly or indirectly associated with open space may generate significant expenditures and provide an important source of revenue for businesses and state and local governments: hunting, fishing, hiking, bird watching, nature photography, snowmobiling, skiing, and mountain biking (ibid. p.14)." (HOS): e.g. The qualitative hospital's outdoors have to be well maintained, which provide some of business opportunities for the firms which offer these services. Also, the qualitative outdoor spaces attract users (patient, staff and visitors) to spend time there, which always attract various services (fast food, small markets, pharmacies, flower shops, accommodation facilities, and so on) to be allocated in immediate surroundings.

Intangible Values of Open Space: (OS): "Earlier 'types' of values, which was focused only on open space values of high interest to humans, and which came from humans, are the only values that can be expressed in economic terms. However, it is important to note some of the intangible values of open space. Below are several suggested by Rolston (1988, in Fausold and Lilieholm, 1996a p.15): a) scientific value - understanding nature, and how it came to be; b) aesthetic value - appreciating the beauty of a natural feature independent of its utility; c) genetic diversity value - maintaining the capacity to adapt to environmental changes; d) historical value - understanding ourselves by understanding our natural heritage; e) cultural-symbolization value - the contribution of geomorphic, faunal or floral features to our sense of identity; f) character-building value - the opportunity to test and learn one's limits and abilities; g) stability and spontaneity values - nature is both constant and infinitely variable; h) dialectical value - the value that derives from overcoming oppositional forces; i) spiritual value - the deep introspection inspired by wildlands as sanctuaries (ibid. p.15)." (HOS): e.g. In the hospital's outdoors: a) scientific value - understanding how the hospital's outdoors and natural surroundings are related to the people's health and what kind of impact they provide for the healing, therapeutic processes; b) aesthetic value - appreciating the beauty of an outdoor feature attract people to spend time there independent of its utility; c) spiritual value - the deep introspection, inspired by "nature fascination" (Kaplan, 1973, 1983) amplifies the therapeutic effects, d) cultural-symbolization value - the contribution of faunal and floral features to our sense of identity, enhancing our strengths to cope with troubles, upsets, grief and illness at all; etc.

Some authors recognized some hidden values after all. E.g. Kaplan (1980) noted that the value of an open space lies partially in the knowledge that it exists, can be seen from some angles and is there to be used if required. For some people it is just as important to have a park present as a resource as it is to physically use it (Kaplan in Wooly, H., 2003). Thereby, the value of 'knowledge of having it there' doesn't mean that it is necessary 'to use it' at all. Presence of possibility 'to use it' it is quite valuable for some people, even they will never use it at all. Moreover, there are, a wide range of variables which determine the value of open spaces, such as connectivity and accessibility, geographical location and the prestige of the address (Roger Madelin in Almeida, J. et al., 2011).

Added value

Open space is the vivid system, all the time with constant changes. As the system is changing, its values are changing too. Nowadays, those changes are carefully monitored and mostly well planned and managed - means controlled. Regarding to the fact that open spaces are one of the main representatives of the public goods, the main aim of these activities is to protect public goods, means public interest (but private interest too), and to offer new opportunities for getting new, increasing benefits for the future. Open spaces are providing a wide range of opportunities to reach desirable benefits as much for the community, that much of the private sector. "Open space doesn't just add value, it can create it." (Newsum, J., in Gensler and ULI, 2011, p.9). For example: presence of the atractive open space, pleasant and well mainained, with natural beauties and wildlife, atract people to visit it and to spend time there; presence of incresing number of people usualy become to be attractive for business and market on the way that the business and market subjects become to be attracted to alocated their offers and venues near to these kind of places, which will increase demands for realestate; presence of increasing demands for realestate will increase value of the local realeastate wich will have a good impact to the local economy; increasing price of the realestate and increased business and market will increasing the tax revenue which will have good impact to the local community; and so on (19). Helen Woolley, Sian Rose and Matthew Carmona (CABE, 2004, pp.6-7) named the elements of this sort of 'chain' such as: a) The positive impact on property prices, b) Good for business, c) Being close to public space add economic value: d) Creating tax revenue. Beside of that, the same authors are underlined some more valuable benefits which appeared from a good open (public) spaces: benefits for children and young people; reducing crime and fear of crime; social dimension of public space; movement in and between spaces; value of biodiversity and nature (ibid. pp.12-31) ; but most important for the case of the matter of health spaces and hospital's outdoors, about which discuss in this paper is: the impacts on physical and mental health, i.e. the health benefits of walking; green spaces and long life; a place for sport; the importance of nature and 'green exercise'; the environment and mental health (ibid. pp.8-11).

'Good urban design' (20) is one of the most powerful tools for adding the value to the open space. A respectable research of CABE (2001) 'The value of urban design' claims that good urban design indubitably adds the value by increasing the economic viability of development and by delivering social and environmental benefits. In the matter of 'economic value', CABE (2001, p.8) claims that good urban design adds vaue by: a) producing high returns on investments (good rental returns and enhanced capital values); b) placing developments above local competition at little cost; responding to occupier demand; c) helping to deliver more lettable area (higher densities); d) reducing management, maintenance, energy and security costs; e) contributing to more contented and productive workforces; f) supporting the 'life giving' mixed-use elements in developments; g) creating an urban regeneration and place marketing dividend; h) differentiating places and raising their prestige; i) opening up investment opportunities, raising confidence in development opportunities and attracting grant monies; j) reducing the cost to the public purse of rectifying urban design mistakes. In the particular matter of the hospital's outdoors is also notable that the well designed open space, which decrease the stress of users, and provide a better condition of services (entrance, way-finding, ambulance, deliveries, and so on) is more acceptable for all and accordingly, patients and visitors are coming to the hospital more willing than usual. On that way, well designed hospitals outdoors which facilitate a wide range of the hospital working routines, highly improve most of hospital's business capacity and become to be a supportive environment as much for the healing that much of the hospital 'good business'.

Beside of 'good urban design', which is usually very expensive, there are other, more simple and cheap possibilities of adding the value to the open spaces: improved old or added some new particular infrastructure (e.g. enlightening, fountains, public solar recharge equipments, public toilets), improving the maintenance (e.g. gardening, landscaping), public art, land art, place of particular importance for some temporary social happenings (e.g. cultural, folklore, religion, productive, fun, competitions), even the accidental occurrence that cost anything, which makes the open space becomes a place of sort of pilgrimage (e.g. theophany, famous film sites, accidental event related to the very famous person, sites of political meetings with particular meanings and importance).

Openess for investment

There are many studies on the 'openness' of the open spaces for different kind of the money investments (public, private, public-private) (21). Related to the ownership status of the open spaces, the studies have mainly presented investors from the public or private sector. Both of those actors are more than aware of the huge potentials for getting benefits, but from different points of view. While the public sector is mainly focused on social and community benefits, and only after that to earning money, the private sector is predominantly oriented to the profit and the fiscal benefits. Investors came from different fields in which the beneficiary opportunities of the investments' are obvious: "a) Public authorities benefit by meeting their obligation to deliver a well-designed, economically and socially viable environment and often by ripple effects to adjoining areas; b) Investors benefit through favorable returns on their investments and through satisfying occupier demand, although the full pay-off may not be immediate; c) Developers benefit by attracting investors and pre-lets more easily and hence from enhanced company image. If they retain a stake in their developments for long enough, they also benefit from good returns on their investments; d) Occupiers benefit from the better performance, loyalty, health and satisfaction of their employees and from the increased prestige that well-designed developments command with guests and clients; e) Everyday users and society as a whole benefit from the economic advantages of successful regeneration, including new and retained jobs, and also through access to a better quality environment and an enhanced range of amenities and facilities; f) Planners and designers benefit because developing and improving of the open spaces is crucially dependent on their input" (CABE, 2001, p.9).

The studies discussing investments in the field of public open spaces are mostly related to the public investments. It seems logical, because the public authorities (state's, regional, city's, municipality's) are more than the prevailing investor of the public open spaces. But it is no so rare situation that some of private money appeared in investments of the public open spaces matter: Public private partnership (PPP), Privately owned public spaces (P.O.P.S.), charitable trusts and foundations, philanthropic donors, but also and individual volunteers, as well.

Over the past years, as a result of the increasing financial crisis, most investigated financial sources were the Public-private partnership (PPP) investments in the funding, construction, renovation, management or maintenance of public open spaces (22). Even, the PPP is most researched in theory with theoretically very promising outcomes, there are still many mistrusts between public and private actors in practice. Comprehensive research of Gensler and ULI (2011) (23) reveals that despite the governments have a long tradition in the preservation of certain open space lands, because of their high importance to the community, the new impetus for the open space creation and preservation is coming from the private sector (Gensler and ULI, 2011, p.3). The study reveals a few main reasons for this kind of assertion: "a) 95% of our respondents not only believe good open space adds value to commercial property, but are prepared to pay at least 3% more to be in close proximity to it (e.g. with these 3% more, London budget would be filled with £1.3 billion of additional capital); b) 84% of those surveyed believe that both the public and private sector should be responsible for the development of open spaces (i.e. this percentage increases to 100% among developers); c) 69% of respondents believe open space should be maintained through a combination of efforts from both the public and private sector; d) 73% say that open space could act as a crucial catalyst for economic development; and e) 82% would be prepared to invest more in open spaces if there was a financial incentive" (Gensler and ULI, 2011, p.3). The results of the study obviously indicating a clear willingness of the private sector to be a visible partner to the public authorities in the development of open spaces.

'Big' players from public and private sector, there are numerous 'players' more who invest on a daily base. Open field of open space is an extraordinary stage for many of the "ordinary people" who, very often, invest a bit of a sort of 'no money investments': their knowledge, goods, influence, advocacy, time, and over the all, a voluntary work (maintaining, gardening, planting, raking, weeding, pruning, caring for wildlife, feeding animals, repairing, cleaning, but also teaching, training, guiding, even performing art) (24). Aggregating, these activities are saving such remarkable expenses, but they are even more important from the point of view of solidarity and social-cohesion. Each of those activities is the crucial personal investment not only for the open spaces, but for the entire community at all, although it often looks like an 'insignificant caprice of a personal mood'. On the other hand, these efforts, united, associated and well organized, could reach together a respectable economic and even better social effects.

In the field of health open spaces, the situation is a slightly different. From country to country, public-private partnership is on a different level of development and cooperation. Hospitals in EU countries are mainly in public ownership and under the umbrella of public investment. They are often symbols of the welfare state and civic pride (Rechel et al., 2009, p.12). But, there are two opposing forces nowadays, which have deep impacts into the public investments in the matter of health: increasing awareness of people in health generate increasing of investments in the field of health, but oppositely, omnipresent financial crisis causes drastic measures of austerity in the same field. The only way to satisfy both of the forces is to find some external (non public) source of financing. Donations of the charitable trusts, foundations and philanthropic donors, although huge sometime, are unpredictable, not sufficient enough and it is not possible to plan it in forward. One of the possible solutions to escape this sort of the financial trap could be the wider using of the public-private partnership regulated by contract obligation between public and private partners, which can offer to the private sector to build, manage and maintain some of health facilities and certain services within a limited time frame. After all, these kind of practice is the key feature of the Private Finance Initiative (PFI) in the United Kingdom, the country at the forefront of this kind of procurement (McKee, Edwards & Atun 2006, in Rechel et al., 2009, p.19). But, obviously, in many of other countries, there is still visible a lack of trust between public and private sector. Authorities, burdened by the importance which they have in health care providing, as much as by increasing public awareness on health matter in general, forcing them to intensify measures of control of all levels of the investments, construction, renovation, management or maintenance of the health care facilities. To be more complicated, the lack of research on hospitals, in general, is even more pronounced when it comes to the question of capital investment (Rechel et al., 2009, p.3) and therefore, public authorities deprived of well developed theoretical and scientific support for improving their own capacity in decision-making practices.

On the other hand, awareness of public authority for the public capital investments in the health sector, is reasonable, because the total amount of annual costs is pretty high. E.g. In the World Health Organization (WHO) European Region, the hospital sector typically absorbs 35-70% of national expenditure on health care, thereby the capital investments in the health sector typically only account for 2-6% of total health care expenditure in the same countries of the WHO European Region. But development of a hospital predestines a large stream of operational and medical costs for decades to come - roughly the equivalent of the original capital costs every two years. (WHO - Regional Office for Europe 2008, in Rechel et al., 2009, p.4) (25).

Discussion

Nowadays, hospitals are on the threshold of the fundamental transition, although they are highly resistant to change both structurally and culturally (McKee & Healy 2002e, in Rechel et al., 2009, p.5). The ageing of the population, higher levels of chronic disease and disability, tremendous developments in medical technologies and pharmaceuticals, rising public expectations and new financing mechanisms, have exerted an upward pressure on redefining desirable role and tasks for the hospitals in the future. Accordingly, recent research which was mainly related to analyze "how hospitals work", shifted their interests to the topics related to "how hospitals should work". It starts to appeared theoretical and practical-design works with slightly new visionary thematic focuses such as: "2020 vision: our future healthcare environments" (CABE and RIBA, 2000) "Future Hospitals: competitive and healing"(Boluijt, 2005); "Core Hospital, Anywhere" (Leistra, 2005); Investing in hospitals of the future (Rechel et al., 2009).

These studies anticipate a future in which health care will be 'home care' based with sharing, traditional hospital activities with the urban surroundings and private sector on base of about 50%/50% with using of wide range of improved "SF" technologies: sensors, remote monitoring, e-health, tele-medicine, tele-dermatology, 'smart' communications, nurse-led minor injury treatment, walk-in services... some of them are even already in testing use such as Tele-dermatology (Source: Primary Care Today in CABE and RIBA, 2000, p.7). But, there is almost no single word about the hospital outdoors, even maybe two particular exceptions: 1) Health, social, and community health centres should provide welcoming public area (not specified that it is outdoor) and to create a diverse therapeutic environment (not specified that it is outdoor) with user control and a sense of being connected to the outside world (whatever does it means, it suggest that users are in indoor space); 2) Public buildings of community care and specialistic care centres should to be a significant landmarks with local character that are intimate in scale and contribute both physically and socially to the regeneration of the local community, easily identified and located on central city sites and well connected to the public transport network (CABE and RIBA, 2000).

Over 100 health and design top professionals participated in focus groups and discussions over several months in the realization of this study. Judging by worldwide known names which was included in the works, the team was more than respectable. Among about 70 paragraphs with about 2300 words, barely 4 paragraphs and 90 words in the original text, were devoted to the open spaces ... partly.

Instead of conclusion - my personal view

Nobody likes hospitals.

No one likes to go to the hospital. The hospital is not the desirable space. Even if the hospital is the remarkable architectural masterpiece and a prideful cultural heritage, even it is obvious that it isn't a lovable place.

Usually, ordinary people go to the hospital only in the final stage of the emergency; only if they are afraid; only if there is no any other possibility to solve the problem they have.

Very often, kids play 'the doctor' games, but they never play 'the patient' games. Nobody wants to be sick. No one wants to be a patient. This is not only because of the distribution of 'the power', about which kids always like to play, but also because 'weakness' is more than an undesirable condition in their social and cultural environment.

Even nowadays, in some of cultures all around the world, it is still absolutely unacceptable to be sick. Somewhere, weakness could be a fatal condition for a social status of a human being. Ill members of some of communities, are often socially marked, stigmatized, isolated, and finally exterminated from their own community. Therefore, sickness is always hidden, as long as it is possible to hide it.

In the English language, to be 'ill' mean different things. According to different English dictionaries, an adjective 'ill' has a different, mostly, threatening meanings: sick, morbid, bad, diseased; but also: spiteful, vicious; but also: naughty, miserable; but also: evil, mean, wicked, malicious; and finally: enemy, hostile, unfriendly, adverse, inimical... No one of those meanings is acceptable for any kind of community all over the world. Check your own language.

One of my neighbors doesn't want to go to the hospital, even when she knows that she has some suspicious changes in her breasts. "Everyone needs a serious reason to die! Something has to kill me!" she said, while she planted flowers in a pot.

Some of the administrative staff of my faculty doesn't want to go to the annual health care control. "I don't want to know" they said.

My uncle, a farmer, was really proud that he has never been at the hospital, before he died in his 80's.

Once upon a time, my doctor told me ominously:"Congratulation my dear; last time, you had been here a seven years ago". "I didn't have a reason to come" I said. "Everyone has a reason to come to the doctor - every year, at least - but not at last" the doctor concluded.

This is the meaning.

Notes

(1) Maslow (1954) has been suggested one of possible frameworks of human needs: physiological, safety, affiliation, esteem, actualization, cognitive and aesthetic.

(2) Sitte, (1889); Howard, (1902); Le Corbusier, (1923); CIAM, (1933); Jacobs, (1961); Rossi, (1963); Venturi, Izenour and Scott Brown, (1972); Koolhaas and Mau, (1995); Florida, (2005); Burdett and Sudjic, (2008); Whyte, (1958); Lynch, (1960); Cullen, (1961); Hall, (1959); Newman, (1972); Sorkin, (1992); Goldsmith, Elizabeth and Goldbard, (2010); Goffman, (1963); Hall, (1966); Sommer, (1969); Gehl, (1971); Whyte, (1980); Marcus and Francis, (1990); Bosselmann, (1998); Alexander, Ishikawa, and Silverstein, (1977); Appleyard, (1980); Jacobs, (1985); Jacobs, (1995); PPS, (2000); Gehl, (2010); Ulrich, (1986); United Nations, (1987); Barton, (2000); Hillier, (1984); Gehl, (2007).

(3) Ulrich (1979, 1984, 1986, 1999, 2008); Verderber (1986); Honeyman (1987); Hartig et al. (1990); Kaplan (1973); Kaplan and Talbot (1983); Kimball (1983); Ewert (1990); Greenway (1990, 1993); Carolyn and Cooper Marcus (1991); Barnes (1994); Cooper Marcus and Barnes (1995, 1999); Hosking and Haggard (1999); Woolley (2003); Sternberg (2009); Stanley et al. (2012). This short list of the chosen authors and their works hasn't any ambition to be comprehensive in the matter of the hospital's outdoors, but it has an intention to be as much adequate for our research's approach as it possible.

(4) Some examples of green roofs it is, available at: http://www.epa.gov/heatisland/mitigation/greenroofs.htm, 19 August 2015 and http://www.epa.gov/heatisland/resources/pdf/GreenRoofsCompendium.pdf, 19 August 2015.

(5) Some examples of urban farming on roof terraces, it is possible to see in: http://www.fiveboroughfarm.org/urban-agriculture/

(6) Some examples of the vertical greenery, it is possible to see in: http://web.peralta.edu/das/files/2012/03/Green-Walls-Intro-908b_c2.pdf and http://www.sciencedirect.com/science/article/pii/S1364032114005073

(7) Some examples of the urban pockets, it is possible to see in: http://issuu.com/urbego/docs/urban_pockets-reclaiming_the_public/1 and http://worldlandscapearchitect.com/student-project-urban-pockets-of-belgrade-belgrade-serbia/

(8) Some examples of the mural programs, it is possible to see in: http//www.muralarts.org/ and http://www.promotionandarts.org/arts-council/baltimore-mural-program

(9) See note (3).

(10) Ibid.

(11) "The lack of research on hospitals in general is even more pronounced when it comes to the question of capital investment" (Rechel et al., 2009), but on this matter will be discussed in the later chapters of this article into the frame of "Economical approach".

(12) Elden (2004) explains that elsewhere Lefebvre suggests that there were oeuvres in the urban environment before industrialization. See Lefebvre, H.: 1) La droit a la ville, pp. 1-3; 2)

Writings on Cities, pp. 65-6; 3) La proclamation de la commune, Paris: Gallimard, 1965, p. 31.
(13) See: Wilbert M. Gesler and Robin A. Kearns (2002) Culture/Place/Health, London, Routledge.

(14) Particularly: Ulrich (1979, 1984, 1986); Verderber (1986); Honeyman (1987); Hartig et al. (1990); Kaplan (1973, 1983); Kaplan and Talbot (1983); Kimball (1983); Ewert (1990); Greenway (1990, 1993); Francis and Cooper Marcus (1991, 1992); Barnes (1994); Cooper Marcus and Barnes (1995).

(15) Ibid.

(16) "Throughout the Western world, there is an increasing pluralism in health care practices and perceptions of health itself. Much of this pluralism involves place - cultural preferences may take people to different places for health care and places are also perceived as healthy or unhealthy. Internationally, there is a growing interest in the relationships between human health and the experience of place, which has been driven by developments in social and cultural theory, as well as observed health concerns. The way that places are shaped by culture will influence the way culturally contested sites, including bodies, clinics and healing places, are perceived by different people." (Gesler and Kearns, R. 2002). i.e. "It is also important to recognize the wide diversity that exists throughout Europe, a diversity which results from different histories, cultures and political trajectories. Not only do health systems differ in terms of funding, organization and governance, but the term 'hospital' covers many different types of institution, stretching from 'super-sized' university hospitals comprising several thousand staff to health facilities barely recognizable as 'hospitals'. Throughout Europe, there are different definitions and understandings of what 'hospitals' are, and this makes comparisons difficult." (McKee & Healy 2002b; McKee & Healy 2002e in Rechel et al., 2009)

(17) It is notable, unfortunately, that in the resources which have ambitions to offer a comprehensive review, classification and systematization of the recent works in the matter of the 'open spaces', but 'hospital open spaces' as well, there are almost no one which refer to the works from the field of the 'economic value' of these urban phenomena.

(18) Because of numerous variations in approaching to the research of the "value of open spaces", it would be impossible to list all important research inside of the limited volume of this short chapter. Because of that, among all, we decide to address to a very few of very instructive reviews of numerous recent studies on this matter, which is possible to find in: a) Charles J. Fausold and Robert J. Lilieholm (1996); a) "The Economic Value of Open Space: A Review and Synthesis"; b) Virginia McConnell and Margaret Walls (2005) "The Value of Open Space: Evidence from Studies of Nonmarket Benefits"; c) CABE and DETR (2001) The Value of Urban Design, London Thomas Telford.

(19) Helen Woolley and Sian Rose and Matthew Carmona, 2004 in their research 'The Economic Value of Public Space' (CABE, 2004) pointed several extraordinary examples: a) The positive impact on property prices: In the towns of Emmen, Appledoorn and Leiden in the Netherlands, it has been shown that a garden bordering water can increase the price of a house by 11 per cent, while a view of water or having a lake nearby can boost the price by 10 per cent and 7 per cent respectively. A view of a park was shown to raise house prices by 8 per cent, and having

a park nearby by 6 per cent. This compares with a view of an apartment block, which can reduce the price by 7 per cent. Luttik, J. (2000) 'The value of trees, water and open spaces as reflected by house prices in the Netherlands'. Landscape and Urban Planning, Vol. 48, pp161-167. b) Good for business: Well-planned improvements to public spaces within town centers can boost commercial trading by up to 40 percent and generate significant private sector investment. DoE and The Association of Town Centre Management (1997) Managing Urban Spaces in Town Centers - Good Practice Guide. London, HMSO. c) Being close to public space adds economic value: In 1980, 16 per cent of Denver residents said they would pay more to live near a greenbelt or park. By 1990 this figure had risen to 48 per cent. The Trust for Public Land (2001) Economic Benefits of Open Space Index (online). New York, The Trust for Public Land. d) Creating tax revenue: Proximity to the Golden Gate Park has been known to increase property prices from $500 million to $1 billion, thus generating between $5-10 million for the state in annual property taxes. 'The Value of Parks'. Testimony before the California Assembly Committee on Water, Parks and Wildlife. May 18 1993..

(20) The definitions of urban design are many and various. Among many of them, we choose two which was quoted in "The Value of Urban Design" (CABE 2001). Perhaps the simplest of recent definitions is quoted by Cowan (2000) as 'the art of making places' (in CABE 2001). The more comprenhensive is this one which undeline that "urban design should be taken to mean the relationship between different buildings; the relationship between buildings and the streets, squares, parks and waterways and other spaces which make up the public domain; the nature and quality of the public domain itself; the relationship of one part of a village, town or city with other parts; and the patterns of movement and activity which are thereby established: in short, the complex relationships between all the elements of built and unbuilt space" (DoE, 1997, para. 14, in CABE 2001). Additionally, in contemporary theory and practice, urban design is defined as a disciplinary subset of urban planning, landscape architecture, architecture and / or various other disciplines. The theory of urban design primarily engaged in the design and management of the public open spaces (i.e. The "public domain" or "public property"), as well as the way it is perceived, experienced and uses.

(21) See note (18).

(22) Public-Private Partnership (PPP) refers to the forms of cooperation between public authorities and the world of business, which aim to ensure the funding, construction, renovation, management or maintenance of public goods or the provision of a service. A main characteristic of PPP is the relatively long duration of the relationship. Public-private partnership, in different resources refers to acronyms PPP, P3 or P3. (This definition is based on the Expert Panel on Effective Ways of Investing in Health 'EXPH', 2014).

(23) This report presents the findings of a survey of 350 real estate developers, investors, consultants and public sector workers across Europe conducted by global design firm Gensler and the Urban Land Institute, aimed at discovering the value of open space in Europe's cities. (Gensler and ULI 2011).

(24) See: http://www.centralpark.com/guide/get-involved.html; https://bouldercolorado.gov/

osmp/volunteer-program; http://www.cabq.gov/parksandrecreation/programs-lessons/open-space/open-space-volunteer

(25) E.g. To be calculable, it would not hurt to note, that only in Germany alone, capital investment in the health sector amounted to purchasing power parity (PPP) US$ 10.3 billion in 2005 (WHO Regional Office for Europe 2008 in Rechel et al., 2009).

References

Alexander, C. Ishikawa, S. and Silverstein, M. (1977), *A Pattern Language Towns, Buildings, Construction*, Oxford University Press, New York.

Ansel, W. (ed.) (undated), *A Quick Guide to Green Roofs*, International Green Roof Association (IGRA), available at http://www.igra-world.com/links_and_downloads/images_dynamic/IGRA_Green_Roof_Pocket_Guide_2014.pdf, 19 August 2015.

Appleyard, D. (1980), *Livable Streets*, University of California Press, Berkeley.

Baltimore Arts (undated), *Baltimore Mural Program*, available at http://www.baltimorearts.org, 18. August 2015.

Barnes, M. (1994), *A Study of the Process of Emotional Healing in Outdoor Spaces and the Concomitant Landscape Design Implications*, MLA thesis, Department of Landscape Architecture, University of California, Berkeley.

Barton, H., Tsourou, C. (2000), *Healthy urban planning - a WHO guide to planning for people*, London, E&FN Spon.

Barton, T. (2000), *Healthy Urban Planning*, Taylor & Francis, London.

Boluijt, P. (2005), *Future Hospitals: Competitive and Healing: Competition Report*, College bouw ziekenhuisvoorzieningen.

Bosselmann, P. (1998), *Representation of Places*, University of California Press Berkeley, CA.

Burdett, R. and Sudjic, D. (Eds.) (2007), *The Endless City: The Urban Age Project by the London School of Economics and Deutsche Bank's Alfred Herrhausen Society*, Phaidon, London.

CABE and DETR (2001), *The value of urban design*, London, Thomas Telford.

CABE and RIBA (2000), *2020 vision: our future healthcare environments*, London, Building Futures.

CABE, (2004), *The Economic Value of Public Space*, London, CABE Space.

Carolyn, F. and Cooper Marcus, C. (1991), *Places People Take Their Problems*, Proceedings of the 22nd Annual Conference of the Environmental Design Research Association. Mexico.

City of Belgrade (2014), *Predstavljen projekat restauracije fasada, poziv donatorima da učestvuju u obnovi zgrada koje su spomenici kulture*, available at http://www.beograd.rs/cms/view.php?id=1626370, 16. August 2015.

City of Belgrade (2015), *Uručene nagrade i zahvalnice u akciji „Za zeleniji Beograd"* , available at http://www.beograd.rs/cms/view.php?id=1686572, 16. August 2015.

Cooper Marcus, C., and Barnes, M. (Eds.). (1999), *Healing gardens: Therapeutic benefits and design recommendations*. New York: John Wiley & Sons, Inc.

Cooper Marcus, C., and Barnes, M. (1995), *Gardens in Healthcare Facilities: Uses, Therapeutic Benefits, And Design Recommendations*, Berkeley, The Center for Health Design, Inc.

Cooper Marcus, C. and Carolyn, F. (1990), *People Places. Design Guidelines for Urban Open Spaces*. Van Nostrand Reinhold, New York.

Cowan, R. (2000), *Placecheck, A Users' Guide*, London, Urban Design Alliance.

Cullen, G. (1961), *The Concise Townscape*, London, The Architectural Press.

Cvejić, J. (2015), *Adaptation of cities to climate changes by using the green architecture*, Lecture, Faculty of Architecture University of Belgrade.

Daley, R. (undated), A Guide to Rooftop Gardening, Chicago, City of Chicago/ Chicago Department of Environment, available at http://www.artic.edu/webspaces/greeninitiatives/images/GuidetoRooftopGardening_v2.pdf, 18 August 2015.

Dee, C. (2001), *Form and fabric in landscape architecture: A visual introduction*. Oxon: Spon Press Design Trust for Public Space (undated) Five Borough Farm, New York, Design Trust for Public Space, available at http://www.fiveboroughfarm.org/urban-agriculture/ 18 August 2015.

DoE (1997), *Planning Policy Guidance Note 1: General Policy and Principles*, London, The Stationery Office.

Đukanović, Z. (2011), *Umetnost u javnom prostoru: ekspertska studija prostorne provere užeg gradskog jezgra Užica za potrebe umetničke produkcije u javnom prostoru*, Beograd.

Academica - Akademska grupa, available at http://www.publicart-publicspace.org/publications/books/public-art-in-public-space, 18 August 2015.

Elden, S. (2004), *Understanding Henri Lefebvre - Theory and the Possible*, London, Continuum.

EPA (undated) *Green Roofs*, United States Environmental Protection Agency, available at http://www.epa.gov/heatisland/mitigation/greenroofs.htm, 19 August 2015.

EPA (undated) *Reducing Urban Heat Islands: Compendium of Strategies* / Green Roofs, United States Environmental Protection Agency, available at http://www.epa.gov/heatisland/resources/pdf/GreenRoofsCompendium.pdf, 19 August 2015.

Ewert, A. (1990), Reducing Levels of Trait Anxiety Through the Application of Wilderness-based Activities. *The Use of Wilderness for Personal Growth Therapy and Education*. General Technical Report RM 193, Ft. Collins, CO: United States Forest Service.

Expert Panel on Effective Ways of Investing in Health (EXPH), (2014), *Health and Economic Analysis for an Evaluation of the Public-Private Partnerships in Health Care Delivery across Europe*, Brussels, European Commission.

Fausold, C. and Lilieholm, R. (1996a), *The Economic Value of Open Space: A Review and Synthesis*, Cambridge, Lincoln Institute of Land Policy Research Paper.

Fausold, C. and Lilieholm, R. (1996b), *The Economic Value of Open Space*, Land Lines: September 1996, Volume 8, Number 5.

Florida, R. (2005), *The Rise of the Creative Class: The New Global Competition for Talent*, Basic Books, New York, NY.

Gehl Architects (2007), *Public Space Public Life Sydney*, City of Sydney, Sydney.

Gehl, J. (1971), *Life between buildings*, Van Nostrand Reinhold, New York; 1987, reprinted by Island Press.

Gehl, J. (1987), *Life Between Buildings: Using public spaces*, New York: Van Nostrand Reinhold.

Gehl, J. (2010), *Cities for People*, Island Press, Washington D.C.
Gensler and ULI (2011), *Open Space: an asset without a champion?*, Gensler and ULI - the Urban Land Institute.
Gesler, W. and Kearns, R. (2002), *Culture/Place/Health*, London, Routledge.
Goffman, E. (1963), *Behavior in Public Places*, Free Press of Glencoe, New York.
Goldsmith, Elizabeth and Goldbard, (2010), *What We See. Advancing the Observations of Jane Jacobs*, New Village Press, Oakland, California.
Greenway, R. (1990), An Eighteen-Year Investigation of 'Wilderness Therapy.' *The Use of Wilderness for Personal Growth Therapy and Education*. General Technical Report RM 193, Ft. Collins, CO: United States Forest Service.
Hall, E. (1959), *The Silent Language*, Anchor Books/Doubleday, New York.
Hall, T. (1966), *The Hidden Dimension*, Garden City/Doubleday, New York.
Hartig, T. et al. (1990), Perspectives on Wilderness: Testing the Theory of Restorative Environments, *The Use of Wilderness for Personal Growth Therapy and Education*. General Technical Report RM 193, Ft. Collins, CO: United States Forest Service.
Harvey, D. (2008), The Right To The City, *New Left Review 53, September-October 2008*, p. 23-40
Hillier, B. (1984), *The Social Logic of Space*, Cambridge University Press, Cambridge, UK.
Honeyman, M. (1987), *Vegetation and Stress: A comparison study of varying amounts of vegetation in countryside and urban scenes*. MLA thesis, Department of Landscape Architecture, Kansas State University, Manhattan, KS.
Hosking, S. and Haggard, L. (1999), *Healing the Hospital Environment: Design Management and Maintenance of Healthcare Premises*, London, E. & F.N.Spon.
Howard, E. (1902), *Garden Cities of To-Morrow*, MA: MIT Press, Cambridge.
Jacobs, A. (1985), *Looking at Cities*, MA: Harvard University Press, Cambridge.
Jacobs, A. (1995), *Great Streets*, MIT Press, Cambridge Mass.
Jacobs, J. (1961), *Death and Life of Great American Cities*, Random House, New York.
Johnson, B. (2009), *Open space strategies - Best practice guidance*, London, Commission for Architecture and the Built Environment and the Greater London Authority.
Kaplan, R. (1973), Some Psychological Benefits of Gardening, *Environment and Behavior*.
Kaplan, S. and Janet T. (1983), Psychological Benefits of a Wilderness Experience. *In Behavior and the Natural Environment*, edited by I. Altman and J.F. Wohlwil, New York: Plenum.
Kimball, R. (1983), The Wilderness as Therapy, *Journal of Experiential Education 3*.
Koolhaas, R. and Mau, B. (1995), *S,M,L,XL*, O.M.A. Monacelli Press Inc., New York.
Le Corbusier (1923), *Vers une architecture*, Editions Flammarion, Paris.
Le Corbusier (1965), *Atinska povelja*, Organ kluba mladih arhitekata, (Originaly published in Franch, CIAM (1933), La charte d'Athènes).
Lefebvre, H., (1968), *Le droit à la ville*. Paris, Anthopos.
Leistra, M. (2005), Uitgekleed ziekenhuis valt in de prijzen', ZorgCentra en bouwen aan de toekomst, vol. 1, p. 6-9.
Lynch, K. (1960), *The Image of the City*, MIT Press, Cambridge MA.

Maslow, A. (1954), *Motivation and Personality*, New York: Harper and Row.

McConnell, V. and Walls, M. (2005), *The Value of Open Space: Evidence from Studies of Nonmarket Benefits*, Washington, DC, resources for the future.

McKee M, Edwards N, Atun R (2006), Public-private partnerships for hospitals. *Bulletin of the World Health Organization*, 84:890-896.

McKee M, Healy J (2002), The significance of hospitals: an introduction. In: McKee M, Healy J. *Hospitals in a changing Europe*. Buckingham, Open University Press:3-13.

Newman, O. (1972), *Defensible Space, Crime Prevention through Urban Design*, Macmillan, New York.

Powell, I. (2015), *Rapid urbanisation*, PWC - Price Waterhouse Coopers, London, available at http://www.pwc.com/gx/en/issues/megatrends/rapid-urbanisation-ian-powell.jhtml, 18 August 2015.

Project for Public Spaces, (2000), *Inc. How to Turn a Place Around: A Handbook for Creating Successful Public Spaces*, Project for Public Spaces, Inc., New York.

Rechel, B. et al. (2009), *Investing in hospitals of the future*, Observatory Studies Series No 16, Copenhagen, World Health Organization, on behalf of the European Observatory on Health Systems and Policies.

Rolston, H. III. (1988), *Environmental Ethics: Duties to and Values in the Natural World*. Temple University Press, Philadelphia, PA, p.391.

Rossi, A. (1963), *The Architecture of the City*, MA: MIT Press, Cambridge.

Shackell, A. and Walter, R. (2012), *Greenspace design for health and well-being*, Edinburgh, Forestry Commission.

Sitte, C. (1889), *The Art of Building Cities*, Hyperion Press, Westport, Connecticut, reprint 1979 of the 1945 version. Originally published in German: Camillo Sitte, Städtebau nach seinen Künstlerischen Grundsätzen. Verlag von Carl Graeser, Vienna.

Sommer, R. (1969), *Personal Space: The Behavioral Basis of Design*, Prentice-Hall, Englewood Cliffs, N.J.

Sorkin, M. (1992), Variations on a Theme Park, in Sorkin, M. (Ed.), *The New American City and the End of Public Space*, Hill and Vang, New York.

Stanley, B. et al. (2012), Urban Open Spaces in Historical Perspective: a Transdisciplinary Typology and Analysis, *Urban Geography*, 33, 8, pp. 1089-1117. Bellwether Publishing, Ltd., available at http://dx.doi.org/10.2747/0272-3638.33.8.1089

Sternberg, E. (2009), *Healing Spaces: The Science of Place and Well-being*, Cambridge, The Belknap Press of Harvard University Press.

Stiles, R., (2009), *Urban spaces - enhancing the attractiveness and quality of the urban environment*, Vienna, Vienna University of Technology.

Ulrich, B. (1986), *Risk Society: Towards a New Modernity*, Sage, London; originally published in German in 1986; *United Nations in 1987, Our Common Future*, Oxford University Press, Oxford.

Ulrich, R. (1979), *Visual Landscapes and Psychological Well-Being*, Landscape Research.

Ulrich, R. (1984), *View Through a Window may Influence Recovery from Surgery*, Science 224, 420-421.

Ulrich, R. (1986), Human Responses to Vegetation and Landscapes. Landscape and Planning 13.

Ulrich, R. (1999), Effects of gardens on health outcomes: Theory and research. In Cooper Marcus, C., and Barnes, M. (Eds.), *Healing gardens: Therapeutic Benefits and Design Recommendations* (pp. 27-86). New York: Wiley.

Ulrich, R. et al. (2008), A Review of the Research Literature on Evidence-Based Healthcare Design, *Healthcare Leadership White Paper Series 5*, Georgia Tech College of Architecture and The Center for Health Design.

UN Task Force, (2015), Sustainable Urbanization in Post-2015 Agenda (1), 11/03/2015, Sudan vision an independent daily Issue #: 3618, Issue Date: 11th August, 2015, available at http://news.sudanvisiondaily.com/details.html?rsnpid=247276, 19 August 2015.

UN, UNCHS (2001), *Urban Millenium*, Special Session of the General Assembly, New York, available at http://www.un.org/ga/Istanbul+5/booklet4.pdf, 19 August 2015.

Venturi, R., Izenour, S. and Scott Brown, D. (1972), *Learning from Las Vegas: The Forgotten Symbolism of Architectural Form*, MIT Press, Cambridge.

Verderber, S. (1986), *Dimensions of Person-Window Transactions in the Hospital Environment*, Environment and Behavior 18.

WHO (2015), *Urban population growth*, Global Health Observatory (GHO) data, available at http://www.who.int/gho/urban_health/situation_trends/urban_population_growth_text/en/, 19 August 2015.

WHO/Europe (1997), *Twenty steps for developing a Healthy Cities project*, Copenhagen, World Health Organization / Regional Office for Europe.

Whyte, H. W. (1958), *The Exploding Metropolis*, Time Ink./Doubleday, New York.

Whyte, H. W. (1980), *The Social Life of Small Urban Spaces*, Project for Public Spaces, New York.

Woolley, H. (2003), *Urban Open Spaces*, London, Spon Press.

02

Regeneration and restoration of the hospital spaces

Ferdinando Terranova

Abstract: The essay proposes a critical path that a designer should follow in designing a meta-project of a hospital. This course is logical and documentary and should take into account: the users, health professionals, and the cost factors relating to the physical structure of the hospital, and the organisation of functional spaces required to carry out healthcare activities. The sources relate to the people whom the hospital must serve and the data collected by direct observation at facilities similar to the one that needs to be designed, in terms of the spaces required and the time frame. The goal is to define design solutions aimed at mitigating environmental pressures.

Landscape design is gaining significant importance. It is the meeting point between an encompassing internal reality that revolves around illness and an external reality that must connote a message of hope, healing, and the quest for normality, as well as hosting the building's premises and marking their division from cities characterised by property bubbles and the detachment of their citizens. A hospital, therefore, is a design blueprint of a cultural-political process of human and social cohesion.

Keywords: social determinants, designing complex entities, technological hospital hub, organisation of interior spaces.

Social Determinants for the Design of a Hospital Entity

The design of a complex structure within a defined spatial context requires a team of specialists from various backgrounds to provide an analytical reading of the area and its urban structure. The internal space must be developed with a constant eye on proximity, connecting routes, and mobility, according a functional development of the physical structure, and in relation to the needs that must be met. In Europe, the contexts are strongly subject to the restrictive laws, both in terms of urban-territorial planning, the environment, and historical preservation. These constraints are supported by strong and often authoritarian technical regulations. The latter, relating strictly to technical and engineering expertise, specifically in terms of hospitals are first and foremost written with the participation of the commissioning party (the State, Regions), construction companies, consulting engineers (design team), and users (health workers). The beneficiaries (patients and their families, medical and nursing students, etc.) are rarely involved. The lack of their contribution strongly hinders the quality of the project and its adequacy. The knowledge of the needs of the beneficiaries, whether particularly vulnerable people (the sick), those waiting anxiously (family and friends), and those subordinate in terms of knowledge and hierarchy (nursing and other staff, students of the medical or nursing professions or others) is essential for the functional structuring and purpose of the hospital spaces. An approach to the way design projects are written has some major limitations that must be addressed in addition to the problems intrinsic to environmental comfort, such as a more human use of hospital spaces. On the other hand in addressing matters of comfort, technical regulations are already at an advanced stage of maturity and experimentation. The question of the 'human approach' is certainly the most complex to be addressed in both design and practical implementation. The major contributors to the team of designers are humanities professionals, who are able to interpret the expectations of the patient and translate these with a view to the design project. While the architectural sciences are able to provide an answer through interior design, the use of colour, lighting, art, and visual installations that are located in the hospital, these answers are only partial and unsatisfactory or otherwise limited. There are fundamentally two expectations of the hospitalised patient: the healing process and its duration. The solution to their expectations can only come from the professional body and its ability to cope with a situation of clinical risk. Since the launch of health insurance systems or national public health systems the role of users is being constantly re-proposed, but with great difficulty. What is evident is the contradiction between the solutions adopted and the degree of change in the hospital environment. These, by setting goals of high productivity - i.e. elevated speed of patient turnaround, do not take into proper account the sensitivities of those who live with disease in the first person. Today, the world of hospital design must address the issue of giving due and adequate attention to the extra-structural expectations of the patient. The only solution would be for all the protagonists of the medical process (medical staff and patients) to take part, along with those who guarantee the feasibility of such an application (engineering companies, construction and infrastructure companies; biomedical equipment and devices manufacturers). The capabilities and authority of the design team is in its ability to mediate contrasting and, at times, even conflicting interests between the different actors. The days of the lone artist, the creative architect, have now passed. Reality requires a design team that would be a careful observer of the human condition of the patient, and of design solutions that enhance the humanisation of the person subject to the medical practices, which are often cruel and dehumanising by their very nature. This view is not yet fully adopted, even if some established professionals, such as Odile Decq, show great sensitivity to the theme of 'humanisation', establishing in Lyon an experimental Bachelor of Science in Architecture entitled *Confluence for Innovation and Creative Strategies in Architecture*. The originality of Ms. Decq's education project is in bringing together neuroscience, new technologies, social engagement, visual arts, and physics to change the meaning and the future of architecture to becoming increasingly trans-disciplinary. The fulcrum of *Confluence* will obviously be architects with strong experience in social architecture, but even more so: critics, artists, thinkers, philosophers, film-makers, neuroscientists, engineers, and craftsmen (Bucci and Decq, 2014). For academics, the hospital is the paradigm of complexity. Relevant aspects that better characterise the complexity of a hospital structure for its proper functioning can be schematically summarised in the following points.

1. Social complexity and, specifically, complexity of a society, determines the organisation of space and the constructed environment, with special reference to its design and partitioning (Kent, cit. da Chiesi, 2010). The hospital as a micro society, a meeting point of the three social protagonists: the professional body, the management, and the patients.

2. The complexity derives from an architectural feature that plays a part in the diagnostic and palliative activities that are inherently extremely diverse. The functions give rise to potentially autonomous and highly functional subsystems. The latter are closely linked to the policies of investment and relative depreciations for the eventual restoration of the physical structure that houses the hospital functions, with the objective of ensuring environment and spatial quality where possible to altogether guarantee efficiency of the structure. Behind the goals of 'quality' and 'efficiency' lies the primacy of the reduction of operational costs, which revolves around innovation, especially in the field of biomedical equipment and medico-surgical devices.

3. The complexity is due to the synergies that have to be arranged between the various subsystems. This is a condition that is also necessary for pursuing the structure-related ends: re-establishing the unity of the sick person their feeling estranged following the many systems of tests and checks involved in the diagnostics - a necessary step to the therapeutic process.

4. Finally, unlike the above-mentioned aspects that, due to their static nature, require long times for the change, an aspect that gives strong dynamics at a hospital, with short times of change, and on occasion even occurring in real time, is the presence inside the hospital of an increasingly invasive biomedical technology. The pace of innovation in clinical settings is incredible. Academics of this complexity affirm that the ever increasing sophistication and interconnection is accompanied by side effects that are not always predictable. This bring us to a somewhat frustrated certainty that some of these systems today are not fully understood (Arbesman, 2014). For example, today we still do not understand the full scope of the curative-palliative potential of stem cells. Will they be able to restore lost brain cells resulting from ageing, to regrow muscles, tendons, and organs? What interpretation should be given to the sequencing of the human genome? Could synthetic photo-receptors be an answer to lost sight? And so forth (Boncinelli, E. et al.).

The primary function performed by a hospital is to diagnose diseases and cure them by starting the therapeutic process. Restoring a person's health is the result of a convergence of knowledge, firstly medical, but and also that of related sciences. The advancement of scientific and technological research in such knowledge requires a constant evolution of the techniques and technologies, as well as of the sites of care, such as hospitals and other principals centres of diagnostics and care outside the hospital. The human condition of the patient requires the adaptation of the places of care to the evolution of neuroscientific knowledge in the superstructural aspects of humans (psyche and culture), humans in a critical condition, or at least in a fragile one, in a context where their dignity as a person might be questioned. These superstructural aspects and the condition of biological imbalance (illness) form a pivot of a complex organisation made up of specialists, reserved communication languages, economic and cultural interests. Generally, the organisation is plagued by a permanent condition of communicative deficits, an elitist aphasia through the prevailing self-referenced and classist attitude on the part of the professional body, incomprehensible to patients and their families. Hospital management performs a function of economic control of the budget (general and administrative management), as well as a dialectic 'disciplinary' one (health department, medical management). These represent the top of a power elite fundamentally based on knowledge and on their practice with a humanity that is fragile and therefore devoid of contractual capacity.

The hospital is a constantly evolving architectural entity. The observations carried out so far corroborate the concept of a permanent and programmed evolution of this entity. The constant acquisition over time of new generations of biomedical technologies, both as equipment and pharmaceuticals, means a permanent conversion of spaces and a re-plotting of the internal architecture.

Some paths faced by designers in attempting to provide rational and comprehensible answers to the users of the hospital's architecture can be identified by the following questions:

- How to make spaces alterable and interchangeable to accommodate the inclusion of a continuous flow of innovative biomedical technologies?
- How to ensure comfort and socialisation of the sick in a highly self-referential structure?
- How to ensure quality and efficiency of the architectural entity?
- How to ensure patient privacy and confidentiality of their biometric and clinical data?
- How to give scope to a site of continuous architectural redevelopment and its coexistence with carrying out medical and surgical practices?

The project designer often works with pre-existing buildings to redevelop and restructure them in an environment characterised by strong spatial constraints.

Other than intrinsic reasons related to architecture and urbanism (1), there are the reasons related specifically to the massive and varied range of biotechnology, capable of understanding the complexities of the human body to deepen the study of the disease, as well as to the continuous innovation that makes this possible. This is alongside the potential deriving from offering a high proportion of bio-tech, which is becoming more widespread. The road is one of duly adjusting to innovation and/or resorting to legal formulas (although the results have so far been anything but brilliant), such as the free loan, leasing and other formulas resulting from the financial culture and the experiences of project financing.

The didactics of the hospital technological hub introduces a prototype of a new regional (territorial) hospital. The challenge of the hospital technological hub will be to keep the functionalist imprint necessary for any complex structure, and at the same time pursue the ambitious goal of humanisation/ socialisation of hospital spaces. While in the past hospitals used to be measured by calculating the number of beds and the types of medical and surgical specialities benchmarked by the foreordained population standards (2), new regional hospitals are measured without fragmentation of individual specialities. A hospital technological hub has undifferentiated patient beds. It's the workforce of specialists that makes the difference, as calculated on the basis of the epidemiology of the reference population, which corresponds to a user base of the population. Behind the user base of the population to be served there is an organisational design for the development of a para-hospital and/or out-of-hospital network in the region. The out-of-hospital part represents a barrier system to the entire inappropriate pathology that tends towards the hospital, and at the same time a system of health and social service offering centred to face the many and chronic illnesses. Its pillars are the rehabilitation with the social reintegration of the individual in his community. The para-hospital network guarantees a system of services that are closely related to healthcare, with the following pillars: day hospital, day surgery, and community hospitals. In some particular territorial situations para-hospitals activities would also include first aid points to address situations that need emergency treatment to limit damage to peoples' health following a belated response to emergency events. The population served is quite numerous, given the concentration of knowledge and technology that lies ahead in the technological hub. Given the high level of investment, hospital technological hubs must be active around the clock. Biomedical technologies becomes obsolete extremely fast; the amortisation to provide for the replacement of such equipment is intense and short in time. Therefore, downtime in their use and maintenance is unacceptable, and contracts must provide for real-time equipment repairs or replacement of parts. Hospital technological hubs are real 'healing machines'. The general hospital environment creates permanent conditions of stress. The devices of biomedical technologies, even if masked or camouflaged, are inherently depressing for patients: they increase their anguish and stress. Any attenuation with any design solution will always be palliative, in terms of the risk-stress. Design solutions aimed at playing down the distressing effects of the activities that go on inside the hospital technological hub are always difficult; some are passable, others unworkable. Only fast treatment turnaround is the solution that really reduces patient's stress; only the creation of a range of pre- and post-hub hospital facilities. This is a strategy for a widespread socialisation in the region, revolving around the needs of the person who is suffering, waiting for a diagnosis or results of therapy. The regional network of out-of-hospital health facilities which operate has as a reference the hospital technological hub. It provides acute care for programmable aspects, such as those related to chronic illnesses. Rehabilitation and social reintegration are two objectives to address disability and mental disorders. In summary, we have:

1. A regional network of out-of-hospital facilities (health homes; associate surgeries of general practitioners and paediatricians; polyclinics; consultations of various kinds) as part of a network that works with reference to the "hospital technological hub", with the following goals:

a) respond to the demand for specialist health services without hospitalisation;

b) respond to the demand for health and social services aimed at the prevention and treatment of disability, chronic illnesses and mental disorders;

c) select and address urgent treatments, suspected or considered as such with the aim of reducing the flow of inappropriate emergencies in the emergency rooms of hospitals.

2. A para-hospital network (day hospitals; day surgeries; community hospitals) integrated both within the "hospital technological hub" and in Health Houses of the regional out-of-hospital network. It addresses programmable aspects of acute care, as well as post-medical and post-surgical treatments.

The design imprint linked to the physicality of the building needs to address not only the structure of interior space depending on the functions and health activities in accordance with the principles of functional proximity, of routes that facilitate the movement of objects and persons present for various reasons within the hospital technological hub, but also of outer spaces, in terms of the immediate surroundings and the relationship with the city. The design is bound by a rhetoric of environmental sustainability which, in turn, is enclosed by a correct relationship between man and environment. A very evocative (at a project design level) meeting point between the superstructure of the person who frequently wonders about disease as the human condition, and the perception of the space of pain. The external projection of emotions surrounding the disease, and medical and surgical practices may be distressing and painful to those who pass by in the area next to the hospital. Thus, the designer's task should be to render the surrounding area less dramatic. The common thread is a path where nature and objects (technology) base their potential in creative socialising: From the green spaces (outdoors) to channelling of natural light into the spaces that normally lack it (indoors). The solutions are many, as are the perceptions of the design team. The goal is to pursue creative solutions that restore dignity to the sick person. In conclusion, the humanisation or, as would be even more preferable, socialisation of hospital spaces must guide the work of designing architects: the hospital is a physical place designed by people for other people that, among other objectives, aims at breaking the alienation and the sense of estrangement that characterises healthcare sites.

Scientific Innovation and Technology Transfer

The latest reports from scientific companies and research organisations presented at various recent events give us a clear picture of what the future of medicine will hold. We can thus speculate on some repercussions in terms of the needs of healthcare sites and the functional cohesiveness of health facilities. The starting point is the lines of research and forecasts concerning scientific and technological research activities in the fields of biomedicine, pharmacology, and bioengineering. Medical and surgical techniques, technologies, and devices are undergoing formidable acceleration in terms of innovations that are quickly transferable in medical practice. These innovations move along certain guiding lines, such as:

1. Bioengineering of surgical robotics and that of medical and surgical devices (for therapeutic treatments and diagnostics), and bioengineering of diagnostic

imaging, where the leading sectors are imaging and ultrasound (for diagnostics);

2. Genetic engineering (for therapeutic treatments);

3. Pharmaceutical technologies (for therapeutics and diagnostics);

4. Medical informatics with imaging transfer (for diagnostics), and telemedicine (for the monitoring of diagnostic and therapeutic processes) (Ruta, 2006).

The first question that must be addressed is the relationship between the time of discovery/invention in one of the medical disciplines, be it a scientific or technological one, and its transfer into medical practice. Specifically, placement of the technological innovation in the hospital technological hub. The second question relates to the time frame of transition into an architectural design project of the container that will host the relevant function and healthcare activities. The third question is the timing of the physical realisation of the container and the arrangement of its surrounding environment. Finally, the fourth question addresses the matters of design and implementation of the network of out-of-hospital health facilities, without hospitalisation. The timing of the design of the hospital technological hub and of the network of out-of-hospital health facilities must be concurrent; equally, the two structures must open for service simultaneously. Up until now, the experience of carrying out a complex public project, such as a hospital has been quite negative in Italy in terms of timeframes. From the moment of the political decision to implement a healthcare project, to the relevant budget allocation for the project launch, but not of full funding, it all in all spans a rather lengthy period of time. As a result, today a hospital facility, is both culturally and technologically obsolete once completed. The project reflects the medical culture and, consequently, the architectural era in which the project tender was originally published. Deficiencies in the design leads the commissioner to make frequent amendments to the project. This results in a corresponding adjustment of the prices of materials and labour costs, as well as a rather lengthy authorisation process. Thus, inevitably, the final product is poor from both a functional and architectural point of view. It is obsolete regarding the spaces and environments intended for health activities, the latter being subject to constant change due to innovations in the biomedical technology. The design project of a healthcare facility, and particularly a hospital, is marked by spatial sub-structuring aimed specifically at assembling a uniform complex of activities that constitute the disciplinary body defined as part of the scientific specialities that fall into the category of instrumental diagnostics for example. A similar reasoning is applied to therapy-related activities. The characteristic trait of such sub-structuring is the need to both constitute a chain of proximity with other sub-structuring, and to create connections and routes made clear through appropriate signage and defined hierarchies. The idea of homogenising the hospital to the extent of an industrial production line, very popular in the 50s and 60s, and mainly linked to gigantic architectural proportions of hospitals of the time, proved unsuccessful. The main difficulty is in managing work areas that have no single manual labour force, as in an industrial assembly line, here, rather, replaced by social protagonists: doctors, patients and their associates, administrators, high-tech field operators such as clinical engineers, physicists, chemists, biologists, etc. - all bearers of knowledge that is at the same time autonomous and necessary to ensure proper health services. The disciplinary fragmentation of the scientific and technical cultures present in the healthcare facility does not help in making it a cohesive community of actors. Indeed, as in all hierarchical organisations, even if professional ones, inside lurks an atmosphere of conflict, however low in actual intensity.

The quality of design composition and the quality of materials and finishes used in the process of implementation are the conditions that will ensuring that the health facility gets integrated into the fabric of the city and becomes a meeting place between the disease and the science for the dignity and health of the individual who experiences the role of the patient. Both design and construction are prey to the negative impact of the lack of medium to long-term planning of activities and related building needs, which departs from the assumption that the high value of the healthcare building or complex of buildings means a life cycle of at least 50 years. This lack results in building adjustment processes, as well as extraordinary maintenance that disrupts daily life and operation of the facility. The hospital is afflicted, as has been suggested, by infinite works, being more like a permanent construction site that awkwardly tries to co-exist with the medical-surgical activities that continue to be provided, as they can hardly be stopped. The design team's role, using mainly the contribution of researchers in biomedical disciplines, is to get in touch with those responsible for engineering the technological trends of new discoveries, from genetics to pharmacopoeia, and especially in the sector of diagnostic and therapeutic machinery. Today, the equipment produced by hi-tech multinationals are large, and the overall dimensional encumbrances are even greater. In the near future, which tomorrow is in the real sense of time, the work of technology scientists will be entirely directed at disciplinary synthesis resulting in generations of increasingly digitised and, essentially, increasingly miniaturised machines. Biotechnology manufacturer provide all metric and volumetric elements related to the overall spaces and dimensions required for dislocation of the machine and its use. The architect-designer can proceed with the drafting of a building plan and graphically transfer the structure's meta-project based on junctures of various functional sets. The dimensions of these sets are calculated based on observation of the handling flows of operating subsystems (staff, patients, visitors), quantified according to the graph theory. This scientific process helps arrive at a more precise idea of the balance between the potentially required and actually available space. Full utilisation of the required space allows the project designer to have areas that are enhanced to create those really required spaces for social harmony. Some academics go further and support the need to represent the actions to which social actors who interact in the hospital give substance, and that remain unsatisfied in the project. Here we are talking about what you can call 'socially produced space'. That is, a set of adaptive practices that are inhabitants' attempt to modify, alter, and, in a sense, "self-design" a space that meets their needs (Chiesi, 2010). This issue has attracted the special attention of some academics of anthropological and philosophical disciplines. The space, as a public space closely connected to the idea of democracy and freedom. Salvatore Veca argues that public space is the place where ideas, beliefs, and conventions, each different, alternative, and, at times, irreconcilable with the others, get a scope to examine one another in mutual contrast, with the objective of achieving adherence and consensus (Veca, 2014; Gregotti, 2011). The hospital is a public space. There are many questions: how to render democratic a strongly identified space when addressing, among other human issues, the issue considered most critical: disease, and possibly death. How to render democratic a space where technical and scientific elite is crucial in tackling the disease. How to render democratic a space dominated a plurality of scientific expertise that often clashes. How to render democratic a space that is strongly hierarchical. We must reflect, today, on the idea of democracy. Does it conform to the market or is it the space of the market that identifies itself with democracy? The 'healthcare market' has burst into the neo-liberal didactics. The latter identifies the most valuable asset of an individual and of a community as an exchange commodity. The market is always looking for added value. How can a market, the one we've known up until now, self-regulate and co-exist with the very idea of freedom? The 'healthcare market', specifically, expresses a power that denies the right to health and to the very existence to the vulnerable, as well as to civilian communities that, in adopting national and universalistic healthcare systems, turn out to be incapable of guaranteeing speculative profits to this 'market' (even if this is not always the case). Think of the super-profits of the pharma industry in Italy! The monopoly of the demand for pharmaceuticals that is the public health service guarantees monopoly conditions for the supply of pharmaceuticals. It is no coincidence that the big pharma are the most tenacious supporters of the national health service. But what is even more serious is opposing and denying the individual the possibility of his projection towards utopia, towards that world that is embodied in the dignity and equality of persons before the disease, which denies, with the violence of real power by those who practice (repression/poverty) and virtual power by those who dominate (media), the legitimacy of the citizenship rights to the same community. A just society governed by social justice is an egalitarian and inclusive society, supported by the cohesive pillar of the welfare state.

Types and Programming of the Hospital and Out-of-Hospital Network

A correct starting point for the designing architect is to have the demand projections for health services in the short and medium range, reasoning mainly on the quality/quantity and distribution of the population to be served: the potential user base. This projection comes from a similar temporal projection of the population. The cognitive tools for such forecasting would be life tables of the population and epidemiological investigations specifically related to the territory corresponding to the user base. The knowledge of numerical consistency of individual illnesses correlated with severity allows access to the frequency with which, in the course of a specified time, such as a year, the population is taken ill with each illness that involves hospitalisation. Diseases that have no severity connotations will be forwarded for treatment to the network of out-of-hospital or para-hospital services, already described above. This also gives access to the average period of hospitalisation for each disease and therefore to how many patients may be hospitalised for each disease that requires hospital treatment. Upstream, policy choices will be made with specific reference to the activity that is selected for further development, both in terms of instrumental diagnostic and specialist clinics. The number of hours of activity of each area will enable evaluation of the potential of these areas, i.e. the number of persons to be treated. At the end of all these cognitive procedures the designer should be able to size the hospital in terms of large areas for diagnostic imaging, clinics for specialist visits, for in-patient hospital stays, and for surgical treatments (surgical unit and day surgery), emergency rooms, cancer treatment areas (radiotherapy), and structure servicing areas (power plants, installations for medical gases, storage areas for special hospital waste, for healthcare materials, and for medicines, the car park, etc.). Over time, the overall sizing of the structure and the size of each area will undergo changes associated, above all, with the policy choices of the management and industrial choices of multinational corporations that produce biomedical equipment and instrumentation. They are able to plan the production of subsequent generations of such instrumentations. At the same time, they are able, even with all the necessary confidentiality dictated by trade secrecy and patent strategies, to indicate the innovative lines of industrial research and time frames of technological transfer. After which, the designing architect has acquired all the necessary elements not only to meet performance, environmental, and technological standards set for the prospective structure but, above all, to quantify and scan over time the supply and demand for a period of time corresponding to the proposed service of the structure. From a meta-project measured only in terms of individual surfaces it is then relatively easy to switch to the integrated project that has all the elements to pass on to its execution, including the element of construction costs, thus opening the road to a tender process with a view to completing the planned structure in the shortest times possible. This is possible today, but guaranteeing financial flows is a pre-requisite. There is, however, a further question that must be addressed. This is not technical, but rather political, aside from the certainty of funding flows: programming of an out-of-hospital health facilities network in the region in relation to past trends and future projections of population and diseases. From the correlation between the composition, structure, and size of the population and epidemiology, it is possible to evaluate health goals and priorities to be achieved today, as well as tomorrow; and, from these, the demand for specialised medical services today and tomorrow. This will facilitate modifying the proposed spaces. Step by step, a health network is constructed, with nodes corresponding to health facilities that are hierarchically organised on the basis of functions that are to be assigned to the various service types characterising the network. Today, for reasons mainly, but not exclusively economic, the regional hospital offering tends to be concentrated in a few physical units. The other reason is to make hospital stays as brief as possible, literally imprinting this brevity on the idea of hospitalisation, starting from the assumption, as already explained, that the hospital environment is by its nature stressful. The concentration tends to perform a function of synthesis of the functions which in the past fell within the exercise of a plurality of hospitals according to hierarchical and dimensional specialisations (3) defined relating to the size of the population and to the frequency with which inhabitants resort to individual specialist services. Within hospitals, one function is always present - that of diagnosis and treatment. The other functions, it was argued, such as training (medical and other) ought to be carried out by the university polyclinics; and scientific research (the new frontiers of medicine) - by both university polyclinics and Scientific Institutes for Research, Hospitalisation and Health Care (Research Hospitals). This very precise division is not so precise in real life, because every structure, be it a hospital, a technological research centre, an industrial enterprise in the health sector (4), an industry that produces intermediate or finished goods (5), or a bureaucratic apparatus that performs management, control or supervision functions, is, in fact, a meeting point of a plurality of knowledge - from medical, to engineering, to management competences, and so forth. The health care system with its facilities is, therefore, an organisation of knowledge transfer and hence of training. The above statement is the completion of an argument that pervades the cultural and political process imprinting the turning points of the conception of a meta-project of hospital care and the ability to develop a construction program that turns into an architectural design project with phases of increasing complexity and adhering to the legislation (Procurement Code and its Implementing Rules, in the Italian case) which regulates the design of public works.

Institutional Structure of Health Protection and Configuration of Interior Spaces

The reference model for the institutional framework of health protection is an exclusively public insurance system or, vice versa, an exclusively private insurance system; or a mixed formula: public insurance with a voluntary supplementary insurance; or a national health service of a universal nature. Each institutional structure plays a decisive role in the configuration of the space and carries with it non-healthcare functions that do not require dedicated spaces, such as labour relations, human relations of the company management, and representatives of the category. These and other instances require spaces for the general and department meetings for a deeper discussion of regulatory issues and work organisation (6), as well as payment aspects (7) - all variables that strongly impact the architectural design of the hospital facility. Therefore, assuming that each region's situation is unique, any interference with the pre-existing facility looks very complex. This is speaking generally. If we are talking about a hospital renovation, the key of the project works cannot be other than bringing in new functions. This looks possible, but difficult. Experience shows results that are on the fringe of being blatantly unsatisfactory. The reasons are to be found, at least in hospitals made before the twentieth century, in a holistic design approach with a uniform architectural texture. Only by the 1900s did designers begin to deal with the problem of functional modules, such as organisation of areas designated to perform single clinical functions, subject to frequent conversions in the view of technological and scientific innovations. Ensuring the possibility of possible future conversions of the interior spaces introduces a concept, which has become a constraint in the new project design: flexibility in spatial organisation. Renovation of the interior partitions, reconfiguration of machinery and facilities, which is almost always accompanied by a remodelling of the spaces housing them, create a legitimate doubt regarding the validity of a hospital conversion-adjustment operation. Innovation linked to the healthcare function that is planned to be introduced; adaptation to mandatory technical requirements in the field of construction appear as an operation at a loss both for the final quality of the building product and for the economic costs of operation. An assessment on advisability of functional recovery of an existing hospital is looking for a serious demonstration of economic viability of the operation on the basis of cost-benefit analysis. In the case of Italy: urban history, population density, epidemiology, and other environmental factors make render a decision to build a hospital from scratch equally problematic, if we take a look at the market of available building sites. To position a hospital site within an urban structure, the value required by the urban land rent does not make up for the final value of the work. Today, the land rent is the main pathological factor in the real estate regime, responsible for its perverse effects on the city, the region, the environment, and the landscape (Campos Venuti, 2010). Today, reasons that are strictly economic and managerial, on the part of both the government and the lobby, have imposed a decisive, strategic path: a purely hospital network becomes a mixed network (hospital and out-of-hospital care). The latter has mainly social care connotations. The hospital network, in turn, will not be 'mono', i.e. composed of structures where the same specialist activities repeat and overlap (internal medicine, general surgery, orthopaedics, obstetrics-gynaecology, paediatrics, ophthalmology, urology, otolaryngology), but a polycentric network that has a hospital hub with a high technological and professional content, differentiated by speciality, in the sense that it contains a comprehensive, if not exhaustive, spectrum of medical and surgical specialities. Around this hospital technological hub that seeks to rapidly treat the programmed acuteness and the one that comes from its emergency room and other sites where emergency cases are treated after stabilisation of the patient, we can speculate about a territorial network of emergency rooms, possibly incorporated into a constellation of out-of-hospital sites and facilities. Some are characterised by a prevalent health component (8), others are constructed to service mainly the social health aspects (9). This constellation is organically functional for the hospital technological hub, it cooperates with the hub on the basis of rigorous programming and at the same time enjoys complete autonomy in organisational and management matters. It is evident that a multi-specialisation structure is itself a centre of training and updating, as well as being a centre for applied research. The solution built around university hospitals and research hospitals appears more complex, which in themselves are, undoubtedly, also hospital technological hubs of excellence. The elitist resistance, expresses mainly by academia of the medical and surgical faculties, is strong, claiming a need for "separateness" from the "health network". Much more profitable, for both the educational process and the research, would be a close and organic collaboration between university clinics and the medical staff who work at the level of hospital technological hubs - a work in tandem in the same place where training and internships take place. A sort of Medical Faculty widespread throughout the region. Universities should remain the centres for training of healthcare, medical, and nursing personnel, as well as that of health technicians in the basic preparatory matters - like biology, anatomy, physiology, etc. - the academic medicine. Such training should be similar for both biologists-geneticists, pharmacists, and psychologists. It may seem utopian (in a possible world) - a vision of a hospital and out-of-hospital health system that is a concentrate of high technical-scientific and humanistic knowledge. But it is the way of excellence in order to implement prevention treatments - one of the most significant aspects of the medical act and one of the pillars of the national public health target. Prevention is a widespread culture in the regions where nature and society exist in closer proximity. The success of this proximity (health) is related to a state of permanent pedagogy (the first pillar), which is completed by the second pillar, that of an action that becomes symptomatology and therapeutic technique. Therapeutic and pedagogical acts are the results of knowledge transmitted by the professional body of medical sciences, either directly or through the mass medium. The legitimacy of knowledge, its impulse, and its support comes through continuous awareness campaigns and cultural insights, supported by the institutions of democratic representation (especially the municipalities and their decentralisation organs).

So far, reference was made, even if without directly citing them, to instruments of regional government that increasingly show their obsolescence: the general plan, area plans, and other planning instruments. In the individual experiences over the last 10-15 years, the interpretation of the planning regulations given by the bureaucracy of the local public administration has been negative. The legal tangle lends itself to a subjectivity of interpretation. The scope given to arbitrary and discretionary power is vast. The urban planning standard and its local regulations have together created a culture of widespread corruption. Urban planning instruments used to limit unauthorised building, depredation of the territory, and landscape havoc have failed miserably. Not only have they failed to safeguard the territory from overbuilding out of various and increasingly extravagant motivations, like the one that gave rise to the so-called 'illegal necessity', but have rendered the expansion of the city so distorted that it already requires urgent building and urban regeneration. What's the alternative? Some propose replacement of the existing planning instruments with an Urban Code that contains some good rules of social coexistence and the freedom of expression of the individual, contained within the limits of non-detailed structural planning (Moroni, 2013).

The yearned for utopia of a non-assertive and prescriptive society? How to counteract, at this historic juncture, a growing twilight of the community spirit? How to create a utopia? Global competition has undermined the values of the community. The crisis unfolds across the board: the crisis of the family; insufficient knowledge of the practical context; rise and crisis of confidence in solutions for emerging from the crisis; fading of the community that in the heat of competitive stress generates less and less solidarity and increasingly - social envy and resentment (Bonomi, 2014). The positive answer to the crisis is that of a recovery of the community spirit, the Utopia: not to surrender to the way things are and fight for things as they should be (Magris, 2001). The envisaged solution is to overcome the narrow areas, such as the physical area of the community, to go to what is called a 'wide area'. Yet it is worth remembering that the rhetoric is directed at problems of production. The wide area is, therefore, an integral part of a commodity chain or of a manufacturing industry sector, but also the way in which different Italian regions (Tuscany, Lazio, Umbria, etc.) have embarked on the path to renewal of their hospitals. The knowledge of the medical professions, knowledge of scientific and technological innovation in biomedicine, and the transmission of that knowledge and skills makes citizens aware of environmental risks and leads them to take part in a mass culture that aims to defeat the disease, disability, chronic nature, and inequality between social classes in terms of health.

The Hospital Technological Hub and the Health Home

The future of diagnostics and treatment processes will be in compliance with the ELC (Essential Levels of Care) at:

1. A multi-specialised hospital technology hub (HTH) with a low number of beds and a high composition of disciplinary knowledge and biomedical technologies, for patients to undergo medical and surgical treatments possible only when hospitalised. Although it may seem radical, the trend in the near future is to move towards a single multi-specialised hospital with a very high technological and professional composition, with a programmed organisation of activities turnover that will be primarily surgical, with a user base (catchment population) of around 400,000 - 500,000 inhabitants and an undifferentiated fleet of beds (not assigned to individual specialities, except those reserved to the ICU), making up a total of around 150-200 units (0.4-0.5 per thousand inhabitants), with an average of 12-15 general and specialised operating theatres. Inside the HTH there is a deployed level I "Emergency Department" (ED), totally independent in terms of workforce, instruments, diagnostics, operating theatres, and beds with bedheads for continuous

surveillance by the central observation desk of the ICU. The ED is the reference point of the emergency rooms throughout the region that are located within some or all of the out-of-hospital structures operating in the area. The concentration of hospitals with the sharp redrafting of the number of beds, on the one hand wishes to move towards a concentration of places of the professional exercise of disciplinary knowledge and, consequently, to a qualitatively higher performance, while on the other conflicting with the question of ensuring citizens' health, wherever they may reside. This proposes an operation dictated by necessity, of the nature opposite to the concentration - that of de-concentration of healthcare services in the out-of-hospital facilities without hospitalisation. The summary of out-of-hospital activities can be distributed across the territory or concentrated in one physical structure - or several structures according to the needs of the inhabited localities served and the existing communication systems with their travel times - called Health Homes, structures designed to ensure health responses and social care to a population of 25,000 to 35,000 inhabitants (Benigni, Fagnoni, Geddes, Giofrè and Terranova, 2007). The choice is closely linked to the territorial diffusion/concentration of the population.

2. Facilities throughout the territory (Health Homes, polyclinics, rehabilitation centres, clinics of various kinds) with medium technological intensity, with prevailing nursing management, health technicians, and therapeutic rehabilitation programmes defined by general practitioners and by paediatricians of free choice, if patients do not require continuous medical surveillance systems (without hospitalisation) for their diagnostic and therapeutic needs. The continuous input of biomedical technology innovations into the diagnostic cycle - the type of technology tending towards progressive miniaturisation - allows the transfer of innovations to decentralised structures that can be placed upstream and downstream of the above cycles. Decentralised structures are potentially alternative to hospitalisation or are able to reduce the length of patient's hospital stay, thus sparing the patient the prolonged stress of hospitalisation and saving the costs of expensive hospitalisation. Health Homes also incorporate emergency rooms (if the population is concentrated in a single urban settlement) or first air points (if the population is distributed in smaller urban/rural localities). These facilities devoted to urgent and emergency treatments are the territorial and functional emanation of the level I Emergency Department ("ED") at the hospital technological hubs of reference. The characteristics of such EDs is that among their on-call (consultancy) staff, beyond

the standard provided by the technical regulations for the level I ED, they have neurosurgery specialists for the treatment of traumas and cardiovascular surgeons for the treatment relative to the obstruction of vessels and arteries (professionals only approved for level II EDs). The proposed solution allows the most frequent risks to be covered, especially concerning road and workplace accidents, and the prevention of neurological and cardiological damage. The network of the Health Homes, if they contain an urgency-emergency area, must guarantee an eventual transfer of the emergency patient to the ED of reference. The maximum time, according empirical standards, is first 45 minutes. After the first 30 minutes after the accident, whether of traumatic or internal nature, the first irreversible damage to the patient begins to appear.

Careful planning, with a view to physical and technical climate factors on the site of the new (prospective) hospital will allow to an appropriate planimetric typology to be proposed. The shape, orientation, and layout of the rooms will have significant influence on energy behaviour of the building. From what has been written, the type of building requires the overcoming of gigantism that characterises current hospital buildings. The site plan of an ideal hospital technological hub is with twin and horizontally oriented blocks, with a significant downsizing of facilities dedicated to vertical movements, that will be replaced by escalators and treadmills, as the volumes containing the various modules do not exceed two floors above ground and two underground floors for parking and storage of hospital materials. The connective system in this type of building acquires great importance, as does the ability to create piazzas and courtyards full of greenery and natural light, as well as covered roads and passages that promote opportunities for meeting and socialising, especially among visitors and ambulatory patients. Due to high energy consumption, a hospital must aim to self-produce energy from alternative sources. The choice is obviously linked to the locally favourable situations (solar, photovoltaic, biomass, geothermal, etc.). The project must dedicate great attention to the building envelope and energy savings, both for reasons of self energy production and of climate change (10). The design of the envelope must respond to these needs and, at the same time, minimise a negative environmental impact.

If the relationship between the architecture of the envelope and the surrounding environment is undoubtedly important, in terms of visual landscape impact this relationship becomes a matter for the short and medium term. Smart reinterpretation of the urban planning is decisive so that climate change does not turn into an environmental disaster. The intelligent solutions depart from urban civil infrastructuring (11), but other equally important solutions may be designed on the level of the actual building (12). The relationship between the building envelope and the environment is not limited to technological solutions of environmental and construction hygiene. Upstream, there is a crucial question of a preventive nature that has the cultural base in the need to bring to reason the designers' arrogance. The latter and their mentors in land speculation continue to pursue the hypertrophy of the architectural development of a globalised capital city. The craze to build an array of super-tall buildings of glass in the desert that consume enormous amounts of energy and do not respond to the housing needs of local citizens has something absurd and irrational about it. The planet is littered with buildings of glass and steel, with the skeleton on the outside of the body, with visible joints and walls that are not orthogonal. The cities have become all the same. They are increasingly boring. At best, you play a bit with the forms, in a rather useless attempt. The result does not change. This architecture is not only not made to measure, but ignores human's dimensions (Rykwert, 2011). If waste and futility connotes urban gigantism, the urban conflict which follows from it constitutes the most worrying aspect. In cities, cohabitation is definitely in crisis. There is a growing sense of not belonging, of disorientation, of rupturing of the social bond. Instead of common spaces there are so many fences. Neighbourhoods where you live armoured. The same shopping centres, like fortresses surrounded by huge parking lots that form the moats (Niola, 2011).

For a continuous science and technology innovation in the biomedical sector, the hospital is subject to an absolute flexibility of spaces. Therefore, inner partitions must be as mobile as possible, with the systems, both functional of the building and biomedical, incorporated in the interior. One aspect that affords some degree of freedom to the designer is a relatively recent conceptual conquest. It's the idea of providing natural light to all areas of the hospital, from the highly technological ones (instrumental diagnostics, ICU) to those considered to be on medium (ED, OR) and low technology levels (hospitalisation). The proposed classification is of course the traditional one that changes along with the introduction of technological innovations in the hospital, such as: operating theatres with robotic technologies; emergency equipment that incorporates the latest generation of diagnostics and therapeutics, such as CT scans, MRI, PET, etc .; instrumental diagnostics with high level of automation in both laboratory analyses and in diagnostic imaging. All research on the presence of natural light in a hospital setting, particularly in areas with a strong presence of innovative technologies, confirms that this factor greatly reduces the risk of stress of health personnel. Window openings in hospitalisation areas directly influence clinical parameters with positive results related to reduced time of hospital stay and reduced use of painkillers. Therefore, for patients the healing process is accelerated. If natural light is one of the design choices seen as essential for the welfare of both patients and health care professionals, the horizontal layout type allows for a favourable positioning of the operating rooms in terms of access to natural lighting. The twin building type also guarantees good natural lighting conditions and reduced length of routes, as well as the ability to expand or reduce the number of beds. The use of natural lighting, of course, leads to a good degree of energy saving.

Functional Modules of Healthcare Buildings for the Performance of Healthcare Services

The hospital (system) can be divided into modules (sub-systems) that are synergistic with one another, as well as possessing their own functional autonomies that can be identified as:

Module 1. Emergency area (Emergency Department, ED) with its own dedicated entrance and reserved routes to the Operating Theatre (OR), the Intensive Care Unit (ICU) and the wards;

Module 2. Area of instrumental diagnostics (imaging, laboratory analyses, endoscopy) and treatments (surgical endoscopy) at the service of hospitalised patients (with a reserved route) and external users - therefore also equipped with a dedicated entrance for the latter and an internal route from the general entrance that does not interfere with the route reserved for hospitalised patients;

Module 3. Surgical and ICU area with internal reserved routes from the emergency area to the hospital wards;

Module 4. Hospital wards area with direct internal routes from the general entrance, as well as dedicated routes from the emergency, surgical, and diagnostic imaging areas.

Beside the emergency area there must be an area reserved especially for dealing with emergencies following disasters, which can be of various types and involve numerous casualties. These disasters may include both natural and man-made ones. Given the high number of people involved in such emergencies, the goal of this area is to alleviate some of the pressure from the standard hospital emergency area; as well as, and this is fundamental, to isolate the possible diffusive and contagious cases due to generated biological agents classified as bacteria and similar organisms, viruses, parasites, fungi, with envisaged containment measures at levels 3 and 4. Such disasters, both natural and man-made, are usually due to the political and administrative choices resulting in the failure of environmental prevention, despite the existence of measures of proven effectiveness. The recurring rhetoric with which these emergencies are identified is that of disaster medicine. Disaster medicine is a branch of medicine that is placed between the culture of medical-surgical emergency and culture of environmental disasters. From a scientific point of view, disaster medicine explores the methods and tools for the implementation of effective medical interventions. The organisational model used is that of wartime medicine. The reserved area is divided into a fully equipped clinic with its operating rooms and beds (pl). The latter are equipped with bedheads for any ICU treatments.

A building module corresponds to each area. If in the past the proximity of some areas was a conditioning factor, today, with dedicated information systems being available (intranet), it has seen a considerable change in dimensions. This allows the designer greater degrees of freedom in the distribution of the modules which in summary are spaces that are positioned according to the orientation but also to the environment. Internet connects the hospital technology hub and the out-of-hospital facilities. The range of health and social health facilities throughout the region also have computerised systems that allow a continuous exchange of information and transfer of materials and laboratory diagnostic imaging in real time (from the Health Homes to the hospital technological hubs and vice versa, as well as within each module of the two health care structures).

Currently, at a scientific and organisational level, there is a growing debate on the best solution to the evolution of disease/healing in the therapeutic environment. Some see a solution in terms of care intensity. The result at the project design level is the identification of hospital sub-modules that are characterised by low risks with low technology levels, by medium risks, and arriving at hospitalisation for treatments with high-risk intensive technology (comparable, in all the effects, to an ICU). The proposed solution creates rigid therapeutic environments, but mostly makes their transfer psychologically (humanly) untenable for patients. In addition to, in case of clinical errors, loss of time and low productivity of the staff. In countries where investment in new hospitals is consistent, experimental research shows a solution for hospital stays which could be called the 'making technology available'. In summary, the proposed solution is that each room can be used for any level of intensity of care, from the lowest and all the way to sub-intensive and intensive care. The only thing that changes are bedheads. The cost of construction may be greater, but not necessarily. The advantages mainly relate to a continuous flow of information on the biometric parameters of the patient with the possibility of medical interventions in real time. This increases patient's "socialisation" in dealing with the professional body, which always remains constant in the course of different therapeutic phases related to the evolution of the disease.

Indoor and Outdoor Spaces

The benefits of an art project that accompanies the architectural design are unquestionable. The works of art and video-art installations bear a significant importance in helping to defuse the hospital environment, to promote the creation of reassuring and classy surroundings. Visually it gives identity to the spaces, it supports the orientation and mobility of those who live the experience of the hospital, as patients, visitors or medical/technical staff. The artistic project metabolises in the interior and/or, as an alternative, in the signage, which is essential for the movements and for finding specific places - that are no longer just anonymous spaces.

Hospital outdoor surroundings, as in any health facility, should not be ignored. On par with the interiors, they play a therapeutic function for patients, and that of relieving work-related stress for the technical and medical staff. A space, outside of the hospital, facing the city, is open to it. But we must ask ourselves, is it really so: Which city? A utopian one, immortalised so well by the Renaissance art, or the real one, a capitalist city? We must note that the current urban concentration turns cities into huge multi-functional machines: perfect in the minds of the designers, chaotic and often unbearable, a source of anguish and alienation, for the people who live in them (Veronesi, 2013). Anguish and alienation is the cultural background that afflicts the humans that revolve around or live a part of their life story within the hospital. The demarcation lines that mark the border between the external, techno-mutant and alienating world, and the internal, pervasively distressing and hyper-technological one are borders, thresholds, passages, official doors from which the invisible barriers of the implied exclusion originate (Augé, 2012): the walls of the prescription, political or criminal control. Inside the hospital, the domain of science, philosophical culture and... unhappiness, an exchange of knowledge, consolidation and upgrading of skills, attitudes and abilities takes place. But then the invisible barriers of exclusion spring up, separating for the sick? Unfortunately it is not so. The Italian context is evidence of this. It was certainly not the intention of the legislators, who in 1978 established Italy's national public health service, to deny the equality of citizens faced with illness. Others, in the delirium of neoliberal ideology that has contaminated the great ideals of solidarity and equality as a condition of the freedom of an individual and of a country, intended to introduce classist measures within the public health service. The justification is always the same: whatever crisis is taking place, whether cyclical or structural, it imposes measures: an erosive universalism of the health service in the face of illness; they are apparently minimalist measures (fees for medicine, specialist visits, hospital admissions). In a final scenario of privatisation of the public health services and a transition that has private subsidiarity as its fundamental pillar, be it a social enterprise, a voluntary association, a non-governmental health protection organisation, a non-profit company, etc. The inequality of citizens that, when faced with illness, can transform a democratic community into an illusory one (Veca, 2014, p.17), which has based its reasoning on the idea that a right guaranteed by the State may be delegated to compassionate private entities (who are nonetheless always careful to profit at the expense of the quality of performance!). The transition to private contains a second pillar: the exercise of freelance professional services within the hospital, with the use of its human and structural resources, its assets and services (intramural). Whoever is prepared to pay for health service has a path reserved for them, a parallel and rapid access service. Waiting lists are no longer a problem. They relate to those who believed in a universal and free health service (the poor, the workers and the middle class: the so-called new poor).

Alongside science, knowledge and responsibility, the hospital environment is dominated by strong communicative aphasia, by authoritarian and self-referential practices, and a colourful range of personalities marked by personal stories of life and suffering. A profound asymmetry dominates the hospital: the sick vs the professional body; the professional body across its hierarchical structure; the sick and the professional body vs the administrative management. Asymmetries that are recomposed on a macroscale to address other issues, fundamental and crucial, for the system(s) of outright power that revolve around health:

- expectations of the local community in terms of ensuring better health of its components;
- results seen in terms of electoral support for political parties who govern in the health sector;
- successes of the trade unions of the professional body in securing employment levels, modern relationships in terms of work organisation and wage rewarding;
- maturation of a culture on the dialectics of environmental determinants that favour or condition and reduce disease processes;
- approach to the determinants of health of local communities using probability methods in population and epidemiological surveys; etc.

Which solution should be accorded to an urban setting, where the city looks more and more like a prison? People, non-existent and with looks of hollow wickermen. An idea of tattered order, an automatic decay. Smog powder is ashen, and its deposits are ubiquitous. The clouds are polluted; the air is ammonia (Genna, 2013). The suburban neighbourhoods, in and out of motorways, ring roads, are alarming, placed under curfew, incendiary. Neighbourhoods where a revolt is hatching. The answer when faced with so much despair is a headlong rush forward: giving the word back to the landscape (Augé, 2012). The landscape as a classless element promoting social integration. A dismissive answer that does not take into account factors that frustrate this line. Who owns the land surrounding the hospital? The legal institution of expropriation for public utility is now impassable for the high cost of land but, above all, for the inviolability of private property, according to the many judgements in its defence by the EU High Court of Justice. Another issue closely related to the first is the need to break the perverse convergence of interests between the land rent (in the hands of manufacturers, duly informed of the directions of urban development under the new planning instruments, even before their approval), the real estate companies (in the hands of financial capital that is forever in search of speculative profit), and administrators of cities (paralysed by the lack of transfers from the State, they see it as a compensatory way to acquire concession fees with the most heinous and destructive political and business planning). Overbuilding of the territory will continue implacably, unless some decisive and subversive political decisions are taken (13). But this is impossible, given the absolute domination, both economic and conscious, exercised with all the tools of violence and persuasion by the State. Capitalism, during the apogee of neoliberal imperialism, needs urbanization to absorb the surplus products that it produces continuously. It is in constant search of territories favourable to the production and absorption of surplus capital. The natural environment is increasingly put under pressure to yield the raw materials needed, including urban development areas, and to absorb the inevitable waste (Harvey, 2013). The crux is - without prejudice to the freedom of personal movement - how to weaken, with a radical 'zero airspace' political choice, the attractive variables of a metropolitan city that, as experience shows, swallows all the surrounding agglomerations, blurring the lines between urban and rural areas. Everything is a metropolitan area. 'Zero airspace' does not mean an asphyxiated construction industry, but rather buildings that operate so that the degraded and inhospitable suburbs become a city but without spreading like wildfire. Instead, through precisely targeted operations, enriching them with the public facilities. Today, rather than explosive, the growth ought to be implosive. We must complete the former industrial, military or railway areas; build on the already built (Piano, 2014). The work of mending that appears minimalist is to be counted today among the most subversive ones, in as much as, specifically, this work is substantiated with another decisive step: the land available for housing development (promptly snapped up by speculators) may well be returned to agriculture. The weakening attraction of a metropolitan city passes through other decisions. The first requires a challenging investment; regarding project financing. That is, a system of rapid rail transits that accommodates mass commuting from residences outside the city to the metropolitan area. The second, a tax reduction and credit lines for redeveloping housing and local welfare (services for children, youth and the elderly, cultural services, health services, social housing and co-housing programs) of minor historical centres to render them more attractive. The third is the development of teleworking and remote assistance (in the case of health care, the "telemedicine") in order to reduce the massive displacement of people to the places of care and increase the culture of self-medication that can be used to deal with some aspects of the demand for health services.

We must bear in mind that the hospital environment is a space marked by suffering, emotion and death. At the same time the hospital is a place steeped in futuristic technology that represents a guarantee, as expected by the patients and the professional body, of a proper diagnosis and an equally correct therapy. The technology of the equipment is not completely neutral, but contains hazardous elements. The materials, on their own or in combination, that are manipulated in the diagnostic-therapeutic processes pose risks of various kinds (14) and with different levels of severity. In summary, the hospital space also contains very serious safety problems, especially for the permanent population of the hospital that is present there for various reasons, but also in terms of possible effects on the outside, on the civilian population (15).

We must reflect on how to safeguard biomedical technologies, especially from damage, theft, and terrorist attacks. In other words, how to ensure safety of equipment, supplies, people who work inside or those present in the healthcare setting for treatment and similar reasons. Security involves monitoring the movement of people from the entrance to the exit of the physical structure. Monitoring which is accomplished by technologically isolating the structure (compartmentalisation for large areas, as written above). A surveillance system is required, featuring filters distributed throughout individual compartments. The various filters must be characterised by their digitization (electronic card) that allows monitoring, tracking, and systematic observation by those circulating inside the hospital space with the allocation of chips for radio frequency identification (RFID, Radio Frequency IDentification) that offer unique identifiers for each individual; the data issued by equipment and medical devices can be easily attached to the chip identifiers that each person carries within the hospital (Bauman and Lyon, 2014). The question raised here is relevant in terms of the ethics of surveillance and the debate launched by the analysis of Jeremy Bentham's Panopticon, by Michel Foucault (Foucault, 1976). Surveillance technologies have reached levels of gross violation of individual and community privacy. It is the triumph of the ideology of protection of the city from the many threats that lurk in the city itself and are born in it. Strongholds of urban insecurity have, over the centuries, become nurseries or incubators of real or alleged dangers, endemic or imaginary. Built with the idea of creating islands of order in a sea of chaos, cities have become more abundant as the sources of disorder and require walls, barricades, guard towers, and bars, both conspicuous and inconspicuous (Bauman and Lyon, 2014).

The gap between the metropolitan city to the capitalist society par excellence is a short one. The age in which we live is pervaded by fear of an unknown future, as well as the fear of unknown foreigners who could come and set off bombs. There is a widespread fear that governments are no longer able to control the circumstances of life. The perspective is our transformation into a 'gated' society, with the aim of keeping out the rest of the world. It is clear by now that governments have lost control of their territories (Judt and Snyder, 2012). Observations that merit further investigation. In the specific case of the hospital setting, the question is how to protect installations, hi-tech and delicate equipment related to the survival of the people? You can not escape, unfortunately, the proposed solution of electronic technologies: today… and tomorrow? This we do not know. A disturbing future. David Lyon warns us of hope: responsibility and acting accordingly (Bauman and Lyon, 2014). No longer a utopia. By now refuge is simple common sense!

The environment surrounding the hospital, the so-called 'surroundings', must be designed to counter the situation of the internal space and, therefore, be friendly, perceived as a place of transit or a meeting place, dominated by the perception of health and well-being, in contrast to that of illness and death in the inside of the hospital. The architect's key role here is in achieving the above by defining the proportions or volumes, the length and width of these volumes (lights), the rhythms, the contrasts, the importance of the materials used for the building and, above all, the adaptation of the volumes that make up the hospital to the site, the location, the sunshine, the climate, the orientation. Hippocrates, in the treatise "Environment", dated between 430 and 410 BC (Vegetti, 1965), examines the problem of the relationship between environmental conditions, the social and historical setting, and the psychological situation of the people. In designing the environment surrounding the hospital, the project architect must reflect on the location of the building, its orientation with respect to the winds and the sunrise, and especially on the continuity, the physical relationship with the city. An environment that must be used by all. Disease is an episode in the life of an individual. Healing is the removal of disease. There cannot, therefore, be an irreversible rift between man in his mental and biological conditions (healthy or sick). In conclusion, the universal design must guide the designer.

Recommendations for project designers can be summarised in the following paragraphs.

1. Developed buildings of very high technological complexity, with the presence of strong professional knowledge and a low number of beds characterise the new hospital building complexes (hospital technological hubs).

2. Continuous inclusion of technological innovations in biomedicine makes the existing hospital structures rapidly obsolete. Today, it is possible to predict the timing of introduction of diagnostics and therapeutics innovations. The slowdown of this obsolescence process is only possible if the design choices are guided by the idea of flexibility of spaces and adaptation of building systems to that idea. Flexibility is accompanied by the idea of modularity, and organisational and management self-sufficiency of every single technical area (module).

3. The 'hospital technological hub' requires large energy consumption for its operation. Without drawing attention to the devastating effects on the soil and the atmosphere, the priority is dictated by the high cost of traditional energy consumption. A solution that requires a 'possible' amount of investment is the use of renewable alternatives to petroleum products, such as solar, geothermal, wind, biogas, biomass, etc. Such sources are found in the nature and are, therefore, low-cost. If this effort is matched by changes resulting from the proper use of insulating building materials, as well as improvements of fixtures to prevent heat loss, and other ingenious solutions, the cost of energy consumption will be considerably reduced.

4. Interior partitions must fully respond to the rhetoric of flexibility and modularity, and cannot be achieved in traditional building. Instead, this solution requires panels produced from lightweight and natural materials, so as to be easily mounted, removed, and installed with all the traditional and biomedical systems (in a way that the devices and installations can always be easily accessed for inspections).

5. The architecture of the 'hospital technological hub' should aim to have an extremely simple (readable) planimetric, so as not to confuse (stress) patients and their visitors or carers. Given the selectivity with which the number of treated cases (the activities of the hub) is programmed and the high speed of patients turnover

that characterises it, yet, at the same time, in a context of total autonomy and self-sufficiency of the urgency and emergency module (Emergency Department) that does not interfere with the planned activities of the hub, the physical structure ought to be developed horizontally, with a sharp limit on the number of the overground floors (max 2 floors, and two underground floors for services). Vertical connections fall under the scope of traditional mechanical-electrical fixtures.

6. The shape deemed best for the form of stay, both in terms of rationality and for full exploitation of the natural light, is the comb-type positioning of the spaces-modules, with a central module for the distribution function.

7. The beds of inpatient module must have the technological equipment similar to those of sub-intensive therapies (bedhead units), which thus eliminate the need for patient transfer in case of aggravation. The patient is monitored by the ICU monitors.

8. Natural light diffused in all parts of the technological hub is the goal that the designer needs to pursue in order to accelerate the healing process and to give greater security to the professional body. Absolute priority is given to technological areas that require greater attention, such as operating theatres, intensive care units, and the emergency room. Specialist design solutions must be developed for the so-called shadowed and dark places, to bring rays of light from the window openings, inner courts, and external routes joining the different modules (buildings).

9. Art works and video-art installations play down the overall environment of the hospital technological hub creating a classy and reassuring environment, giving specific, reassuring and comforting spaces.

10. The building of the hospital technological hub must be designed to withstand climate change that is producing increasingly violent and destructive events. Therefore, glass walls are unsuitable, not only for the high energy consumption, but also for the notable fragility of such a building. The building should be designed using natural (green) or artificial systems for sound, thermal and hydraulic insulation, with the aim of cooling, and creating thermal and environmental comfort.

11. Between the distressing and hyper-tech internal space of a hospital and the external space of the city (chaotic and uninhabitable), the dividing zone is a boundary, most often visible (bars, walls, gates and so on) intended to cordon off and isolate the hospital. During the 1970's, on the emotional wave of the struggle against totalitarian (closed) institutions such as civilian hospitals, the line

of 'de-institutionalisation' of the hospital institutions was pursued towards an open access, free movement and the presence of relatives - essential elements in the healing process, as well as in control of work processes and of negligence of the professional body. In its operation, today the 'healing machine' is facing a society dominated by computer systems, networks where technology has taken precedence over human impetus, or rather it is the means to impose something (hegemonic view; justicialism; populism; pogroms; witch hunt; etc.). The presence of highly expensive and sophisticated biomedical technologies, the complexities of managing them, and the need, as far as is possible, to safeguard the privacy of individuals, requires an approach of closing up the institution to prevent damage, misappropriation of particularly dangerous consumables and potential sources of bio-terrorism, and to protect people from intrusions, beyond lawful ones, on their privacy, to prevent theft of sensitive information that may lead to conditioning and manipulation not only by individuals and criminal organisations, but also by the very same insurance companies. This is prevented using the same enforcement systems, but in the opposing sense. Access to the hospital technology hub will be increasingly subject to authorisation processes, for the purposes of control, tracking, and so on.

12. Thus far, the solutions for hospital outer spaces have been disappointing and obvious: a functional space for the delivery of goods for the operation of the health facility, and a space to be used as parking for staff and visitors, and for the users of medical services. It has been repeatedly stated that this outer space ought to be understood as a link and transit for people of the city to the city. The architectural solution that has materialised so far is a tunnel full of commercial and leisure facilities, with shops, cafés, restaurants, libraries and whatever else, able to attract people not only as health facility visitors, but as consumers. It has been, and still is argued that this aspect - consumerism - makes the environment far less oppressive and dials down the distress and drama of a closed structure, as hospitals are traditionally understood , where one fights a battle for life, against disability and death. Although many new hospitals have received this message of openness, the solution is confirmed as being a palliative one compared to a context where you play the game that calls into question the humanity of an individual. Talking of the hospital technological hub, the humanisation discourse must be addressed not only with architectural solutions but especially with correct relational forms between the professional body and the patients and their families, with the

deployment of powerful biomedical technologies and organisational solutions to speed up the turnover, thus making patients' stay in the hospital as brief as possible. The external environment must be an environment that stands out as a place for stopping and socialising, where a green space prevails that is equipped with numerous commercial and leisure opportunities that makes the hospitalised and the professional body feel like a part of the living world, albeit protected from all those aspects that make life in the city impossible at times - such as pollution of various kinds and the civilisation of machinery. Parking, functional and storage areas ought to be resolved using underground spaces.

In conclusion, there are two final considerations.

a) In terms of recovery and restoration of hospitals built in the 1960s-70s to create hospital technological hubs, the particular construction systems of that era and bad quality of building technologies used at the time make these hospitals unsuitable for extraordinary maintenance and unable to meet the demands of flexibility and modularity. The excessive size of these structures owing to an organisational structure where each individual speciality was granted its own, segregated space, the expansionism due to the hierarchy of micro-organisations (services, sections, divisions), and the relevant functional (hospital beds) and employee standards have had a negative effect on the urban environment - in terms of the buildings' violent visual impact. For large hospitals, the wear and tear of materials that make up the structure of reinforced concrete, and the numerous and complex technical regulations (hospital, seismic, electrical, fire, safety, energy saving standards, etc.) issued in the last 30-40 years, as well as the adaptation of the pre-existing ones to the EU legislation, are such that, at the expert level, the prevalently proposed ideal solution is the conversion of use (provided the planning instruments make it feasible), or otherwise outright demolition. Small general hospitals of local communities should be converted into Health Homes or similar out-of-hospital structures. This entails a light level of operations, to clean up the layers of construction projects that occurred over time while maintaining the pre-existing structural elements and architectural floor plan.

b) Faced with a scenario of a self-referential and authoritarian structure pervaded by biomedical technology, the prerogative of the professional body becomes the problem of returning some form of democracy to its management. The role of the local community, politicians, and intermediate bodies of society, such as unions, is crucial. The entire fabric of society ought to be involved in a continuous action of raising community awareness of the technical and scientific professions aimed at the protection of human health. Only an alliance of the latter with the local community and politicians can remove the air of segregating elitism from the work of the professional body, and reduce the famous lack of communication that makes patients very frustrated.

Notes

(1) Examples include: revisions of building systems in relation to seismic legislation, fire safety legislation, thermal insulation for the purpose of energy saving, wear of materials, both natural and artificial, adaptation of legislation on plants and fixtures, adjustment of the legislation on the areas protected by the Superintendency of Antiquities and Fine Arts, regulations on industrial or productive restricted areas, etc.

(2) Basic hospital for 50,000 inhabitants; provincial hospital for 450,000 inhabitants; regional hospital for 1-1,500,000 inhabitants.

(3) Basic hospital; provincial hospital; hospital of regional and national significance; specialised hospitals; university polyclinics; research hospitals.

(4) Biomedical equipment industry; pharma and blood products industry; industry of medical and surgical devices; etc.

(5) Furnishings; lighting; water purification plants; heating, air and temperature control; etc.

(6) Number of health workers per patient or per bed; service time; hierarchical structuring of the staff; professional updating and training.

(7) Overtime, holiday work and night work.

(8) Outpatient clinics; day surgeries; specialist clinics.

(9) Rehabilitation and functional recovery centres; mental health centres; serviced residences; geriatric centres; dentistry centres; family counselling with attached obstetric-paediatric outpatient clinics.

(10) Which technology solutions should be provided for heat waves, hurricanes, storms, rains, flash floods or water bombs, persistent drought, etc.

(11) Sewage and white water drains; rainwater collection tanks; urban green spaces and urban parks; road drains; reinforced river embankments; dams upstream of the city and engagement of canals and pipelines for relief of large natural pools in agricultural land; etc.

(12) Roofing able to absorb, to a limited extent, solar rays and act as a temperature reducer; foundations turned into large tanks, like the old cisterns, in order to lighten the road system of drainage ditches and then, once the alarm stage is over, empty the content of water tanks into the sewer network.

(13) Incentivising policies to strengthen smaller centres with adequate low-cost housing, social infrastructure, and community initiatives targeted at people. Incentivising policies for remote work and remote assistance; policies to combat the new demographic movement to medium and large cities; several solutions can be employed to lighten the density of urban population, including capping the number of new building permits for an extended period of time, with the exception of maintenance; etc.

(14) Electromagnetic fields; optical radiation; laser radiation; explosive atmospheres; chemicals; carcinogens and mutagens; biological agents; etc.

References

Arbesman, S. (2014), "Troppo complicato", in *Internazionale*, 16 May, p. 56.
Augé, M. (2012), "La città di tutti", in *La Repubblica*, 1 October, p. 37.
Bauman,Z. and Lyon, D. (2014), *Sestopotere*, Editori Laterza, Bari, IT, pp. 18, 92-93, 150.
Benigni, B.; Fagnoni, M.; Geddes, M.; Giofrè, F.; Terranova, F. (2007), *La Casa della Salute*, Alinea, Florence, IT.
Boncinelli, E. et al. (2014), "La medicina del futuro", in Le *Scienze*, maggio.
Bonomi, A. (2014), "L'area vasta nuova frontiera dei distretti", in *Il Sole 24 Ore*, 27 April, p. 15.
Bucci, S. (2014), "Decq: L'architetto sarà un neuroscienziato", in *Corriere della sera*, 23 April, p. 21.
Campos Venuti, G. (2010), *Città senza cultura. Intervista sull'urbanistica*, in Oliva, F. (Ed.), Editori Laterza Bari, IT, p. 15.
Chiesi L. (2010), *Il doppio spazio dell'architettura*, Liguori, Naples, IT, p. 57.
Foucault M. (1997), "La politica della salute nel XVIII secolo", in Dal Lago A. (Ed.), *Archivio Michel Foucault*, vol.2, n.7, Feltrinelli, Milan, IT.
Genna, G. (2013), *Fine Impero*, Minimum fax, Rome, IT, pp. 25-7.
Gregotti, V. (2011), *Architettura e postmetropoli*, Einaudi, Turin, IT.
Harvey, D. (2013) *Il capitalismo contro il diritto alla città*, Ombre corte, Verona, IT, p. 10.
Judt, T. and Snyder T. (2012), *Novecento*, Editori Laterza, Bari, IT, p. 375.
Kent, S. (2010), op. cit. in, *Il doppio spazio dell'architettura*, Leonardo Chiesi (Ed.), Liguori, Naples, IT, p. 46.
Magris C. (2001), *Utopia e disincanto*, Garzanti, Milan, IT.
Moroni, S. (2013), *La città responsabile. Rinnovamento istituzionale e rinascita civica*, Carocci, Rome, IT.
Niola, M. (2011), "La città senza cuore", in *La Repubblica*, 27 October, pp. 50-1.
Piano, R. (2014),"Il rammendo delle periferie", in *Il Sole 24 ore*, 26 January, p. 40.
Ruta, C. (2006), *Ai confini della Medicina. Verso l'economia dell'essere*, EGEA, Milan, IT.
Veca, S. (2014), *Non c'è alternativa. Falso!*, Editori Laterza, Bari, IT, pp. 17, 87.
Vegetti M. (1965), *Opere di Ippocrate*, Unione Tipografico-Editrice Torinese, Turin, pp. 163-202.
Veronesi, S. (2013), "Roma e le altre, città chiuse", in *Corriere della Sera*, 20 October, pp. 20-1.

For a full understanding of this essay, it is necessary to have a basic knowledge of architecture and socio-anthropological disciplines. In addition to the reference materials cited in the text, on the specific subject of architecture aimed at finding appropriate design solutions to address the issue of protection and promotion of health, we would like to suggest the following texts:

Giofrè, F. and Terranova, F. (2004), *Ospedale e Territorio, Hospital and Land*, Alinea, Florence, IT.
Giombi, D., Lucarelli, M.T. and Terranova, F. (1989), *Igiene Ambientale*, La Nuova Italia Scientifica, Rome, IT.
Terranova, F. (Ed.) (2005), *Edilizia per la sanità*, UTET, Turin, IT.

03

Healing Environments Design

Nađa Beretić

Abstract: The paper researches a gap between urban open spaces and health care facilities. In common for a sure, they have a stress of all users and doubtless are proved therapeutic effect of green open spaces presence. This paper symbolically presents green spaces as health promoters, but considered balance among all other types of urban open spaces based on the design inputs for health and wellbeing. The urban open spaces of healthcare facilities are considered as a productive supplement in the interior areas, but not only in healing purpose rather to provide a restorative space of well-being for all users, healing rather than curing (as visitors as the parents and staff, and all others) – positive outdoors, restorative environments. If we have been once in the hospital, we can always clearly recognize the smell of it. Then, why we cannot recognize the smell or sound or some other sense as a quality of urban open space within healthcare facility? What are the possibilities of the design inputs to contribute? People relate emotionally to their physical surroundings and environments affect their behaviour and social activities. Healing places must highlight the social dimension of design: social, physical and psychological benefits to be set up as a goal during the design process. Aesthetic and perceptual goals will help designing to shape the environment, but always considered user preferences and ecological needs (contextual issues).

First research question cope with existing researches from related fields, disciplines and participants, who and how can contribute to the design process of healing environments.

Reflected through design, these facts opening the main related question to address papers results: what are the design inputs (patterns and needs) on relation people, environment and interaction (behaviour) in order to provide healing place?

Keywords: healing environments, urban design, open space, green space and landscape patterns.

Introduction

The paper researches a gap between urban open spaces and health care facilities, in order to overcome this gap by clarifying design inputs.

Urban open spaces in general are natural and cultural resource of society, opened in social terms and don't bordered in three physical dimensions, which are dedicated to people activities and pleasure and, important for psychological and social relieving a society. More particularly, the ones within healthcare facilities must stress out stress, not as the only one present specificity, but the overwhelming present and, present among all users (as visitors as the parents, workers and staff, and all others). The urban open spaces of healthcare facilities in this paper are considered as a productive supplement in the interior areas, but not only in healing purpose rather to provide a restorative space of well-being for all users – healing environments. Rather, healing than curing. A recent book (McCullough et al., 2009 p. 45), generally considers healing environment as a place to heal the mind, body, and soul, as "a place where life, death, illness, and healing define the moment and the building supports those events or situations". With a difference due to a statement, for this paper environments are considered as the one who supports; then, 'do' as well. The topic of the natural environment, people, and the relationship between them, it's not an innovation of the paper. One of the first research-based analyses showed the psychological perspective and how various natural settings of environment impacts on people (of diverse ages and cultural heritages), have been done in 80s, by Kaplan & Kaplan. Accordingly, the benefit of natural patterns which foster tranquillity and well-being are exists. The main hypothesis of the paper to be examined is healing environment design as a tool for creation of the restorative character of space, healing environment place, positive distraction. Positive distraction is anything causes a positive emotional response (McCullough et al., 2009). Accordingly, which are the ways to design and interpret environments to enhance its beneficial influences within healthcare facilities? Is it possible to define landscape patterns for design which can be not only more beneficial to healthcare facilities, than recognizable as well?

Ending the past century, the topic of healthcare outdoors became a focus of many researchers, and it is contemporary interest and, nowadays is possible to find more that 1000 papers, books, proceedings and other types of literature. It exists also 'online library' created by Therapeutic Landscape Network (1), which gathers all the literature related to environmental therapeutic effects on people, arranged by alphabet. This database is a multidisciplinary community of designers, health and human service providers, scholars, and gardeners who emphasis on evidence-based design in healthcare settings. Multidisciplinary is a contemporary approach, but this act clues also a necessity for more research in common.

All the sources have been observed in this paper includes Western countries, European and North American literature. Healing and therapeutic gardens are the most present topic, observed from a huge spectrum of different backgrounds. One of the possible reasons is the complexity of the topic, because design seems to be a subcategory of the health (basically, health belongs medicine related sciences). Speaking about its outdoor spaces, the design should be leading field, or tool, to act. Starting from the personal background, both, landscape architecture and urban planning and design, this paper contribute to the theories of urban or landscape design within healthcare facilities, respecting and including contributions of all related disciplines.

The structure of the paper is built by two main sections: Preceding research and Design inputs. First section is organized in defining, classifying key notions (creation of the relationship graphics: human – healing environments – design) and observations on historical conception of outdoor spaces within healthcare facilities. Design inputs section presents extracted conclusions on previous sections and final result of the paper, healing environments design formulation graphics.

Finally, as introduction started with 'stresses relax' trough nature, as an individual, overwhelming present need of all users within healthcare facilities and its environments, to believe and hope, to have feeling of security and sense of belonging are desirable, space attendees, positive distractions. Respectively, I would like to conclude and begin with the sentence of Frank Lloyd Wright: "Study Nature, love nature, stay close to nature. It will never fail you".

Preceding research

This chapter is devoted to defining the key notions and present theories dealing with the research of urban open spaces within healthcare facilities. It researches the notions trough two lenses. The first is a review of existing literature about defining the main theories in the field of healthcare outdoors, and the second one observes historical and cultural conception of outdoor spaces within healthcare facilities.

The first subsection relies on existing and use the knowledge from other fields contributes to understanding and classifying the benefits in common. Later, benefits will be specified and set up as a goal in the process of design. There is already a lot written, than hence the classifying is more appropriate for, than defining already developed. But, using knowledge from the other fields is only appropriate for the writing of the paper. Wider contribution is to understand and include all other possible participants from a wide range of experts to be involved in the proses of design (previously counting on the direct and indirect users of healthcare institutions). Participatory design is not only contemporary approach, deliberating urban open spaces within healthcare facilities, and then it is a necessity. Like to reach features contributing personal benefits of wellbeing, as primary to know what you must not to do. For instance, as the medical personnel know the qualitative and quantitative, both positive and negative effects of some substances, landscape architect knows which species promote them (e.g. which are toxic or not), reflective to use it or not but joint decision and etc.

The second subsection contributes to understanding, reviewing, former and current approaches of professional practices to the urban open spaces within healthcare facilities.

Defining and classifying key notions

Starting with going multidisciplinary interests in a huge field of healthcare related topics, the section is oriented to find an appropriate approach for defining key notions, as present potential to be used for the design inputs of open spaces within healthcare facilities. The method contains three main steps. The first phases was collecting existing literature, and then categorize it into main disciplines which research the field of health, health environments and which are in relation with urban open spaces. The second step was to understand the differences of the used notions among disciplines, choosing and classifying the chosen literature. Finally, the connections among them are clarified and presented graphically (Fig. 1). The graphical result is not a literature review. It is review on chosen literature selected by multi-criteria. Its author's work of collecting, understanding and connecting the main present literature about design of urban open spaces within healthcare facilities, the relationship: human – healthcare environments - design.

Roots of relationship: human – healing environments – design

Collection of the existing literature is included research by four groups of key words. The first one includes terms in relation with healing environments and urban open spaces of healthcare facilities: healthcare environments, hospital environments, outdoor hospital environment, external environment, exterior environment, healthcare open spaces and healthcare green spaces. The second group is health effects related to the landscape: landscape and public health, landscape and environmental stress, restorative urban open space, restorative landscape, landscape and recovery, spaces of wellbeing, natural patterns in hospitals, healing environments, healing landscape, therapeutic landscape, experience of landscape and gardens in healthcare facilities. The third group is used as a 'control layer' to put all material in the relation to the field of design: health design, healthcare outdoor design, landscape patterns, landscape perception, and planting design; the supplement to this group is the main literature from the perspective of urban design expertise in urban open spaces design and production of space theory. But, the process was not linear; oppositely, it was pretty iterative. One of iterations is a fourth key word group, created after studying all literature collected in advance, when the main categories are already created. It served to fill up 'the holes', to complement the knowledgebase according to previously categorized main notions of interest: landscape design metrics, medical geography and cultural geography, environmental psychology, healing gardens, health & wellbeing, biophilia, ecological design and green spaces, urban open spaces design metrics.

The selection process of presenting literature is accomplished by multilevel criteria, sometimes by deductive and other ways by inductive process. In just a few days, according to explained key word groups, the result was few hundreds of references found, and the number was constantly growing. The first excerpt criteria were relevance of the author (number of papers he has been cited) and type of paper (books, than scientific research papers, at first). Secondly, reduction continued by criteria of the author's contribution to the topic, for example, if, he defined notion or he is its interpreter; the creators first. But, this criteria includes not only defining, interpretations with the qualitative benefits of the general topic, also (like criteria of innovation). For instance, Edward Wilson (1984) in his book *Biophilia* set up the biophilia hypothesis, but Heerwagen (1998) in her research paper *Design, productivity and wellbeing: What are the links?*, put it in relation to design. Further, the selection process eliminated books where the chapter is more specific; e.g. Cooper Marcus is respected author and expert for the field on health outdoor spaces, but from her book (1997, co-editor with Francis, C.) *People Places: Design Guidelines for Urban Open Space* is extracted the particular chapter *Hospital outdoor spaces* of Robert Paine. Some literature is added as representative of the book synthesizes few main categories, e.g. is the book *Healing Gardens: Therapeutic Benefits and Design Recommendations* (edited by Cooper Marcus, C. and Branes, M., 1999). The book is categorized in the field cultural geography because its historical and cultural overview present in the first part of the book, but it consists also chapter explains design issues, moreover, in the context of environmental benefits to well-being and written by Roger Ulrich who is representative of environmental posology. This characteristic is included as a qualitative advantage comparing to the book *Gardens in healthcare facilities: Uses, therapeutic benefits, and design recommendations* (Cooper Marcus and Barnes, 1995) where historic overview and the typology of outdoor spaces in healthcare facilities is previously written about. The criterion of diversity was permanently present, addressing to the goal to collect disciplines and theories exist around the topic of healing environments design, as much as it is possible. Correspondingly, some divergent and recent literature is added; an example is the paper *Urban open spaces in historical perspective: A transdisciplinary typology and analysis* (Stanley et al., 2012); or spatial border exception unit: *Regional Public Health Information Paper* (2010) - New Zeeland.

Once the choice and categorisation were maddening, full definitions of the main notion are presented (Table 1: Definitions of key notions). Aiming to point out representatives creates complex relation of human interaction with healing environments, result is the graphic solution shaped it distinctively and easily-readable (Fig. 1: Roots of relationship: human – healing environments – design).

Eight main categories created and observed are: design metrics - landscape, medical and cultural geography, environmental psychology, healing gardens, health & wellbeing, biophilia, ecological design and green spaces - urban open spaces design metrics. The first and the last category are the beginning and the 'final touch' sparkles, as the personal research interests. The differences are starting points; initial aspect was landscape architecture, or other times the inception was urban design. In general, design metrics are in common, but the typology of spaces is defined in different ways. The landscape approach is a starting point, according to the specific topic and scope category: health and wellbeing (the field of measuring the qualities of life). The landscape approach has a historical dimension in terms of healthcare facilities, while the notion urban design is a much younger discipline (2). Healing gardens are taken as an indispensable concept to be considered; the field of testing, generally (un) known and present in the researches. Environmental psychology is the field of relations and effects on human health and its surrounding, and the discipline the most scientific papers were found. Medical and cultural geography are disciplines putting those relations in historical, spatial, social and symbolical context. Biophilia is recent theory ('80s), widespread in literature, based on the importance of nature for the human wellbeing. Ecological design is category of current intent based on natural processes. It's counted as a possibility doesn't as a necessity. Biophilia is considered as one stream of theories to follow it or don't (other categories are developed disciplines, except the scope category).

The Roots of relationship: human – healing environments – design (Fig.1) every category is pictured by own colour. Bold lines distinct literature with the main category, while the tinier associates bordering examples. If thinner lines touch the bold one, case is akin to the category. Thinly lines of the same colour relate also the literature unites with affiliated concepts. If the same colour lines are discontinued, they don't have connections in common. Double coloured, dashed line exemplifies common fields and diverse initial perspectives.

CATEGORY key terminology	definition
DESIGN METRICS pre-determined characteristics, standards	Pre-determined characteristics, "performance guidelines, the intention of which is not to tell the designer what to do, but rather to provide reminders of recommended qualities and elements" (Cooper Marcus and Barnes, 1999, p.24). Oriented to measure quality, they are standards.
LANDESCAPE language of space perception of landscape	The landscape architecture is foundation field; in relation with design metrics are considered a pattern language and perception theories; and evidence based design as the most influential in the outdoor healthcare design approaches.
EVIDENCE BASED DESIGN physical enviroment effects on health and well-being person's needs therapeutic landscape healing garden	Base design concept of healthcare facilities since the mid-1990s. It is defined as "...the physical environment matters to people's health and well-being and that the health and well-being of the whole person needs to be addressed rather than just the disease." (Cooper Marcus and Sachs, 2014). It is not presented in the graphic 1 and 2 as separated category even though that is affirmative approach, it is rather knitted trough other categories. First reason, nowadays it has a name evidence based design, but the idea is also ancient, and secondly, it is often related to notion 'therapeutic' what this paper is not oriented.
CULTURAL GEOGRAPHY experience of landscape historical perspective of relationship people-nature	A branch of human geography whose all aspects include: "cultural, social, developmental, economic, political, and health geography" (English Oxford dictionary). The cultural geography definition is: "the study of the impact of human culture on the landscape" (Dictionary.com's 21st Century Lexicon). The main concept of landscape is: stress reduction and increased levels of individual comfort (emotional and/or physical) is possible to reach trough landscape experiences; aiming to explore "positive, healing or therapeutic characteristics of place" (Velarde et al., 2007, p.200).
MEDICAL GEOGRAPHY healing sense of place (healing lanscape is place identity based) 4 dimensions of therapeutic landscape: natural, built, symbolic and social environment	It was firstly established at American universities in the 1970s as product of Jacques May (*The Ecology of Human Disease*, 1958) and the discipline has deepened by the influence of Melinda Meade (*Medical Geography and Human Ecology*, 1977), linking with time population, environment and culture (Brown, 2001-2011). In terms of health environments, the field of medical geography gains importance in the 1990s by research of Wilbert Gesler. The landscape concept was taken from cultural geography. It introduced for a first time the concept 'healing landscape' as the idea of place identity, to use particular place with natural or historic features for the maintenance of health and wellbeing (Velarde et al., 2007, p.200; Jiang, 2013, p.142). Four dimensions of therapeutic landscapes explored are: natural, built, symbolic and social environments. The main aspects of the healing concept are addressed to: multidimensional character (physical, mental, spiritual, emotional and social), wholeness (connectedness or integration), healing from within, an on-going process with meaning in one's everyday life and, healing is humanistic approach; in particular "healing sense of place" (Gesler, 2003).
ENVIRONMENTAL PSYCHOLOGY therapeutic landscapes and healing gardens restorative environments cognitive (experience, perception and behaviour)	Two main theories exist: Attention-Recreation Theory – ART and the restorative environment (set up by Kaplan and Kaplan in the book *The Experience of Nature*, 1989) and psycho-evolution theories and healing gardens (creator is Roger Ulrich, explains in two his works: *View through a window may influence recovery from surgery*, 1984 and Ulrich et al., *Stress recovery during exposure to natural and urban environments*, 1991). Environmental psychology is a second stream of therapeutic landscape theories. Its researchers are engaged about the effects of physical environment to cognitive processes and emotions (experience, perception and behaviour). Environmental psychology is the disciplines the highest number of scientific papers are found.

definition	CATEGORY / key terminology
Ancient and modern concept, as the widely explored notion, very diverse defined. The definition of it depends on historical and cultural context as the background field of researchers. Notions related are: therapeutic gardens - places designed with therapeutic intervention in order to improve health, engaging the therapeutic activities, the therapeutic team and the clients (Cooper Marcus and Barnes, 1999); restorative gardens (or restorative environments) environments beyond the hospital buildings that provide opportunities to reduce direct attention fatigue (Kaplan, 1995), in some literature, synonyms used for restorative environments are healing, therapeutic and supportive environments; and horticultural therapy garden - therapy engage plants for the curing of specific disease, often sensory gardens. This paper approach is rather healing than curing: Healing gardens are green urban open spaces as complements of healthcare facilities, natural-like settings where individual can experience physical and/or emotional wellbeing.	HEALING GARDENS healing gardens and therapeutic gardens horticultural therapy sensory stimulation
The term well-being is used to denote the quality of life (Dasgupta, 2001). It connects all other categories aiming to discover role of nature in quality of live. Health and wellbeing as joined strategy comprises (Rudge, 2013): mental – to be happy (the mind: to be happy and develop and grow learning skills), fiscal – to be healthy (the body: condition), social – aspiring (the heart: to aspire, to have friendship, love and/or engage on someone) and spiritual – in common (the spirit: to have sense of community, to have sense of meaning, to contribute) health and wellbeing.	HEALTH & WELLBEING how physical environment affects the quality of life mental, phisical, social and common health and wellbeing
It has become as derivate to promote health and wellbeing uniting researches from different perspectives (psychology, biology and sociology). A young theory introduced by Edward Wilson in his book *Biophilia* (1984), uphold an instinctive bond between human beings and natural living systems. Biophilic design dimension are naturalistic, structural, cognitive and emotional; the design and process are natural (e.g. connections are generic, forms are natural etc.).	BIOPHILIA human beings and natural living systems design dimensions are: naturalistic, structural, cognitive and emotional
Ecological design it's a response to present environmental crisis not as a style but as "form of engagement and partnership with nature" Çelik (2013, p.326). It is on the intersection of major sets of design, ecology and sustainability with main characteristics: holistic, responsive, dynamic and intuitive. The choosen to be present because of its pervasive aspirations of all other fields (not only health related).	ECOLOGICAL DESIGN design regards for natural processes; holistic, responsive, dynamic and intuitive
Urban open spaces are primar subject of urban design, by Consil of Europe defined as "a public living room for the locality" (1986). They are natural and cultural resource of society, opened in social terms and don't bordered in three physical dimensions, which are dedicated to people activities and pleasure and, important for psychological and social relieving a society. Green spaces are its subcategory (other is grey spaces). Design dimensions are: morphological, perceptual, social, visual, functional and temporal.	URBAN OPEN SPACES design dimensions: morphological, perceptual, social, visual, functional and temporal
Type of urban open spaces with 3 primary functions: ecological function and environmental conditions (integrated and diversity), social function (availability and accessibility - very sensitive tasks for the healthcare enviroments) and structural and aesthetic functions. Benefits they service are social, health, environmental and economic advantages and opportunities. Economic benefits are necessary to be present (stores of medical equipment, café etc.) but this paper is not concentrated in it.	GREEN SPACES urban open spaces

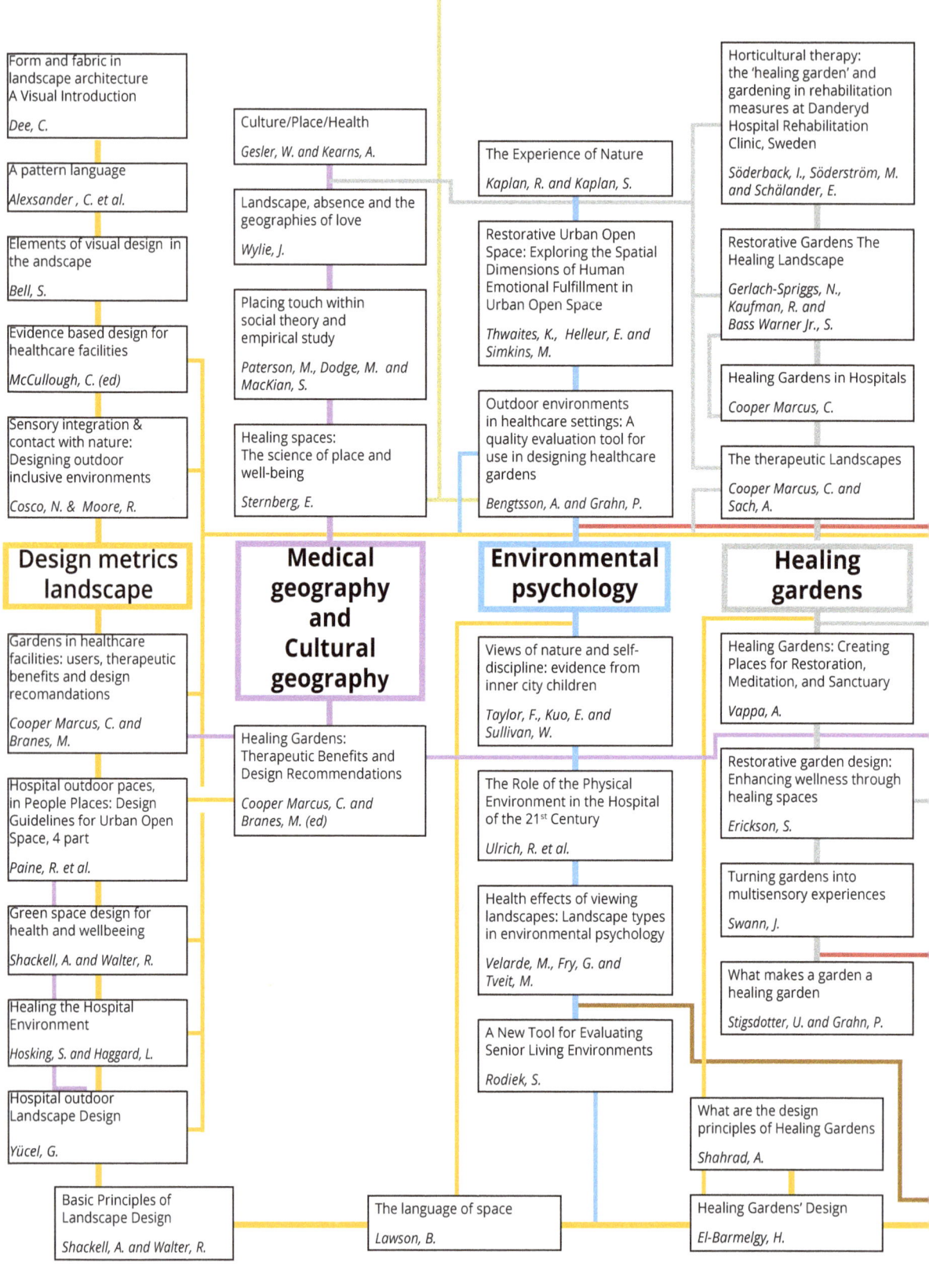

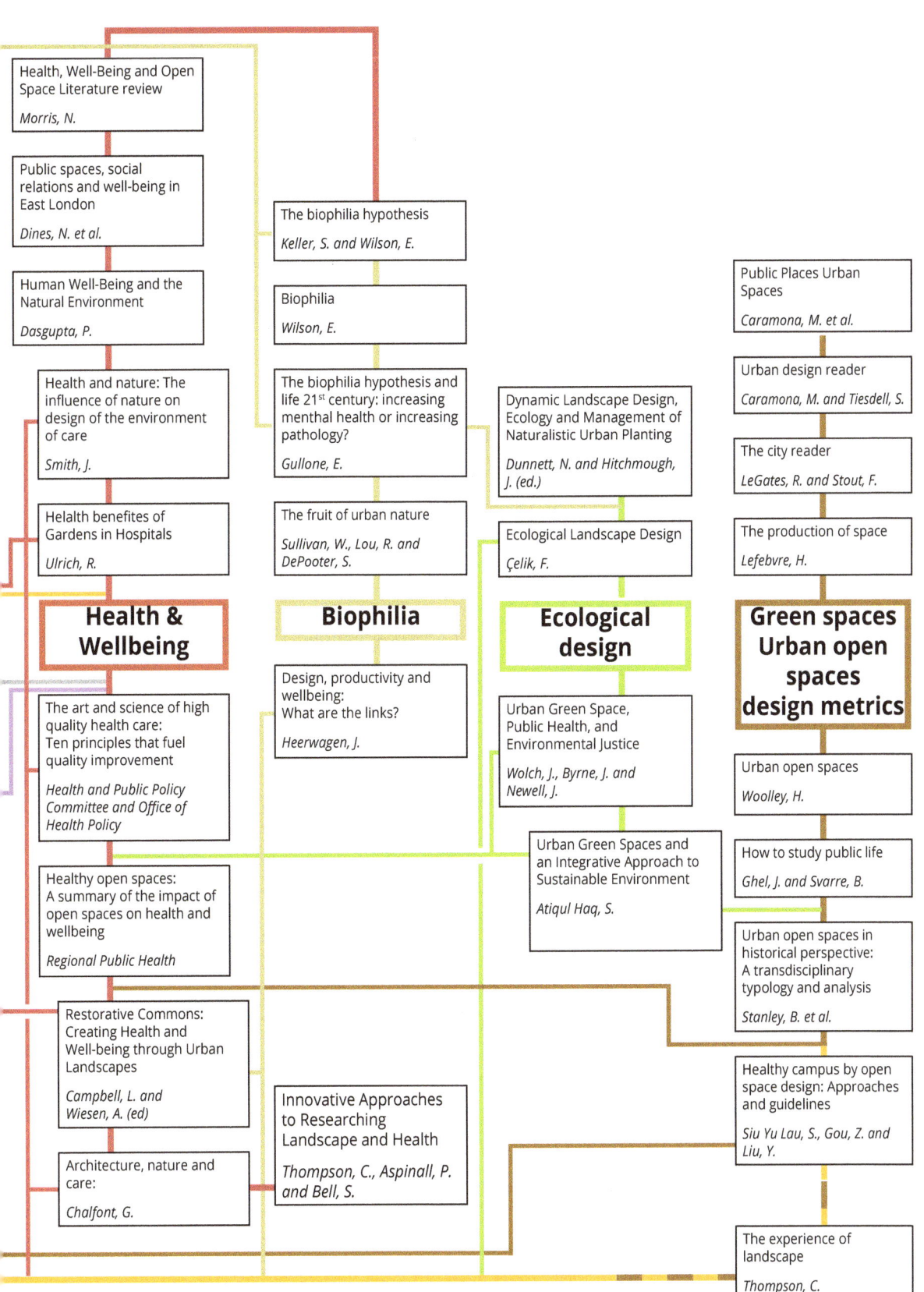

Figure 1: Roots of relationship: human – healing environments – design

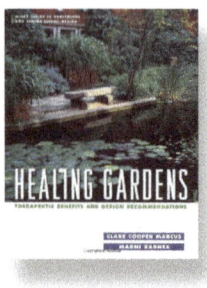 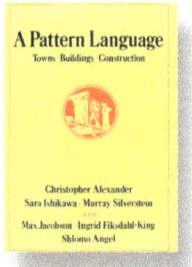 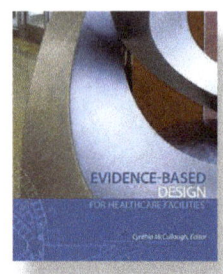
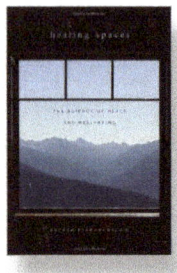 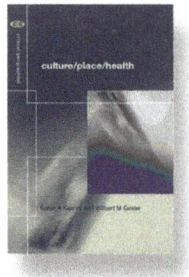 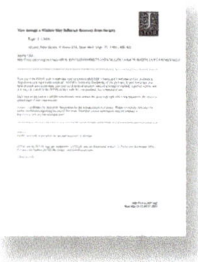
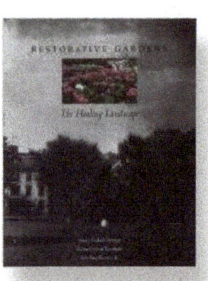 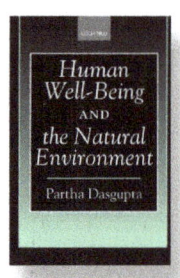 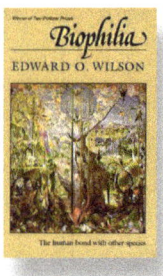
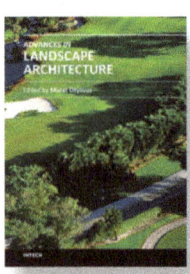 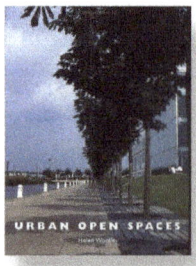 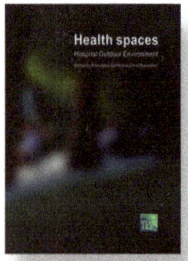

Figure 2 : Diverse approaches to research of health spaces (hospital outdoor environments), (impacts on creation of the relationship: human - healing environments - design)

Observations on historical conception of outdoor spaces within healthcare facilities

While the main focus of the paper is the meaning and use of design in healthcare facilities is important to place this account in historical context. This section will provide short historical (and cultural) overview the relationships of urban open spaces and healthcare facilities. It aspires to illustrate a link between design features of urban open space as natural environments and its benefits to healthcare facilities and medical outcomes. Period under observation includes span from ancient Greece to the present ones.

The garden (a few times called courtyard) is the term has been used as a notion to define open spaces of healthcare facilities. There is a time gap in terminology, but the main function of the spaces (if it existed) have been always related to recovery as a fundamental aspect of patient care, to enhance human well-being. On historic discourse, Warner (1994) explains garden in healthcare facility was ever in the medical focus of the facility. Gardens have been usually absent when the role of a facility was to cure or treat the symptoms of an illness, but healing or recuperate was considered the primary function of the healthcare environment and incorporated to enhance the healing process.

Garden design has been intuitively recognized the value of gardens as places of healing and repose, by societies. Depending on the social, historical and geographical context various cultures through history created gardens to engage and satisfy all the senses. The research supporting this observation has been done in 1984 by the Roger Ulrich (3).

Asclepius, was the god of medicine and healing in ancient Greece, to whom were devoted healing centres or *Asclepieia*, at least since the fourth century B.C. to the sixth century A.D. *Asclepieia* places were spread all over the ancient world; nowadays one of the most known is the sanctuary at Epidaurus in the Eastern Peloponnese, south of Athens, listed in UNESCO (United Nations Educational, Scientific and Cultural Organization) World Heritage Collection. The design of the buildings (included a temple, loggia and theatre) was focused to ensure awareness of the surrounding landscape. It demonstrates a unique configuration of buildings and green space where mindful attention was given to the relationship between the topography and natural landscape, because they were considered as very important for the creation of a healing environment. Second important part of the healing environment design was its contemplation as a sacred place. "For over a thousand years people came to the Epidaurus, believing that Asclepius would appear in their dreams while they slept at the site and heal them." amounts Butterfield (2014, p. 40). Major design features in this period are human aspirations who embodied interaction of architecture with nature, between buildings and open space; a place of strong body and mind experience and storytelling where the building is secluded spot in beautiful and live landscape scenario.

The first enclosed gardens (4) with restorative qualities as treatment in Europe occurred with the twelfth century. The qualities recognized by the writings of St. Bernard (1090-1153) are sunlight and a place to sit or stroll amongst seasonal plantings (Cooper Marcus and Barnes 1995, 1999, Pain et al., 1997, Butterfield 2014 & Barnes 2004). During the middle ages the enclosed garden in medieval monastery hospices was concentrated on courtyard. The courtyard was a place provided physical and spiritual comfort to pilgrims, the homeless, the sick, the insane and the dying. The place was often incorporated an arcaded courtyard allowed "degree of shelter, sun, or shade they desired in a human-scale, enclosed setting" (Cooper Marcus, and Barnes, M. 1995, pp.7-9). Gardens served as a common place to take care of the weak and sick and were integral to the daily routines and rhythms of institutions. The relationship between health and the environment was very close. Enclosed gardens emphasized control and order, providing the viewer with an ideal perspective of nature, with special attention to the changing of seasons (cycles of planting). Garden design was a deliberate attempt to evoke a reflective mood of the nature, natural harmony and tranquillity was believed to keep calm and comfort of the patients as a source of enjoyment, contemplation and social exchange. The design role of open spaces was based on believe that gardens can refresh the senses; it can ensure spiritual sense of peace and hope. This sensorial dialogue was established at first trough keeping the hygiene of place, clean air which was managed by plenty of greenery. Medicinal and aromatic plants enabled plenty of fragrances and, were used in therapeutic purposes. Colours have been thought to have a profound effect upon mind and body and green was widely believed to relax and refresh the eyes and lawns and meadows (who were in monastery property, as the large amount of books) have been contemplated as a place sit in grass turf to study, argues Butterfield (2014).

As described by Warner (1994), the significance of the meditative/restorative garden decline during in the 14th and 15th centuries, with deprivation of their religious content and also public health care appeared in the large urban centres. Marcus's and Barnes's observations in 1995 (cited in Warner 1994) quoting, that open spaces attached to hospitals became accidents, if they even consisted. Open spaces within and surrounding the healthcare facilities became less valued. Nevertheless, Warner (1994) mentioned some gardens remained in hospitals with number of courts planted with rows of trees. He remarked out an example from Spain (Zaragoza), where the hospital included a vineyards, gardens and orchards for the patient's treatment. But, important fact is that this is mental hospital and that we are speaking about treatment now as a primary one and as a primary function, not about respectfully place for relax, refresh, enjoy, odour, believe, harmony, tranquillity… This paper doesn't develop this type of treatment in scientific purposes, it tend to evoke the place with its sense (without intentions about sacral role, appropriate to current society, but yes as a place of believing, hope and peaceful respect). The trend of therapeutic landscape will continue during 18th, 19th century, until present times, and will be argued more.

The concept of design for healthcare facilities didn't existed, according to Pain et al. (1997) "only the deadly ill or the very poor, unable to afford home care, went to the hospital where they most often died". The Romantic Movement's influence in 18th century was reborn the concept of nature as places for bodily and spiritual restoration (Warner, 1994). Patients and the outdoor environment were usually included sitting in the sun and fresh air, and more often reappearance was related to healthcare facilities for veterans. Sense of open space was occupied by special attention to prevent the spread of infection, its tasks were "hygiene, fresh air, and cross-ventilation" explain Marcus and Barnes (1995).But design of the physical form of the healthcare environment was sought for the once during medieval period where the sense of well-being would be enhanced in a pleasant environment. With advanced improvements in medical techniques and treatments in public health, ending of 18th and beginning of the 19th century, many typologies of healthcare buildings and it open spaces are created: sometimes rooms were in sequence that can have the view on inner yard, than pavilion types and psychiatric ones who needed special design to be separated by greenery from the outer public. As reported by Warner (1994), grounds and plantings which were protecting patients 'landscape vistas' were developed to enable also therapeutic experiences, and patients took a part in farming and planting activities as a therapy. To note again, the paper doesn't concentrate on the therapeutic landscape, but the importance of being involved, of interaction with nature is a qualitative criteria of the urban open space in healthcare facilities. At the other hand, open spaces paid a lot of intention on view of nature, fresh air and exposure to sunlight, commonly. These big development changes brought also first roof gardens, usually designed with few flower boxes for a short break (Pain et al., 1997). From previous concepts of landscape and healthcare facilities (counting from antigen Greek to medieval), we can stress out that not only perception of landscape has been changing, than a scale was a crucial factor. Diversity of green open spaces has arisen; very probably one of consequence is high-arisen density of the cities. However, this is one precondition for still present struggles in urban open space design.

End of 19th and 20th century (parallel to fast social changes) emphasis on purity, hygiene, fresh, air and sunlight, while the architectural modernism produces innovative designs, in short. Doesn't matter if the architects were embittered or fascinated by the industrial revolution, the causes and motives were the same: purity, hygiene, fresh, air and sunlight. Also, the solutions were similar concerning landscape as a place for living, but people, place and nature were not always the subject of sympathy. Warner (1994) explains this as a consequence trough transformation of the pavilion type of building into high-rise construction. Green spaces became "space left over planning" (5). After World War II, horticultural therapy programs with special-purpose were progressing in diverse horticultural therapy programs. 20th century trends in healthcare "changed from caring to curing" (Barnes, 2004). By the 1970s, came the period of 'sensory deprivation' as Butterfield (2014) says. She continues: "indoor spaces were designed for hygiene and clinical efficiency and outdoor spaces primarily for parking" Butterfield (2014). For the period of the 1990s, the image of the entrance was important, setback from streets and very rarely stresses reduction, as explained, Marcus and Barnes (1999): "Landscaping is often seen as a cosmetic extra". Like that healthcare environments distinguish between the term healing and curing.

However, we can stop here, because further, arguing is very case dependable in terms of urban open space distribution, quantities and qualities.

Design inputs

This section summarizes on perviousness, extracting already proven relations of people, environments and its relations (behaviour), from different expertizes previously presented and concerning learned lessons from historical conceptions existed. The synthesis is oriented to results with design inputs for urban open spaces within healthcare facilitates, as final result of the paper.

Environments are context that surrounds us; the habitat of all living systems participate and interact. They are including physical space as well as cultural, psychological, socio-ecological and historical influences.

Healing environments are environments that surround the healthcare facility; prioritizing to take care, healing rather than curing. Practitioners of 'everyday life' are patients, family, client, doctors, workers, stuff, students...and community. They repose fiscal space and internal space; spatial manifestation of people with individual (and communal) physical, mental, emotional, social and spiritual characters. Landscape patterns and processes as design inputs can support those interaction; addressed to treat healthcare outdoors as extensions of facility, place to take care.

Design framework is essential to be set up in the beginning. It is always consisted of the process and proposed steps to be followed, oriented to balance requirements and needs with capacities of dispatcher and receiver, to improve quality of life. The design process of healing environments within healthcare facilities differs any other design process is that is has two layers of objectives. In the cognitive layer, lie the healing objectives (e.g. to provide stress relief), alleviation of physical symptoms and improvement in the human overall sense of wellbeing (El Barmelgy, 2013). Mainly, all literature related to design and health, point out awareness that specific design features may elicit a positive or negative response, depending on the symptoms of the patient's illness, infers a key design consideration. But, usually, it is concentrated in therapeutic effects of design; a design input of the paper occupies by evoking a positive response and improving mood, restorative effects of all users.

A first design stage is inventory phase, starting with questions what to know about users and site. Here the participation process starts as well, usually with interviews or queries, or some other participative tools with more direct or indirect engagement (and participation should last always parallel to all design stages, but it will not be discussed because of its own complexity and particularity in context of healthcare facilities; it exists). Based on results of previous phase, the next is developing ideas and setting up goals, with evaluative criteria (indicators). There is much iteration before implementation and meditation stage.

Summary of design process of healing environments presents Fig. 3. Colours used are related to previous graphics, about relationship of notions and theories, human – environments - design (Fig.1) showing impacts of other knowledge in the design possess and mutual consequences.

On the first hand design process is presented, on the other are readable fields of its impact and components creating it, reading and evaluating. Correspondingly, next part of the paper presents its key components.

Starting with set up goals according to user need, and finishing with percentage of their satisfaction, while the middle is created of their behaviours, cultural and socio-ecological patterns and norms denoting the design people needs are first design criteria. Further are synthetized environments needs and interaction or behavioural patterns (see Table 2). Features are summarized on researches from environmental psychology analysis, health and wellbeing, medical and cultural geography and design metrics.

From antiquity to our day, healing landscapes draws on the constitutive link between bodies, wellness, and place. Practices of storytelling transformed these spaces into places of memory, meaning, denoting and long term pilgrimage. Nowadays it's not appropriate to think about healing landscapes as pilgrimage, but storytelling is wiled characteristic of it to evoke links and to produce positive distraction. One of possible design approaches based on landscape architecture is a language of patterns. Once again, this approach of using design patterns is one possible approach, before all previous steps were in common while designing healing environments.

Design patterns "describes the field of physical and social relationship which are required to solve the stated problem, in the stated context" (Alexander, 1977, p. xi). Alexander (1977) explains that each design pattern stand is an element of the language of design, they are the individual words or phrases that when joined form the final story. Design patterns are not closed list, on the contrary, it has to be a continuous updatable list based on designers 'experiences' and the special design conditions of each case (environmental, social, and economic).They aim to assist the designer in achieving goals.

It is chosen because it is already examined, but in therapeutic scope, and because of its flexibility; every case has its language. The language constituted for the paper is based on typology of landscape constitutive forms and fabrics, as approach used in landscape architecture for experienced environmental design. Experiences design is found suitable for healthcare outdoor spaces concerning that all of them are space to wait; dead or curing, or lunch break, or to wait, positive distraction is welcome. Therefore entities are adapted to healthcare environments. Main categories of landscape patterns are: spatial patterns (subcategories: typology of space and character), paths patterns, hard landscapes, foci and details (see Table 3).

In order to examine design goals and pattern language of landscape design, as conclusion, each of defined 52 patterns are matched selected 31 needs and presented graphically (see: Healing environments design formulation graphic, Table 4). The result serves as data base of possibilities. Next design step should be election of patterns serves to particular case.

Each blade of grass is a new discovery, a new beginning. Every case is challenge for designer to balance, as every environment has its health needs. The paper presented optimum design inputs. The design is a primer tool of creating healing environments, as it was since ancient times but, contemporary challenges of society changed it goals according to its development. Healing environments design formulation graphic is one possible contribution to contemporary practice with ancient intensions of role of healing environments as positive outdoor of healthcare facilities.

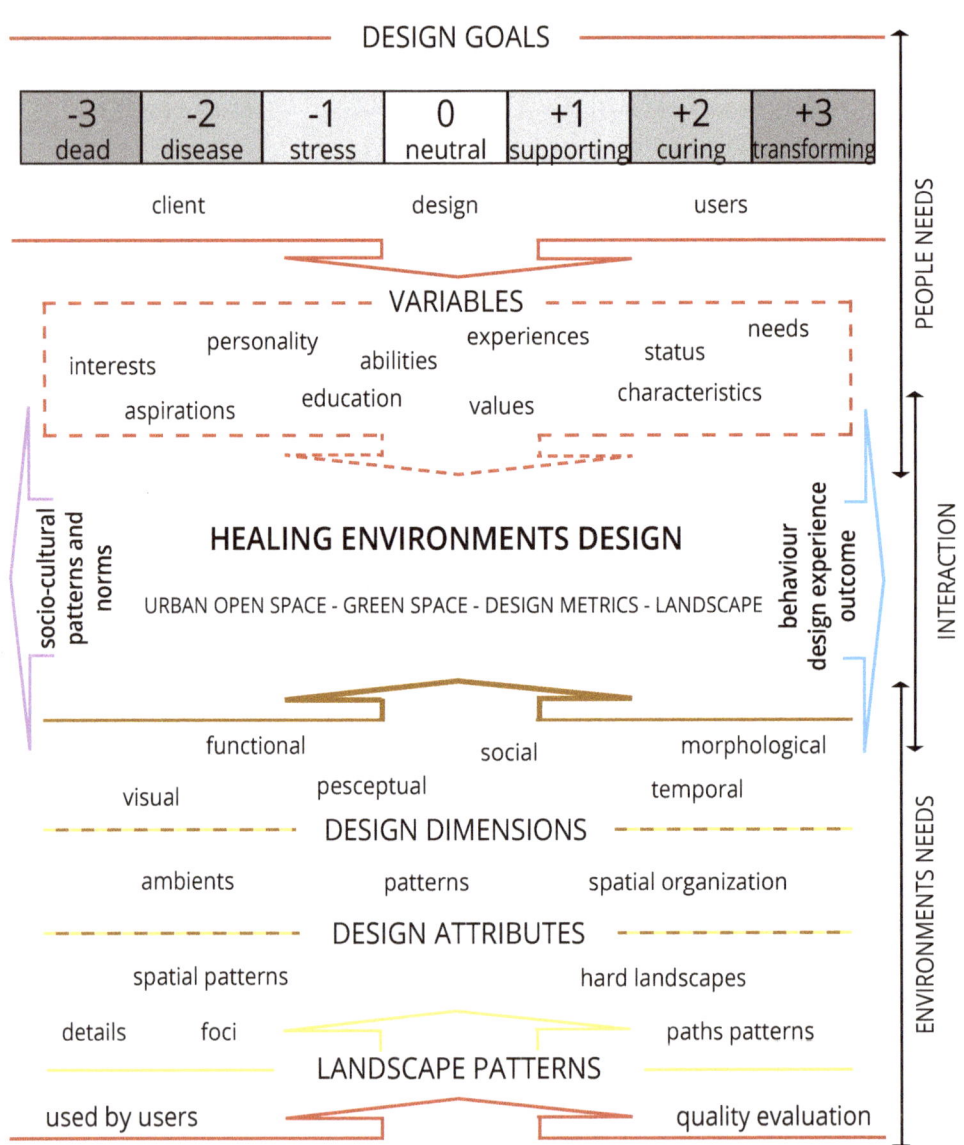

Figure 3: Design process of healing environments

CODE	NEEDS CATEGORIES
PN	**PEOPLE NEEDS**
PN 1	Closeness and easy access
PN 2	Enclosure and entrance
PN 3	Safety and security
PN 4	Orientation and way finding
PN 5	Variety (and different options in different times, kinds of weather)
PN 6	Independence, choice and freedom
PN 7	Perception of privacy
PN 8	Beauty and satisfaction
PN 9	Place to interact
PN 10	Control
PN 11	Physical – movement and exercise
PN 12	Mental/to be happy (the mind: to be happy and develop and grow learning skills)
PN 13	Social/aspiring (the heart: to aspire, to have friendship, love and/or engage on someone)
PN 14	Spiritual/in common (the spirit: culture, sense of community, sense of meaning, to contribute)
PN 15	Organization: leadership, teamwork, technology, service, ownership, evaluation
EN	**ENVIROMENTS**
EN 1	Integration with surrounding (the world beyond facility); make it accesible
EN 2	Integration in-out door
EN 3	Microclimate
EN 4	Habitat for all
EN 5	Natural – compensation to nature
EN 6	Time - Seasons changing in nature, as the day and night...
I-B	**INTERACTION - BEHAVIOUR**
I-B 1	Clarity and spatial orientation
I-B 2	Interactive place (physical and experience)
I-B 3	Positive distraction / environment experience: nature, light, artwork, material, senses
I-B 4	Magic, Dreams, Healing, Destination, Journey, Sanctuary (example, *Epidaurus*)
I-B 5	Attractiveness, Mystery and Enjoyment
I-B 6	Observation, balance and relaxation
I-B 7	Variety of activities and abilities
I-B 8	Familiar tasks (work, care, study, recreation)
I-B 9	Expectation, hope, understanding, belief
I-B 10	Compassion, communication, social support, empathy

Table 2: Needs categories

	CODE	PATTERN NAME	EXPLANATION
SPATIAL PATTERNS — TYPOLOGY OF SPACES	P 1	Lansdcape grounds	green areas between buildings, link with walking paths
	P 2	Lansdcape walls and sky	one ambient to another with sky plane; natural when it is possible
	P 3	In-between spaces	transition space with very elastic measures; to wait, to view...
	P 4	Entery garden	located near healthcare facility entrances; representative
	P 5	Courtyards	most used spaces in hospitals 'everyday life'
	P 6	Plazas	typically paved and furnished spaces with few plant, often planting pots
	P 7	Terace	usualy smal size open space, alternative planting
	P 8	Roof garden	long term economic, mulitilevel benefits, green 'oasis'
	P 9	Healing garden	gardens in curing purposes: teraphcutic, meditationsensory, horticultue
	P 10	View garden	enclosed gardens with limited acces; water, sculptures, topary plants
	P 11	View/walking garden	atrium type of gardens, acces can be controled or not
	P 12	Eatable garden	fruit and vegetable gardens (it's not neccesay to be separate garden)
	P 13	Childrens garden	equiped specialy for childrens interaction with surrounding
	P 14	'Giardino segreto'	place for intimacy, storyteling, smells...
	P 15	Activity pocket	if the primary function is studing, dinnin area...it can be 'mixed' with other ty
	P 16	Wild life	habitat for all (it supports positive distructions, helps to feeling of emphaty...
CHARACTER	P 17	Country town	integral part of the city as its own entity
	P 18	Positive outdoor	related to healthcare facility, but to heal rather than cure
	P 19	Diversity and hierarchy of spaces	from square to isolated spaces, but with view on the larger one
	P 20	Public outdoor room	comfortable time
	P 21	Mosaic of subcultures	to coexist in the same space (activities, enviroments...)
	P 22	Mistery, legibility, complexity, coherence	qualities influence people's experience (proven by: Kaplan and Kaplan, 1989)
	P 23	Life cycle	settings to support any stage and passing from one stage to another
	P 24	Street cafe	a place where people can sit lazily, legitimately, view the time goes by
PATHS PATTERNS	P 25	Acces path (and road)	must be distinguished, easy accesable and readable to reach faclity
	P 26	Axial path	the shotest route
	P 27	Meandering path	alternative route
	P 28	Loop path	distinguished from the more frequently used pathways
	P 29	Waterway	paths folowing (and crossing) the water body/bodies
	P 30	Forest path	route troug groups of trees
	P 31	Mound path	gives different view points
HARD LANDSCAPES	P 32	Connection with nature	when it is possible, integrate green areas with surrounding ones
	P 33	Gatheways, entrance and fences	marking to be 'in' the healthcare facility open space
	P 34	Parking	shiled, it's not nessesary to be visible
	P 35	Emergence entrance and space	standards of the faclity, distinguished and secured
	P 36	Stop-by places	sequences of path's expansions
	P 37	Canopy	open space for different weather conditions
	P 38	Furniture	to exist adequate (signs, seating, litter bins, lighting)
	P 39	Illumination	sense of security and aestetics
	P 40	Sequence of sitting	arranged to give possiblity for different types of socialization
	P 41	Garbage disposal	to prevent any desease (not only medical garbage-particulary sensitive topic)
FOCI	P 42	Type	spece to gatger, edge, focal space, landmark, public sculpture, building
	P 43	Form	vertical foci, scale foci, hidden foci (rare: e.g. springs or holles)
	P 44	Signature	experience of foci helps us to orient
	P 45	Artworks	form that marks a place of spiritual, cultural or social significance
	P 46	Vegetation foci	an 'event' in the landscape assist orientation (single tree, group of trees on la
DETAIL	P 47	Colours and light (and shading)	shaping experience; richness, diversity and complexity as simplicity and coherc
	P 48	Patterns	to identify or create order; geometry, natural forms and process, with patterns c
	P 49	Textures	intimately related to light; natural as much as possible
	P 50	Vegetation, Water	as earht or rock they can interact with all senses
	P 51	Touch, smell, sound, view, taste	provides 'immediate' sensory experience of landscapes
	P 52	Time	planting! maintance, evaluate, upgrade

Table 3-4: Landscape patterns within healthcare outdoors and healing environments design formulation graphic

	PEOPLE NEEDS	ENVIRONMENTS NEEDS	INTERACTION - BEHAVIOUR NEEDS
	PN 1 / PN 2 / PN 3 / PN 4 / PN 5 / PN 6 / PN 7 / PN 8 / PN 9 / PN 10 / PN 11 / PN 12 / PN 13 / PN 14 / PN 15	EN 1 / EN 2 / EN 3 / EN 4 / EN 5 / EN 6	I-B 1 / I-B 2 / I-B 3 / I-B 4 / I-B 5 / I-B 6 / I-B 7 / I-B 8 / I-B 9 / I-B 10

■ in relationship ▨ relationship is possible ☐ without relationship ⊠ not in congruence

Notes

(1) The Therapeutic Landscapes Network is a knowledge base and gathering space, a website, about healing gardens, restorative landscapes, and other green spaces that promote health and well-being. The idea of a virtual space as bibliography was born in 1999. at the annual ASLA (American Society of Landscape Architects) Healthcare and Therapeutic Design Professional Practice Network Meeting in Boston, aiming to keep in touch all the works on related topics from different backgrounds and to be continuously uploaded. The website is created in 2004. when it won an ASLA Professional Communications Award of Merit, and in 2009. it became interactive.

(2) Urban design is notion dating from 50s of last century, borne from the *City Beautiful Movement*; a little bit earlier was used *the notion civic design*. The literature of landscape history refers to garden history, starting with the Hanging Gardens of Babylon (500-600 BC).

(3) Dr. Roger S. Ulrich is Professor of Architecture at the Centre for Healthcare Building Research at Chalmers University of Technology in Sweden, and is adjunct professor of architecture at Aalborg University in Denmark. He was co-founding director of the Center for Health Systems and Design at Texas A&M University and he was from 2005-2006 senior adviser on patient care environments for UK (Britain's National Health Service), served to create scores of new hospitals. He is the most frequently cited researcher on the topic evidence-based healthcare design. He demonstrated, in his 1984 research, that patients with a view of nature had a faster rate of recovery, needed less medication for pain, even that they were ready to be discharged from the hospital sooner than patients in rooms that looked out on a brick wall (Ulrich, View through window, pp.420-421).

(4) Enclosed garden, lat. *hortusconclusus*, is the notion derived from the Roman courtyard and used in the history of gardens in general. It appeared even in Roman gardens which first period of creation and development flowered with the reign of Emperor Cicero (from 106 until 43 BC). Greek garden creators who were importing the knowledge and made Roman gardens succeed to convey Greek form, plastic of the models, poetic sense of nature and the unique connection between building and garden. Enclosed garden emerged with an idea to be a peacefully quiet and calm breathing space separated from the chaos of unhealthy city life or the healthy but unsafe countryside.

(5) Space left over planning - SLOAP, is the notion in general use in the landscape architecture and urban planning as a practice characterized 20th century, where the priorities during city planning are given to traffic and buildings, then green space on the remaining surface.

References

Alexsander, C. (1977), *A pattern language*, Oxford University Press, New York.

AtiqulHaq, S. (2011), "Urban Green Spaces and an Integrative Approach to Sustainable Environment", *Journal of Environmental Protection, SciRes*, Vol. 3, pp.601-608, (online), available at http://www.scirp.org/journal/jep (accessed 14 January 2015).

Barnes, D. (2004), Healing Gardens in Healthcare Facilities: Linking Restorative Value and Design Features, *Unpublished dissertation(MSc)*, Department of Architecture, University of British Columbia, Vancouver, BC Canada.

Bell, S. (2004), *Elements of Visual Design in the Landscape*, 2nd ed., Spoon Press, London & New York.

Bengtsson, A. and Grahn, P. (2014), "Outdoor environments in healthcare settings: A quality evaluation tool for use in designing healthcare gardens", *Urban Forestry & Urban Greening*, 13, pp.878–891 available: Science Direct (accessed 23 January 2015).

Brown, N. (2001-2011) *Melinda S. Meade: Medical Geography and Human Ecology, 1977 By Nina Brown*, Center for Spatially Integrated Social Science – CSISS (online), available at http://www.csiss.org/classics/content/39 (accessed 27 January 2015).

Butterfield, A. (2014), Resilient places? Healthcare gardens and the Maggie's centers, *Unpublished dissertation (PhD)*, Falmouth University, University of Arts (UAL) London.

Campbell, L. and Wiesen, A. eds. (2009), Restorative Commons: Creating Health and Well-being through Urban Landscapes, *General Technical Report*, U.S. Forest Service, Northern Research Station, Meristem.

Carmona, M. and Tiesdell, S. (2007), *Urban Design Reader*, Architectural Press, Oxford, UK.

Carmona, M. et al. (2003), *Public Places Public Spaces: The Dimension of Urban Design*, Architectural Press, Oxford, UK.

Çelik, F. (2013) "Ecological Landscape Design" in Özyavuz, M. (Ed.), *Advances in Landscape Architecture*, INTECH (online), available at http://www.intechopen.com/books/advances-in-landscape-architecture/ecological-landscape-design, pp.325-350.

Chalfont, G. (2005) *Architecture, nature and care* (online), available at http://www.chal.fontdesign.com/media/Architecture_Nature_Care.pdf (accessed 07 February 2015).

Cooper Marcus C. and Barnes, M. (1995), *Gardens in healthcare facilities: uses, therapeutic benefits, and design recommendations*, Martinez, The Center for Health Design, CA.

Cooper Marcus, C. and Barnes, M. (1999), *Healing Gardens: Therapeutic Benefits and Design Recommendations*, Wiley, New York, NY.

Cooper Marcus, C. and Sachs, N. (2014), *Therapeutic Landscapes: An Evidence-Based Approach to Designing Healing Gardens and Restorative Outdoor Spaces*, Wiley, Hoboken, New Jersey and Canada.

Cosco, N. and Moore, R. (2009), "Sensory integration and contact with nature: Designing outdoor inclusive environments", *NAMTA Journal*, Vol. 34 No. 2, pp.158-177.

Dasgupta, P. (2001), *Human Well-Being and the Natural Environment*, Oxford, NY.

Dee, C. (2001), *Form and fabric in landscape architecture A Visual Introduction*, Spoon Press, London & New York.

Dines, N. et al. (2006), Public spaces, social relations and well-being in East London, Policy Press for Joseph Rowntree Foundation, Queen Mary, University of London.

Dunnett, N. and Hitchmough, J. eds. (2004), *Dynamic Landscape Design: Ecology and Management of Naturalistic Urban Planting*, Spoon Press, London and New York.

El-Barmelgy, H. (2013), "Healing Gardens' Design", *International Journal of Education and Research*, Vol. 1 No. 6 pp.1-20, (online), available at www.ijern.com (accessed 14 January 2015).

Erickson, S. (2012), "Restorative Gardens design: Enhancing wellness through healing spaces", *JAD*, No. 2, pp.89-102, New Haven: Yale University Press.

FirdevsYücel, G. (2013) "Hospital Outdoor Landscape Design" in Özyavuz, M. (Ed.), *Advances in LandscapeArchitecture*, INTECH (online), available at http://www.intechopen.com/books/advances-in-landscape-architecture/hospital-outdoor-landscape-design, pp.381-398.

Gerlach-Spriggs, N., Kaufman, R. and Bass Warner Jr., S. (2012), *Restorative Gardens: The Healing Landscape*, Yale University Press.

Gesler, W. and Kearns, A. (2002), *Culture/Place/Health*, Routledge, London and New York.

Gesler, W.M. (2003), *Healing Places*. Rowman & Littlefield, Oxford, UK.

Ghel, J. Svarre, B. (2013), *How to study public life*, Translation by Karen Ann Steenhard, Island Press, US.

Gullone, E. (2000), "The biophilia hypothesis and life 21st century: increasing mental health or increasing pathology?", *Journal of Happiness Studies*, Vol. 1, pp.293–321, Kluwer Academic Publishers, Netherlands.

Health Thinking (2013) *Constructing Plymouth's Joint Health and Wellbeing Strategy* (online), available at http://healthservant.blogspot.it/2013/01/constructing-plymouths-joint-health-and.html (accessed 27 January 2015).

Heerwagen, J. (1998), Design, productivity and wellbeing: What are the links?, *Paper presented at: The American Institute of Architects Conference on Highly Effective Facilities*, Cincinnati, Ohio.

Hosking, S. and Haggard, L. (1999), *Healing the Hospital Environment: Design, management and maintenance of healthcare premises*, E & FN Spon, London, UK.

Jiang, S. (2014), "Therapeutic landscapes and healing gardens: A review of Chinese literature in relation to the studies in western countries", *Frontiers of Architectural Research*, 3, pp.141–153, available at Science Direct (accessed 23 January 2015).

Kaplan, R. and Kaplan, S. (1989), *The Experience of Nature: A Psychological Perspective*, Cambridge University Press, New York, Port Chester, Melbourne, Sydney.

Kaplan, S. (1979), Perception and Landscape: Conceptions and Misconceptions, *Submitted to the National Conference on Applied Techniques for Analysis and Management of the Visual Resource*, Incline Village, Nevada.

Kellert, S. and Wilson, E. eds. (1993), *The biophilia hypothesis*, Island Press, US.

Kony, H. and Kony G. (2013),"The Perceptual-Based Design Model: A Conceptual Framework to Designing Constructive Individuals' Experiences Based on the Perceived Attributes of the Settings", in Davis, J. et al. (Eds.), *Proceedings of the 44th Annual Conference of*

        the Environmental Design Research Association, Rhode Island, May 29 – June 1, The Environmental Design Research Association – EDRA, McLean, VA, US, pp. 79-86.
Lawson, B. (2001), *The language of space*, Architectural Press, Oxford, UK.
Lefebvre, H. (1991), *The production of space*. Translated from French by Donald Nicholson-Smith, Blackwell publishing: Malden US, Oxford UK, Carlton, Victoria Australia. (The original published 1974. and 1984.).
LeGates, R. and Stout, F. eds. (1996), *The city reader*, Routledge, London and New York.
McCullough, C. (2010), *Evidence-based design for health care facilities*, Sigma Theta Tau International, Indianapolis, US.
Morris, N. (2003), Health, Well-Being and Open Space: Literature review, *OPENspace: the research centre for inclusive access to outdoor environments*, Edinburgh College of Art and Heriot-Watt University.
Moughtin, C. and Shirley, P. (1996), *Urban design: Green dimensions, 2nd ed.*, Architectural Press, Oxford, UK.
Oxford English Dictionary (2005), *Human geography 2nd Ed.* Oxford: Oxford University Press.
Paine, R. et al. (1997), "Hospital outdoor spaces" in Marcus, C C. and Francis, C. (Ed.),
People Places: Design Guidelines for Urban Open Space, Vol. 4, Van Nostrand Reinhold, New York, NY, pp.311-320.
Paterson, M., Dodge, M. and MacKian, S. eds. (2012) "Introduction: Touching Space, Placing Touch" in Paterson, M. and Dodge (Eds.) M. *Touching Space, Placing Touch*, Ashgate Publishing Group, UK, pp.1-28.
Regional Public Health Better Health for Greater Wellington Region (2010), Public Open Spaces: Spaces: A summary of the impact of open spaces on health and wellbeing, *Regional Public Health Information Paper*, Lower Hutt, New Zeeland.
Royal College of physicians and surgeons of Canada, (2012), The art and science of high-quality health care: Ten principles that fuel quality improvement, *Royal College position statement on quality improvement science*, Health and Public Policy Committee and Office of Health Policy, Canada.
Shackell, A. and Walter, R. (1991), "Basic Principles of Landscape Design", *Environmental Horticulture Department, Florida Cooperative Extension Service,Institute of Food and Agricultural Sciences*, Florida, (online), available at http://edis.ifas.ufl.edu (accessed 13 January 2015).
Shackell, A. and Walter, R. (2012), *Green space design for health and well-being: Practice guide*, Forestry Commission, Edinburgh.
Shahrad, A. (n.d.), *What are the design principles of Healing Gardens*, American Horticultural Therapy Association, (online), available at http://www.protac.dk/Files/Filer/What_makes_a_garden_a_healing_garden_Stigsdotter_U__Grahn_P.pdf (accessed 21 January 2015).
Siu Yu Lau, S., Gou, Z. and Liu, Y. (2014), "Healthy campus by open space design: Approaches and guidelines", *Frontiers of Architectural Research*, 3, pp.452–467
        available: Science Direct (accessed 23 January 2015).

Smith, J. (2007), Health and nature: The influence of nature on design of the environment of care, *A Position Paper for the Environmental Standards Council of The Center for Health Design*, The Center for Health Design, Columbus, OH.

Söderback, I., Söderström, M. and Schälander, E. (2007), "Horticultural therapy: the 'healing garden' and gardening in rehabilitation measures at Danderyd hospital rehabilitation clinic, Sweden", *Developmental Neuro rehabilitation*, Vol. 7 No. 4, pp.245 – 260, (online), available at http://dx.doi.org/10.1080/13638490410001711416 (accessed 27 January 2015).

Stanley, B. et al. (2012), "Urban open spaces in historical perspective: A transdisciplinary typology and analysis", *Urban Geography*, 33, 8, pp.1089–1117, (online), available at http://dx.doi.org/10.2747/0272-3638.33.8.1089 (accessed 02 February 2015).

Sternberg, E. (2009), *Healing spaces: The science of place and well-being*, Belknap press, Harvard University Press, Cambridge, Massachusetts and London, England.

Sullivan, W., Lou, R. and DePooter, S. (2004), "The fruit of urban nature: Vital Neighbour hood Spaces", *Environment and behaviour*. Sage Publications, Vol. 36, No. 5, pp.678-700 available: Science Direct (accessed 23 January 2015).

Swann, J. (2006), "Turning gardens into multisensory experiences", *Nursing & Residential Care, Practical series*, Vol. 8, No. 4, pp.171-174.

Taylor, F., Kuo, E. and Sullivan, W. (2001), "Views of nature and self-discipline: evidence from inner city children", *Journal of Environmental Psychology*, Vol. 36, pp. 1-16, (online), available at http://www.idealibrary.com (accessed 23 January 2015).

Thompson, W., Aspinall, P. and Bell, S. (2010), *Innovative Approaches to Researching Landscape and Health Open Space: People Space 2*, Routledge, Milton Park, Abingdon, Oxon.

Thwaites, K., Helleur, E. and Simkins, M. (2005), Restorative Urban Open Space: Exploring the Spatial Dimensions of Human Emotional Fulfilment in Urban Open Space, *Landscape Research*, Vol. 30, No. 4, pp.525-547 available at Taylor & Francis Online (accessed 23 January 2015).

Ulrich, R. (2002), Health Benefits of Gardens in Hospitals, *Conference paper: Plants for People*, International Exhibition Floriade.

Ulrich, R. et al (2004), The Role of the Physical Environment in the Hospital of the 21st Century, *Report to The Center for Health Design for the Designing the 21st Century Hospital Project*, (online), available at https://www.healthdesign.org/chd/research/role-physical-environment-hospital-21st-century (accessed 25 January 2015).

Ulrich, R. S. (1993) "Biophilia, Biophobia, and Natural Landscapes" in Kellert, S. R. and Wilson, E. O. (Ed.), *The Biophilia Hypothesis*, Island Press, Washington DC, pp.73-137.

Vappa, A. (2002), Healing Gardens: Creating Places for Restoration, Meditation, and Sanctuary, *Unpublished dissertation(MSc)*, Landscape architecture, College of Architecture and Urban Studies, Virginia Polytechnic Institute and State University.

Velarde, M., Fry, G. and Tveit, M. (2007), "Health effects of viewing landscapes: Landscape types in environmental psychology", *Urban forestry & Urban greening*, Vol. 6, pp.199–212, available at Science Direct (accessed 22 January 2015).

Ward Thompson, C. (2010). The experience of landscape – understanding responses to landscape design and exploring demands for the future, *Presented for the Degree of PhD by Research Publications*, The University of Edinburgh.

Ward Thompson, C. Aspinall, P. and Bell, S. eds. (2010), *Innovative Approaches to Researching Landscape and Health Open Space: People Space 2*, Routledge, London and New York.

Warner, S. B. Jr. (1994), "The Periodic Rediscoveries of Restorative Gardens: 1100 to the Present", in Francis, M., Lindsey, P. and Rice, J.S. (Eds.), *The Healing Dimension of People-Plant Relations, Proceedings of a Research Symposium*, University of California, Davis Center for Design Research, Davis, CA, pp.5-12.

Wilson, E. (2003), *Biophilia*, Harvard University Press, US.

Woolley, H. (2003), *Urban Open Spaces*, Spoon Press, London.

Wylie, J. (2009). "Landscape, absence and the geographies of love", *Transaction Institute of the British Geographies*, Royal Geographical Society (with IBG), pp.275-289, (online), available at http://lepo.it.da.ut.ee/~cect/teoreetilised%2seminarid_2010/maastiku_uurimisr%C3%BChma_seminar/Wylie_2009.pdf (accessed 23 January 2015).

Zborowsky, T. and Bunker-Hellmich, L. (2010), *The Role of Design in Creating Optimal Healing Environments Conference*, Aprile, 30th, Society for the arts in Healthcare, AECOM company, Ellerbe Becket.

04

Observation as a way of knowing and measuring open hospital spaces

Fabio Quici

Abstract: To speak of open hospital spaces is to explore, first and foremost, their identity, as well as their role and their function in practical terms. Can they be considered 'places'? Can it be said that the open spaces of today's hospital structures present characteristics sufficient to qualify them as public spaces?

The public that frequents hospital structures has a well-defined identity, consisting of patients, visitors and medical staff, each with its own specific needs and expectations. The spaces in question are not those traditionally found in urban areas, such as squares or streets, nor are they traditional urban parks. The first step towards understanding the nature and the function of open hospital spaces, in order to be able to plan and design them adequately, is to investigate the behaviour and the expectations of the users of such spaces. What is needed is a 'survey' of the current conditions and uses of the existing structures, in the form of a critical examination of the behaviour of the people who deal with the distribution of time and spaces in hospitals on a daily basis. Using the approach to analysing human behaviour in open spaces developed by Jan Gehl, an attempt is made to calibrate this methodology to the distinctive characteristics of open hospital spaces, in order to arrive at an understanding of their dynamics and, as a result, succeed in adequately fine-tuning the objectives of their design and planning. Quantifying the users in light of their different activities, determining the various categories, identifying the areas where individuals tend to concentrate, observing the activities that predominate in order to gain an understanding of real needs, recording the duration of such activities: these are the goals of a 'survey' carried out through an attentive observation and collection of the available data.

A number of recent experiences point to a radical change in outlook in the design and planning of hospital structures, with the starting point for such change tied to the increased attention paid to the therapeutic component of their outdoor spaces. An example is what has been done at the John Hopkins Hospital in Baltimore, as well as recent projects in Europe where the design of open spaces played a key role in the overall planning and design strategies.

Keywords: survey, behavior, outdoor, hospital.

Introduction

«Public spaces consist of open spaces (such as roads, sidewalks, squares, gardens and parks) and covered spaces built not for profit, but for the common good (...). Both types of spaces, when they possess a clear-cut identity, can be considered "places". The ultimate goal is for all public spaces to become places". So states point 8 of the Charter of Public Space drawn up on the occasion of the Biennial of Public Space in 2013. But can the outside spaces of today's hospital complexes be considered places? And, even more importantly, to what extent can these spaces be characterised as public? The fact that the term 'open spaces' is used with regard to their design does not necessarily mean that they are 'public spaces', much less that they constitute locations. The evidence is there for everyone to see. Hospital complexes are often isolated from the surrounding urban context by barriers, or they are found in areas landscaped as generic greenery, based on a modernist tradition that seeks to combine the functional efficiency and hygienic condition of the buildings with extensive open spaces. In the case of the buildings, the space that separates them from the surrounding barriers serves as an interstice interpreted first and foremost in infrastructural terms (access ways for vehicles and pedestrians, parking facilities, utility installations etc.), with any stopping or lingering viewed primarily as an impediment to the frenetic motion of the hospital. In the case of the large lawns or planted fields, they place the spectre of illness at a remove, relegating it to functionalist cathedrals that society appears to wish to banish from its day-to-day existence. In both cases, we are dealing with what, according to Peter Buchanan, should be an open space, or an 'architectonic event', and therefore a 'place'. But in actual fact, open hospital spaces, for the most part, are not eve addressed as an urban-planning or landscaping problem. To what extent can they be considered public? They are spaces frequented by the public, but were they really designed with the public in mind? Were they planned for the types of individuals and activities that actually put them to use? The public that frequents hospital facilities presents well-defined characteristics. It is made up of patients, visitors and medical staff, each group with its own specific needs and expectations. We are not dealing with traditional urban spaces, such as squares or streets, that attract all types of people and are capable of accommodating and encouraging all the traditional activities that take place in a public space. Nor are we taking about urban parks, with their leisure-time activities. An outside hospital space, when designed with its users in mind, so as to meet their actual needs, is a space arranged in different settings geared towards guaranteeing mobility, privacy and places of rest or pause (1). Areas of greenery are established as filters, to separate the hospital from the road. Porticos are built with roofs or awnings to mark off the areas where vehicles stop to let off passengers, and they hold seats or benches, signs providing directions and various services. In the case of hospitals that consist of a number of different pavilions, the green areas (landscape grounds) with pedestrian walkways and sites for pausing and stopping can be used both as connections between the buildings and for moment of waiting or recreational pauses. The designs that work hardest to ensure the physical and psychological comfort of patients can include 'gardens for convalescence', meaning healthful sites for meditation and healing, planned to host both active and passive activities: contemplating the garden from a window, sitting in it, eating, reading, walking, exercising etc. But apart from the customary procedures that establish the zoning of an open hospital space, the planning and design of these settings should start with the use of what is an indispensable tool for any architect of outdoor spaces,

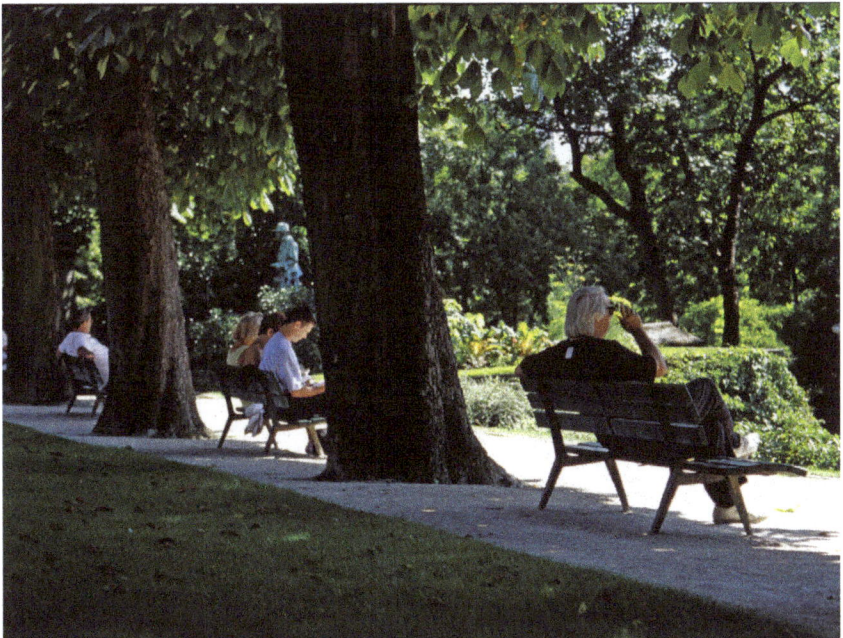

Figure 1: The observation of the use of public spaces as fundamental parameter for their design

and namely a knowledge of the actual behaviour and expectations of the users (which can differ from country to country, or even from region to region), something that can obtained only through close and attentive observation.

'Surveying' the use of outdoor spaces

The operation of surveying – and, therefore, gaining knowledge of – an urban space, in the same way as the surveying of architecture, is a specific process whose objective is to arrive at «a critical, scientific knowledge (meaning knowledge that is focused, analytical, verifiable and transmittable), together with an ordered documentation, of the quantitative and qualitative dimensions (physical-spatial, metric, historical, regarding the state of use and preservation etc.) of its archaeological, architectonic and landscaping assets, all of which the survey itself contributes to defining» (Ugo, 1994). This objective is normally achieved through the establishment of 'models' based on the different disciplines drawn on for the operations of measurement. But while there is no question that the notion of 'measurement', in connection with public spaces, is of key importance in determining the components and proportions that configure and give form to the physical space, it is not equally suited to observing the use that is made of the space. An analysis of the use of public spaces centred on people's behaviour – spontaneous and/or brought about by the environmental conditions or the planned space – would allow us to assess the quality of urban spaces, so as to obtain parameters of use in fulfilling the expectations of the users of such spaces. It follows that another type of 'measurement', together with other operating instruments, must be brought into play if we are to fully appreciate this aspect which, though so readily apparent, proves difficult to 'measure' and transcribe. One of the more attentive, as well as innovative, experts on public life is Jan Gehl (2). His analyses take their bearings from earlier studies, such as those carried out in the field of urban design by Gordon Cullen, or the sociological observations of Jane Jacobs, plus the thinking of Aldo Rossi on cities, together with the studies of Las Vegas done by Robert Venturi, Steven Izenour and Denise Scott Brown, as well as Kevin Lynch's work on the principles of perceptive orientation in cities. The thinking and analyzing method developed by Jan Gehl across the years begin with his design practice and it is returned in a systematic way at first in the book *Life Between Buildings* (1971), then in *Cities for the People* (2010) and more recently in

How to Study Public Life (2013). The aim of Jan Gehl's analyses is to arrive at a form of urban planning on a human scale, grounded in the activities and behaviour of actual people, and therefore reflecting the activities habitually carried out in open public spaces. Any design operation should be preceded – as Jan Gehl sees it – by an analysis of human behaviour. Such an analysis revolves around the realization that design, gender (male-female), age, financial resources, cultural background and any other factors determine how we use, and how we do not use, public spaces. The main instrument for studies of life in public spaces is direct observation. "The study of the behaviour of individuals in public spaces can be compared to the study and structuring of other forms of living organisms. Whether animals or cells are involved, the total number is counted, the speed at which they move under various conditions is observed, and an overall description of how they behave is arrived at through systematic observation" (3). Based on these considerations, Gehl has listed what he considers to be the five main questions to be answered through the observation of human behaviour in public spaces:

- How many? A quantification of the individuals who move through a space, or who spend time in it, is the first variable that can and must be evaluated. In this way, for example, the dynamics of the flows can be understood and the predominant activities can be quantified.

- Who? The second priority is to understand who the primary users are and what groups of people (measured according to a variety of parameters, such as gender and age) use a given public space.

- Where? The third focus of observation and evaluation are modes of behaviour; consideration must be given to where people usually go and where they prefer to stop and spend time (along the boundaries of a space or at its epicentre, or do they distribute themselves indifferently throughout the space? Do they prefer spaces that are public, semi-public, private etc.?).

- What? The fourth observation evaluates what takes place in the urban space, what are the primary activities to which it gives rise: walking, stopping, sitting, playing, interacting, remaining by oneself etc.

- How long? The fifth question entails measurement of the temporal dimension, meaning the amount of time that people devote to the different activities. A place that is inhospitable or otherwise inadequate, for example, leads people to pass through quickly, whereas a well-proportioned, welcoming place encourages people to stop and linger.

These observations, which are elementary in appearance alone, can aid in arriving at an understanding of the spontaneous or conditioned behaviour of individuals, together with their needs and expectations. The questions posed can help reach an understanding of the role of a place where design and planning work shall be done and of the primary behaviour patterns of the types of individuals who shall be the final users. At the same time, a behavioural analysis always proves to be the most effective tool for evaluating, after the fact, whether or not a public space has been properly designed.

Now we shall try posing these same questions with regard to a generic open hospital space.

How many? This is the primary question in the case of areas pertaining to hospital facilities, as well as the one used, in practical terms, to set the main design and planning guidelines. The evaluation of the number of users and the related flows of movement determines the positioning of the pedestrian and vehicle access points, together with the related paths of circulation, which are differentiated in accordance with whether they carry medical, public or logistical traffic (4). Hospital design would still appear to respond to this question above all others when it comes to deciding the forms of outdoor spaces. But what if we are looking to give to a portion of these spaces features and functions that make them viable settings for a public considered not only to be merely passing through? In this case, steps must be taken to quantify the large number of people who, in addition to moving through the outside spaces, also manifest a need to stop and spend time in them, even if the spaces are not equipped for such use. Whoever has spent any time in a hospital structure – even to simply visit or accompany a patient – is familiar with the vital need (both physical and psychological) to go outside and "get some air" on a nearly periodic basis throughout the stay. Nevertheless, this concern is usually neglected during the planning and design work, or it is addressed by assuming that a few seats or benches placed without following any particular criteria constitute an adequate response.

Who? Who are the users of open hospital spaces? Normally this is considered a generic classification that covers visitors, patients and medical staff. But a more accurate examination of how these spaces are utilised could result in the identification of subcategories presenting different needs. Visitors, for example, include individuals accompanying patients, who are often obliged to remain inside the hospital, or in its outside spaces, for medium-long periods of time, while smokers must necessarily use the outside spaces (5), in addition to which there are children and old people: both those able to move under their own power and others unable to do so. Patients' needs also vary widely, depending on their health, their pathologies and the length of time they are hospitalised. This is why optimal planning and design work makes provisions for 'healing gardens', meaning sheltered, healthful sites set aside for psychophysical relaxation and healing. In the case of the personnel as well, even though they have limited time to use the outdoor spaces, there is no mistaking the tendency to seek and to consider contact with the outside as an indispensable element in improving working conditions.

Where? Observing where people are likely to go or stop and spend time within an urban context (be it a street, a square, an entire neighbourhood or a generic empty urban space) can provide the dimensions and parameters of the logic underlying the movements of people as they use public spaces, together with their levels of satisfaction. In the areas bordering on healthcare facilities, and within their areas of pertinence, the main directions considered under planning and design work are those consisting of entry and exit movements. If observation is also made of where people are accustomed to stop and spend time, then it will become apparent that their decisions, under the most frequent conditions, are influenced by the scarcity of spaces set aside for waiting or for other types of recreational activities designed specifically to be carried out in outdoor spaces. The highest concentrations of presences will be recorded in and around the entry points to the structures or in the vicinity of the zones offering food service and refreshments (normally found inside the buildings, near the entrances) or where there are seats or benches, even if these are found in isolated, 'leftover' areas of the outdoor design, along connecting roads or amidst parking areas. In such cases, the observations recorded may have little real meaning, given that the directions of movement and assembly may be influenced by the layout of the locations or by the fact that the sites available leave little room for free choice. Still, based on the behaviour patterns that people are led to follow, considerations can be formulated for corrective work or for a full reformulation of the overall planning of the areas set aside for public use.

What? This is the single most important question that can be answered by observing the activities that occur in outside hospital areas; close observation of the main activities engaged in by users can prove to be of fundamental importance in good

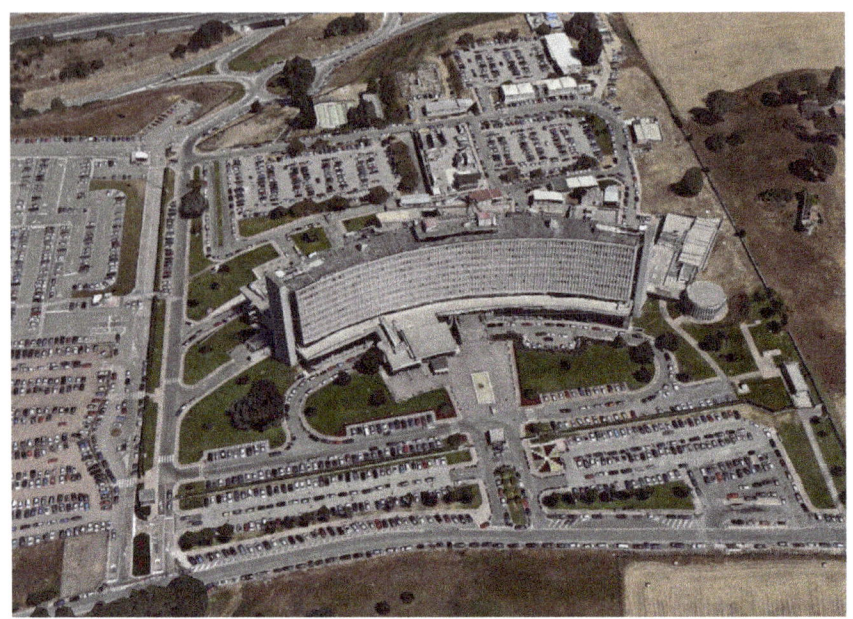

Figure 2: Open areas next to Rome's hospitals become marginal and residual areas. Sant'Andrea Hospital (above) and Gemelli General Hospital (below)

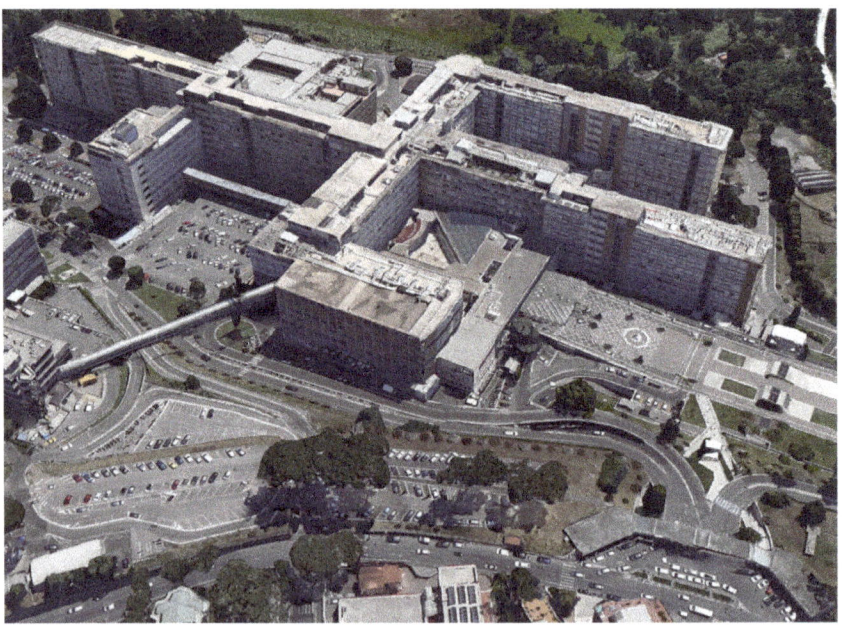

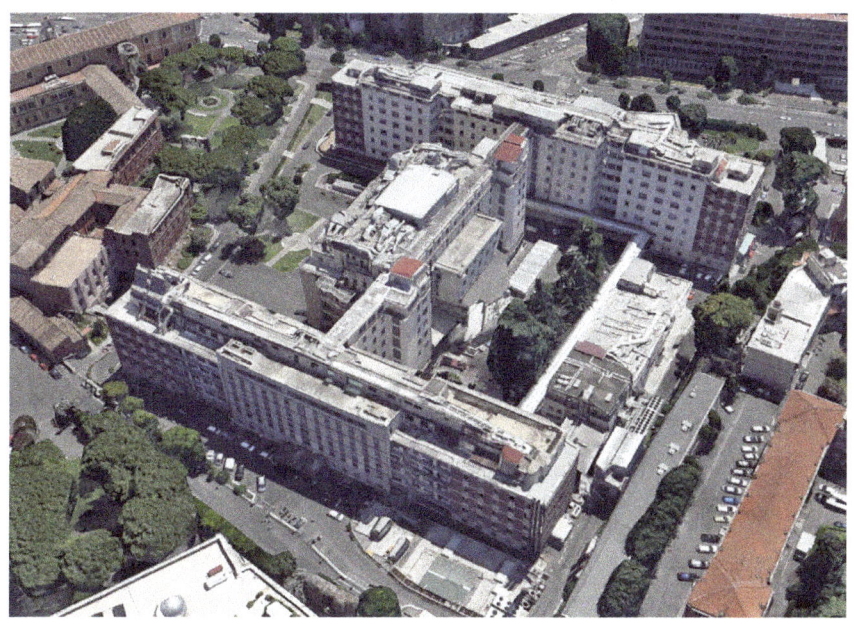

San Giovanni Hospital (above) and San Camillo Hospital (below)

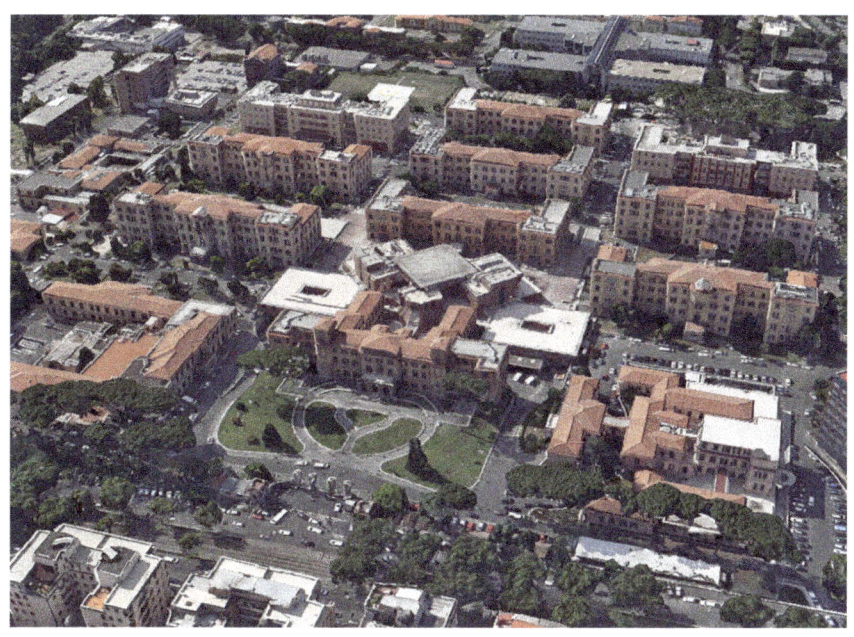

planning and design. First of all, it can be determined whether or not those spaces satisfy the all important function of facilitating the efforts of visitors to orient themselves, and therefore move about. All too often this activity is left to be carried out by a redundant superstructure of ambient graphics (signs and signals) that do not always do the job effectively. Secondly, it can be noted that most people who are obliged to frequent hospitals (patients and visitors) spend the bulk of their time merely waiting. Apart from the appropriately outfitted waiting rooms, the areas of distribution, the rooms for the patients and the spaces for food service and refreshments, a large part of the time is spent in some connection with the outside spaces. This relationship can be said to be established even through nothing more than the simple visual link sought out from the inside, through the windows, during waiting times. It is during the time spent waiting that a great many of the other activities that can be observed take place. There are people who wish to be off by themselves (one of the needs given the least attention), while others seek out interaction in order to exchange experiences or simply make contact with people willing to listen to them; others feel the need to move about constantly; while still others are merely looking for a place to sit and watch the activities going around them, as a simple but invigorating form of distraction. When children are present, the outside space proves all the more important in terms of providing opportunities for entertaining activities, even when there is no equipment specifically designed for the purpose. To accommodate all these activities, there is often nothing more than a few seats and benches arranged without any particular criteria or, when all else fails, low walls, stairways or portico that serve as stopgap measures to meet these needs. When patients are involved, the outside spaces are often the scene of the first rehabilitation movements they make on their own, or such spaces represent their sole contact with the 'outside world', or their initially contact following a lengthy period of hospitalization.

How long? The duration of the activities – meaning the evaluation of the time factor – measures the extent to which them outside spaces meet the users' needs (6). If it is found that too much time is needed to reach the wards and the clinics, then it is common practice to introduce corrective measures, seeing that the parameter in question influences the level of efficiency aimed at by the healthcare structures. On the other hand, when the environment and the structures of the outside areas do not favour the activities referred to above, his consideration would not appear to be given an equal amount of consideration. It is no accident that, in many Italian hospital structures, the day-to-day rhythm is linked to the frenetic pace of hospital operations. What is more, the fact that the hospital is often experienced as a negative setting, with its connotation of illness, appears to keep the public from staying or lingering. And yet the time spent waiting to visit hospitalized friends or relatives, or waiting one's turn for medical examinations and appointments, make these sites the most heavily trafficked, and most vigorous, 'public squares' when it comes to social interaction. What can be done to establish a parameter of efficiency that also takes into account the capacity of outside hospital areas to accommo-date stopping and waiting while exercising their therapeutic and socialising effects? First and foremost, a radical cultural change is needed.

From observation to planning and design. Success stories

Hospital architecture is a field still strongly influenced, in many instances, by the school of modernist efficiency, an introverted approach geared primarily towards the functional performance of the 'healthcare machine', without paying heed to its relationship with its users, the city or the surrounding countryside (7). The conception of outside spaces that results lacks any overall vision, nor does it contribute in any way to achieving the physical and psychological wellbeing that constitutes the general objective which such structures are meant to pursue. In the same way as the 'open spaces' of modern cities, the outside spaces of hospital areas have not been conceived of, codified or theorized in 'concrete' terms, meaning that their planning has not taken into consideration factors of architecture, landscaping, aesthetics or any therapeutic effect; instead it has been defined abstractly, though only in a negative sense, as the empty spaces produced by the layout on the terrain of the architectural plans (8). Still, a number of recent experiences point to the rise of a radical change in the current mindset. The firm of Herzog & de Meuron in Basel, for example, has developed a number of cutting-edge projects meant to renew the very concept of hospital structures, drawing on the experience it gained with the REHAB Rehabilitation Centre (for spinal cord and brain injuries, built in 2003); a two-storey building faced with wood components and designed in close relationship with the surrounding countryside, its area of pertinence – though designed to provide the necessary privacy and tranquillity – is free of any barriers around its circumference or visual obstacles. The new advance represented

REHAB led to the development of projects on a larger scale for the Kinderspital of Zurich and for the NYT Hospital Nordsjælland in Hillerød (Denmark), both of which won their respective design contests, precisely because they proposed a type of hospital design able to represent an alternative to the usual massive structures. The first project was for a three-storey paediatrics hospital structured around a series of courtyards, as if it were a small city looking in upon itself. The wood facing, the horizontal layout of the structure and a use of greenery that, in addition to linking up with the connection to the surrounding city, also occupies roof areas, all contribute to an overall atmosphere characterised by a familiar, human touch. Just a short distance away is a second, cylindrical structure that provides the geometric counterpoint to the hospital, establishing a dialogue with its surroundings as it provides a separate venue housing activities of education and research. The layout used in the design of the Hillerød hospital is horizontal as well, only in this case the distribution of the volumes is organic, running along curved lines that enclose, in their central portion, extensive surface areas rendered as gardens, including both a series of courtyards and a roofing surface designed to be usable as an open

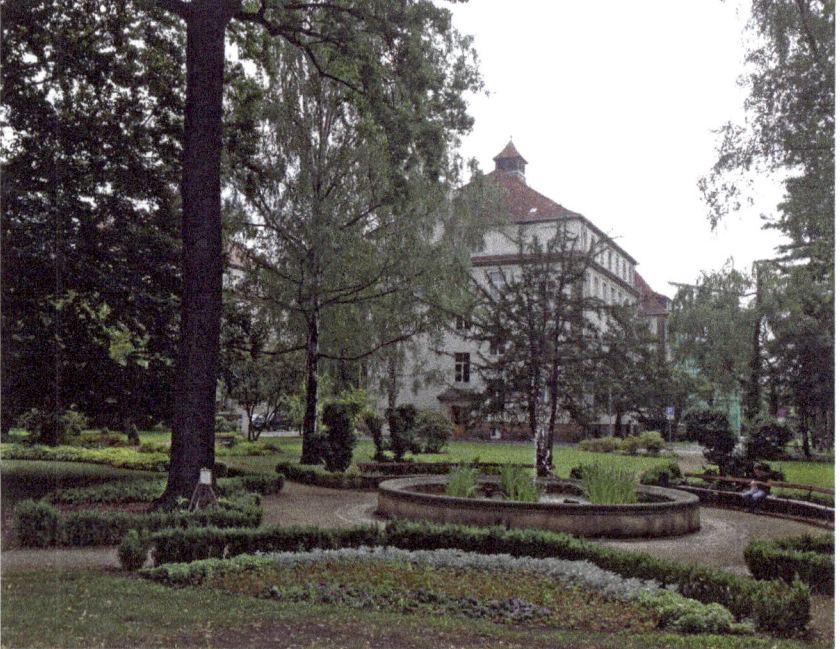

Figure 3: Open spaces designed like a park in the Universitatsklinikum Carl Gustav Carus in Dresden

space. The green core of the building establishes a dialogue, as well as continuity, with the natural surrounding countryside – on which it appears to rest – to the point where the passage from the internal spaces to the outside ones becomes almost imperceptible. The trend that sees terraced floors and roof surfaces used to house gardens in the available open spaces (9) of hospital structures would appear to be confirmed in recent years by the increasingly frequent appearance of such gardens in the United States. Especially worthy of note are the Schwab Rehabilitation Hospital Rooftop Garden in Chicago (arch.: Douglas Hills Associates, 2013), the therapeutical garden (*healing garden*) on 7th floor of the Smilow Cancer Hospital in Yale (arch.: Shepley Bulfinch, 2010), the St. Louis Children's Hospital Rooftop Garden (arch: Mackey Mitchell Architects e EDAW, 2007) and the Rooftop Garden of the Mary Catherine Bunting Center at Mercy in Baltimore (arch: Ellerbe Becket con Mahan Rykiel Associates, 2010). The fact that "Healing Gardens" open both to patients and the public would appear to have become an indispensable prerequisite in the United States (10). Indeed, the Joint Commission on Accreditation of Healthcare Organizations recently introduced the presence of nature and public greenery as a factor in the evaluation of hospital structures (11). A project of particular importance, in light of this trend, would appear to be that developed by the Olin firm for the John Hopkins Hospital in Baltimore. The design laid out and gave form to four different public spaces: the Entry Court Gardens, the Western Courtyard Gardens (containing: the Entrance Garden, the Healing Garden and the Meditation Garden), the Phillips Courtyard and the Little Prince Garden. As stated by Susan Weiler, a partner of the Olin firm, the project has created "a new standard of excellence for patient care and hospital design. The gardens have been designed as places of orienta-tion, respite, rejuvenation and calm, with a visual simplicity that accentuates the aesthetic pleasures of the gardens. The newly conceived circulation pattern allowed us to keep one-third of the enormous football-field-sized site for the courtyard gardens" (12). The spaces were designed with both patients and visitors in mind, in such a way that they can either be experienced directly or provide comfort through the windows of the patients' rooms, simply by being seen. The conceptual work on each detail is meant to enhance physical and psychological wellbeing while facilitating the orientation of visitors and patients by means of an outside space that not only performs in a functional sense but, even more importantly, places the hospital's relationship with the visitors and the patients on a more friendly footing. "The Entry Court is

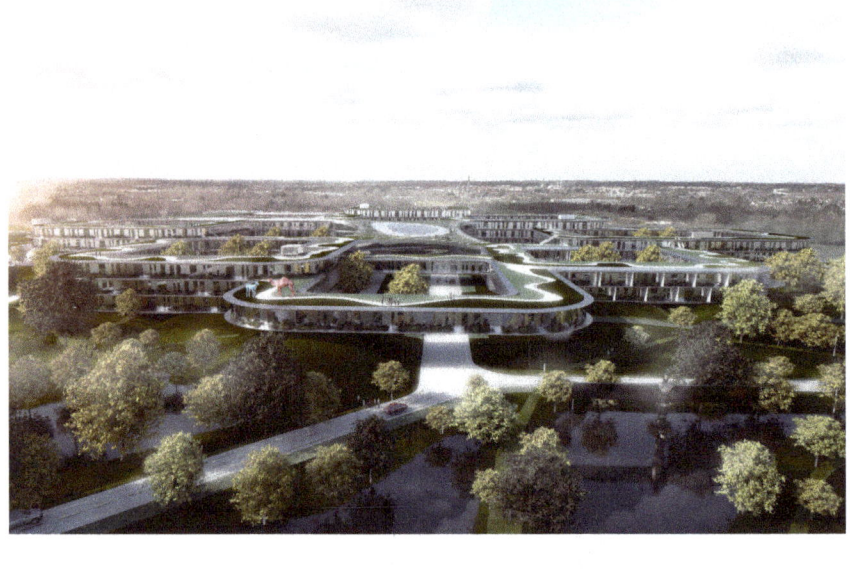

Figure 4-5: Herzog & de Meuron, The design for the Children's Hospital in Zürich, Switzerland

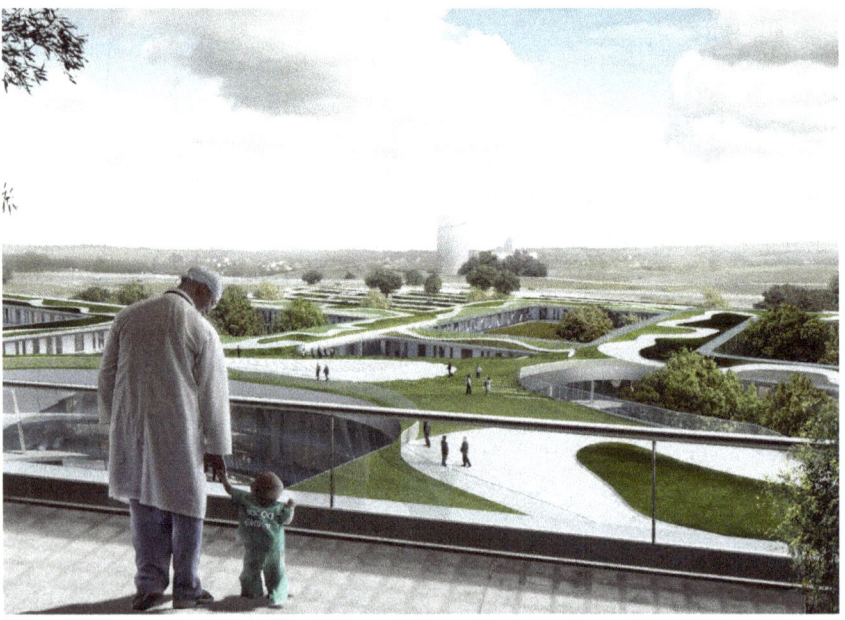

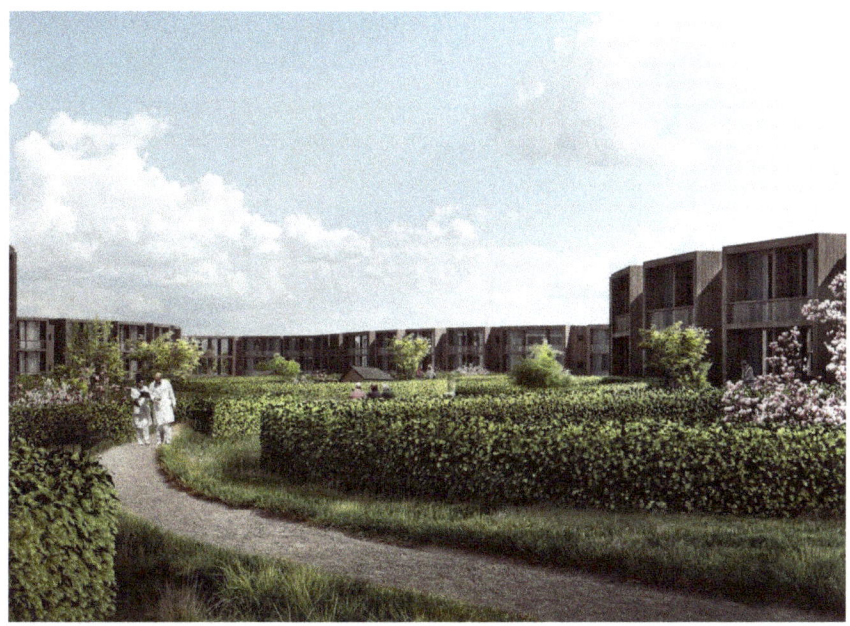

Figure 6 - 7: Herzog & de Meuron. The design for the NYT Hospital Nordsjælland in Hillerød, Denmark (above) and Henning Larsen Architects. The design for the recover and extension of the Hospital in Herlev, Denmark (below)

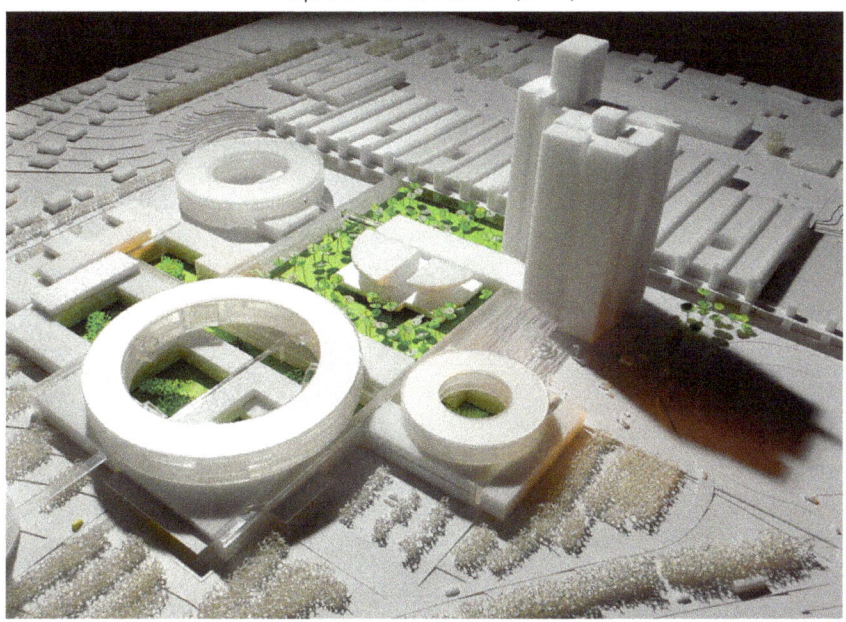

designed to facilitate pedestrian safety as well as to provide ease of movement and clear views for anxious drivers (...) The rich and durable paving palette of bluestone, brick, quartzite and granite will provide visual continuity to the vehicular and garden spaces. This continuity helps to emphasize the patterns and colors of the paving and planting, which is also intended to be viewed from above by patients, visitors and staff". The Western Courtyard Gardens, including the Entrance Garden, the Healing Garden and the Meditation Garden make available different kind of space's experiences through the use of different shapes, articulations, plants, colors and sounds. The plants selected for the Entrance Garden, for example, help mitigate traffic noise, both by serving as a carrier and thanks to the offsetting sound made by their leaves. The Healing Garden consists of two distinct spaces: one more open, and therefore better suited as a site for social relations, and the other more secluded – almost a secret garden. The presence of the water, along with the noise it makes, is inspired by the oriental tradition for endowing each space with the right atmosphere. The Meditation Garden, on the other hand, is designed to be a full fledged oasis of peace and quiet. Decorative elements and plants provide the proper scale, the visual focal points and exactly the right mood for undisturbed contemplation. In order to accommodate recreational areas, as well as a hub of attraction for the external spaces, the plans call for a hospital cafeteria that is to be connected directly to the Phipps Courtyard. Meanwhile the Little Prince Garden is an area set aside for the entertainment of children, inspired by theme and motifs from the adventures of The Little Prince by Saint'Exupéry.

The increasing tendency to ensure that open hospital spaces serve a purpose, including a therapeutic benefit, by paying particular attention to each and every type of user, would also appear to be confirmed by European models, as can be observed in France, Great Britain and Denmark. The Henning Larsen Architects firm recently won an international competition for the restoration and expansion of the Herlev Hospital in Denmark (13). The existing hospital was housed in a 120 metre tower based on a stereometric geometry and isolated from the surrounding context, in accordance with the tenets of the functionalist style. The new proposal calls for the construction of a second complex, adjoining the existing one and designed to mediate and mollify it proportions. The expansion consists of a set of buildings laid out horizontally, with a rectangular base holding three circular structures arranged in such a way as to create numerous small outdoor spaces in the form of courtyards and gardens. Underlying the proposal is the wish to interpret, on the level of design, the well known therapeutic and recreational effect that only the presence of greenery can provide. This quest has dictated the guidelines of the entire project, so "luxuriant courtyards, green roof gardens, and a large, central green heart provide the new hospital with an altogether vibrante and life-affirming atmosphere". The outdoor spaces of the hospital are designed to interact with the public in such a way that they prove attractive, serving as a stimulus for all the senses, even from the inside of the building; "as many of the hospital users have a view of the outside environment through the window of the building, the landscape is designed as a number of 'pictures' varying with the rythm of the hospital and changing seasons".

The need for a change on the design of hospital structures ca be traced, therefore, straight to the demand for a different type of efficiency, meaning one measured not only in terms of the functional performance of the organisational system, the technology and the structures, but also with regard to ties to users, the city and the countryside. The goal is to restore what Renzo Piano refers to as a "humanistic vision of the hospital" by reflecting on the "state of mind of those who experience a hospitalization, either directly or indirectly", so as to, "reduce the trauma caused by such moments to the greatest extent possible" (14). Thus Piano's proposal of an ideal hospital immersed in greenery, structured around volumes with a maximum of four floors, following the model of pavilion style hospitals, to create a structure whose spaces are measures on a human scale, and without winding up isolated from the rest of the urban fabric. The hospital features a ground floor providing all the services that could prove useful to patient and visitors, but which, at present, are often missing (cafes, newsstands, laundry rooms, stores, florists, hairdressers etc.) (15). This ideal design conceived of by Renzo Piano would appear to have reached fruition in the design proposals referred to above, simply taking the form of a response dysfunctional aspects and the unmistakable needs of existing hospital structures. The formulation of the ideal necessarily draws on a knowledge that can be accrued only through a 'survey' of the open hospital space that takes note of the numbers, the identity, the behaviour, the actions and the reactions of the users.

Notes

(1) The design criteria outside hospital spaces should satisfy the following prerequisites: accessibility, visibility, feeling of control, feeling of security, physiological comfort, quiet, familiarity, flexibility, sustainability. The types considered include today: landscaped grounds, landscaped setbacks, front porches, entry porches, entry gardens, courtyards, plazas, roof terraces, roof gardens, healing gardens, meditation gardens, viewing gardens, the viewing/walk-in garden, edile gardens; cfr. Gökçen Firdevs Yücel, *Hospital Outdoor Landscape Design* (cdn.intechopen.com/pdfs-wm/45442.pdf).

(2) Founding Partner of Gehl Architects, Jan Gehl is Professor and Researcher at the Royal Danish Academy of Fine Arts, School of Architecture. Over the course of his career, he has published several books, including, *Life Between Buildings* (Van Nostrand Reinhold, New York 1987), *Cities for People* (Island Press, Washington D.C. 2010), *New City Spaces*, *Public Spaces - Public Life, New City Life* (with Lars Gemzøe, Island Press, Washington D.C. 2008). He is an honorary fellow of RIBA, AIA, RAIC, and PIA. More informations on the site gehlarchitects.com

(3) Jan Gehl, Birgitte Svarre. *How to Study Public Life*, Washington DC: Island Press, 2013, p.3. The activities that contribute to performing this type of "survey" are listed by Jan Gehl: Counting, Mapping, Tracing, Following/Monitoring, Investigating, Photographing, Annotating, Testing/Walking.

(4) As a rule, the outside circuits are catalogued in terms of flows of visitors, patents to be hospitalized, outpatients, emergency room patients, supply of pharmaceuticals, meals and materials and personnel employed by the structure. Each of these flows needs an access point to the building. The first three use the same entrance, while the other three categories should have separate points of entry. Cf. Nicoletta Setola, *Percorsi, flussi e persone nella progettazione ospedaliera*, Firenze University Press, 2013.

(5) The current trend is to prohibit smoking even in open hospital spaces, as is the case at the hospitals of Rovigo, Udine and Prato.

(6) As Jan Gehl pointed out, "registering human activity in relation to the physical environment presents a number of special problems, first and foremost because the question involves processes – chains of events – undergoing continuous change. One moment is not like the previous or the one to follow. In contrast to measuring buildings, for example, time is an important factor in activity studies"; J. Gehl, B. Svarre, cit. p.19.

(7) When the topic of a lack of familiarity and failure to recognise the identity of hospital structures is brought up, at times it regards the relationship with the staff, but quite often the environmental factor comes into play as well.

(8) «While in cities of the past the physical relationship between full and empty volumes was defined in terms of proportions and qualities of perception, in the "open city" of modern times this relation tends to be undermined by the advent of a merely positivistic approach to urban spaces, conceptually considered to be the interval and the spacing between constructed objects» Cf. Pierre-Alain Cro-set, introduction to the section entitled "Modernism and the

Codification of Open Spaces", *Casabella* 597-598, monographic vol. *"The design of open spaces"*, january-february 1993, p.11.

(9) This solution was implemented, in particular, by the existing hospitals found within large urban agglomerations where it is difficult to find undeveloped areas at street level.

(10) See the examples described in the recent book edited by Clare Cooper Marcus e Naomi A. Sachs, *Therapeutic Landscapes: An Evidence-Based Approach to Designing Healing Gardens and Restor-ative Outdoor Spaces*, John Wiley & Sons, Hoboken, New Jersey, 2013.

(11) In 1995 the American Horticultural Therapy Association made a number of recommendations regarding the characteristics that therapeutic landscapes should present: therapeutic gardens in the hospital setting should be simple, unified and easily comprehended places; in the hospital garden setting, it is important to design and program for the widest possible range of user abilities – thera-peutic gardens commonly stimulate the full range of senses — memory, hearing, touch, smell and sometimes taste — as necessary supplements to the visual experience; therapeutic goals focus on mobility, motor skills, social interaction, cognitive ability and emotional status - restorative goals promote general well-being, with focus on play, relaxation, socialization, education and creativity; a profusion of plants and people/plant interactions is essential; edges of garden spaces and special zones of activities within the garden are intensified to direct the attention and energies of the user into the garden; modified features to improve accessibility.

(12) Interview published on «Architect+Artisans», 12 april 2012.

(13) The project won an international competition that was concluded in 2014. Construction is planned for 2017. Together with the firm of Henning Larsen Architects, the team includes Friis & Moltke, Brunsgaard & Laursen, Orbicon, Norconsult, NNE Pharmaplan and SLA. Of particular note are some excerpts from the comments accompanying the jury's award, with respect to the change in outlook evidenced by the approach to hospital construction: "Based on a comprehensive analysis of developments in the healthcare sector and a strong focus on creating a welcoming, clear, worthy and sensuous setting for patients, relatives and staff, the vision of the competition team has been to create a symbiosis between the hospital and its surroundings. A symbiosis where the individual elements form part of a natural cycle and create a "sensory hospital" that will position Herlev Hospital as an exemplary and innovative spearhead in healthcare." "The project powerfully unites building design and landscape into an architectural whole providing patients, relatives and staff with the experience that "focus is on the individual". The project must be emphasised for its high and wellargued ambition level for healing architecture. The healing potential of architecture is consistently translated into sensuous spaces - in an approach characterised by great variation and commitment at many different levels.".

(14) Here reference is made to studies carried out by Renzo Piano in 2001 on a new model for hospital design, on behalf of the Minister of Health, Dr. Umberto Veronesi.

(15) Along with the considerations on the humanisation of hospitals and their integration with the surrounding city, other points on which Piano calls for reflection are tied to the topics

of innovation (or flexibility of structures), reliability (safety in terms of the environment, technical-construction con-cerns, plant engineering and hygiene of sites), research (the presence of departments devoted to clinical-scientific research) and training (the hospital as a site for the training of personnel).

References

Cooper Marcus C., Francis C. (1998) *People Places*, John Wiley & Sons, Hoboken, New Jersey; USA.

Cooper Marcus C., Sachs N.A. (2013), *Therapeutic Landscapes: An Evidence-Based Approach to Designing Healing Gardens and Restorative Outdoor Spaces*, John Wiley & Sons, Hoboken, New Jersey, USA.

Croset P.-A. (1993), introduction to the chapter "Il Moderno e la codificazione degli spazi aperti", Casabella, 597-598, monographic vol. *"Il disegno degli spazi aperti"*, gennaio-febbraio 1993, IT, p.11.

Cullen G. (1961), *The Concise Townscape*, Architectural Press, London, UK.

Firdevs Yücel G. (2013), *"Hospital Outdoor Landscape Design"*, available at cdn.intechopen.com/pdfs-wm/45442.pdf

Gehl J. (1971) *Life Between Buildings*, Danish Architectural Press, Copenhagen, DK.

Gehl J., Svarre B. (2013), *How to Study Public Life*, Island Press, Washington DC.

Jacobs J. (1961), *Death and Life of Great American Cities*, Random House, New York, NY.

Lynch K. (1960), *The Image of the City*, Cambridge (Mass.) Technology Press, Cambridge, Mass.

Rossi A. (1966), *L'architettura della città*, Marsilio, Padova, IT.

Setola N. (2013), *Percorsi, flussi e persone nella progettazione ospedaliera*, Firenze University Press, Firenze, IT.

Venturi R., Izenour S., Scott Brown D. (1972), *Learning fron Las Vegas*, MIT Press, Cambridge, Mass. London, UK.

Fabio Quici

05

Exploring the relationship between outdoor and indoor environments in the hospital design process

Francesca Giofrè

"Architecture, attesting to the tastes and attitudes of generations, to public events and private tragedies, to new and old facts, is the fixed stage for human events. The collective and the private, society and the individual, balance and confront one another in the city. The city is composed of many people seeking a general order that is consistent with their own particular environment."
 Aldo Rossi, 1978, p.22

Abstract: This paper discusses the relationship between the city, the hospital and its indoor and outdoor environments, and aspects that need to be taken into account when planning a hospital complex within a city to create a continuum across them. In particular, the paper deals with issues related to urban and social integration, and the influence that the functional organization of the physical spaces and the typology of the hospital has on the qualities of the outdoor spaces around the hospital itself. The paper argues that the design process does not consider the outdoor spaces as an integral part of the hospital in a proper way, but only as a residual spaces to support medical activities. Against this backdrop, the paper contends that the outdoor spaces need to be integrated as part of the design process through a multidimensional design approach that involves the user groups. In the newly-created 'outdoor related spaces', new categories of activities emerge for the community and the user groups. Overall, the paper offers design considerations that help to create the right balance between the city and the hospital's outdoor and indoor environments.

Keywords: hospital outdoor – indoor environment, supportive design, user groups, design inputs.

Introduction

The hospital traditionally understood as a place of diagnosis and treatment is slowly transforming into a physical environment that promotes health. This evolution is possible on the condition that the hospital becomes one of the hubs of the network formed by the other institutions in the region – medical, civil and production – in a close relationship with the needs of the community served.

"A health promoting hospital does not only provide high quality comprehensive medical and nursing services, but also develops a corporate identity that embraces the aims of health promotion, develops a health promoting organizational structure and culture, including active, participatory roles for patients and all members of staff, develops itself into a health promoting physical environment and actively cooperates with its community." (WHO, 1998). Health promotion is intended to mean the implementation of strategies and actions that address aspects linked to the human condition of people as citizens and workers, as well as traditional diagnosis and treatment activities. This strengthens the link that exists between society and the hospital, between the city and the hospital, and between the community and the hospital, also acting through the relational, organizational and functional transformation of the indoor and outdoor physical environments that constitute it.

Even today it is valid to claim that the hospital represents one of the most complex buildings in terms of design, implementation and management. The morphological, functional and technological configuration of the hospital over time has not been able to anticipate the constant alterations and innovations of the role and the functions that had to be and still have to be defined, increasingly quickly. The appearance and mission of the hospital have changed very slowly in view of the potential offered by constant innovations – in the fields of medical sciences, genomics, biomedical equipment, information technology, and virtual reality – and by the advancement of new requirements to contain operational and sustainability costs and the rise in greater awareness of the centrality of user needs.

Hospital architecture has therefore been the result of the search for a more adaptive and dynamic efficiency, which was achieved in building types that were 'crystallized' through an established design practice (Giofrè, 2002). The very term hospital, from the Latin *hospitale*, a place where guests are accommodated, with the direct reference to beds, is now too generic and obsolete considering that for some years the trend has been to reduce the number of beds and hospitalization times.

Since the end of the '90s in Italy there has been a lively debate on the hospital 'of the future', on how and what it should be and what functions it should perform. In 2001 the architect Renzo Piano wrote the decalogue of the hospital of the third millennium, which was commissioned by the Ministry of Health. It spreads awareness that the hospital must define its role as a specialized place for high-intensity care, capable of delegating medium- and low-intensity care to more economic and modest facilities in the region. The hospital with its mission refined as such takes on a central role of connection between the heterogeneous elements that constitute the healthcare network in Italy. The direct consequence of the points made is the need to design a hospital building that is attentive to the needs of users and suitably equipped from a technological perspective, a veritable container of technologies; it must be integrated in its internal functions and in its connections with the outdoors (Giofrè and Terranova, 2004; Giofrè and Terranova, 2006). A study was commenced on the hubs of the network and the characteristics of the services and spaces of the other satellite buildings of the hospital, such as houses of health, community hospitals, healthcare residences for the elderly, hospices, and Alzheimer's centres.

It is clear, however, how over time the hospital was conceived in building and technology terms as a separate entity, the product of completely independent technical knowledge, as an enclosed, rationally functioning space. Even now there is the need to reconsider the hospital as a subsystem of the city system and its network of services and as a product capable of meeting the challenges that come from its environment and from society as a whole (Falcitelli, Trabucchi and Vanara, 2000), if not anticipate them.

With this in mind the intent is to investigate the relationship that now exists between the city and the hospital and the role and functions that could and must be performed by the outdoor spaces pertaining to the hospitals in connection with the indoor spaces, also in the design development phase. The outdoor spaces that gravitate around the hospital building in the specific Italian context are considered even residual, marginal, in other words 'other' with respect to both the city and the enclosed, rationally functioning environment of the hospital, even though.

Italy is located in the temperate zone with a Mediterranean climate and enjoying the outdoors is an essential factor of individual lifestyle. The outdoor spaces, in particular those of large hospital complexes, represent an important resource to be enhanced and returned to the city and can represent a testing ground for the launch of those strategies given different names, such as healthy city, salutogenic city, green city, smart city.

The hospital that promotes health must, through the representativeness of all of its architecture, outdoor spaces and buildings, transmit in *un unicum* the power of the identity of the health culture, which is the expression of a given society and its continuous transformations.

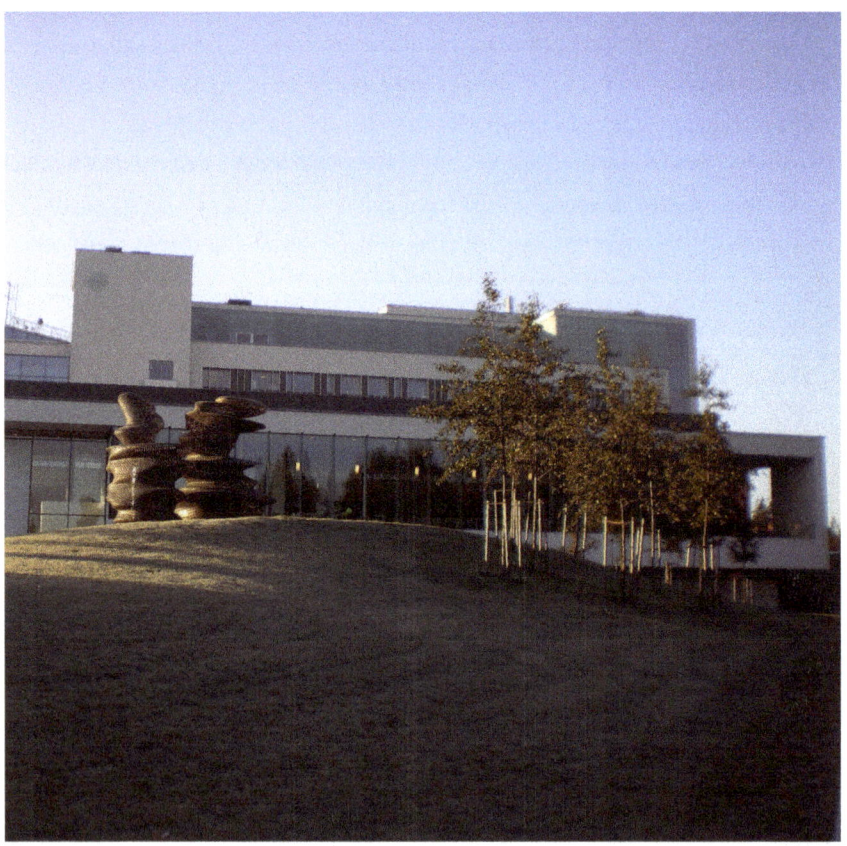

Figure 1: Outdoor spaces, Akershus University Hospital, Oslo, Norway, photo by Francesca Giofrè

Urban and social design integration

In many Italian situations the hospital is located in metropolitan contexts, occupying a substantial part of the territory, and its dimensions vary according to the functions provided and the catchment area served. In some cases the areas where the hospital is located are central and congested, or they have become so over time, and have strong historical characteristics. From a typological point of view it is necessary to distinguish between hospitals that are characterized by being concentrated in one building, with various arrangements of In many Italian situations the hospital is located in metropolitan contexts, occupying a substantial part of the territory, and its dimensions vary according to the functions provided and the catchment area served. In some cases the areas where the hospital is located are central and congested, or they have become so over time, and have strong historical characteristics. From a typological point of view it is necessary to distinguish between hospitals that are characterized by being concentrated in one building, with various arrangements of all the functions, and large hospital complexes. In Italy general hospitals are the example of large hospital complexes, a term used to define those places where different health promoting activities, such as diagnosis, treatment, and research, are carried out in different buildings. General hospitals are small cities within the city, sometimes referred to as a 'city of health', such as that in Turin. Whatever the architectural configuration of the hospital, it must be considered a subsystem of the city and as such it must integrate and contribute to the higher system of the 'city' and its networks, forming a whole. If we consider the city-hospital relational system as a whole, the system is at the same time more or less the sum of its parts and it is also different to that sum. The hospital system is 'small', but not necessarily 'small' in relation to its capacity to significantly influence the higher system of the city, of which it is an integral part. The properties and behaviours of the two systems are not casual, insofar as they are the result of design choices, but in any case it is the people that shape the two systems, sometimes even unpredictably. The search for the adaptive architectural efficiency of the hospital studied from a theoretical viewpoint, as stated in the introduction, is as if it had been able to process information and to form a model, evaluating the 'futility of integration' with the higher system of the city. The link between the hospital and the city is therefore not mechanical, rather it is still engaged in a conflictual dialectic relationship, not of continuity but of breakage and it is also this aspect that leads to a perception of the hospital as a place of power and control (Foucault,1976), segregation and disease (Sack, 1986) and as highly stressful for all categories of users, each for different reasons (Ulrich, et al. 1991; Malkin 1992; Horsburgh, 1995). The osmotic process between the system and the subsystem is interrupted and the types of physical barriers that enclose and delimit the area of the hospital subsystem, where there is a complete absence of a relationship with the surroundings, are a demonstration of this. Although in practice these barriers are crossed on a daily basis by flows of material and immaterial goods and services, people and vehicles, waste of various kinds, and so on. The relationship between the outdoor spaces pertaining to the hospital building and the indoor spaces is also interrupted. Reference should be made to various studies that highlight how the relationship with the outdoor spaces is an important resource that should be enhanced and that is capable of activating processes that promote well-being (Burnett, 1997; Marcus and Barnes, 1999; Ulrich, 2001; Van Den Berg and Wagenaar, 2006). The bordering perimeter of the hospital complex limited by 'barriers' can be treated as a space that can be defined as public and semi-public, shifting established concepts that identify different hierarchical levels of space, a permeable boundary, just as some open spaces inside the complex can assume the same value. The problems mainly linked to forms of controlling accesses for security purposes can be easily resolved through the use of remote control technologies, as can those linked to sources of noise outside the building through appropriate design solutions. In this way the hospital opens up to the city, reactivating an interrupted dialogue and restoring the image of a place forming part of the health promotion system. The Healthy City "is one that is continually creating and improving those physical and social environments and expanding those community resources which enable people to mutually support each other in performing all the functions of life and developing to their maximum potential" (WHO,1998). The hospital, as an infrastructure for health promotion, is a physical and social space of the city and helps to create a healthy city also through the removal of both physical and perceptive barriers.

Aldo Rossi (1995) looks at the city as architecture not only in reference to "the visible image of the city and the sum of its different architectures, but architecture as construction, the construction of the city over time." (...) The city "addresses the ultimate and definitive fact in the life of the collective of the environment in which it lives. (...) The contrast between particular and universal, between individual and collective, emerges from the city and from its construction, its architecture." This contrast "manifests itself in different ways: in the relationship between the public and private sphere, between public and private buildings, between the rational design of urban architecture and the values of locus or place" (p.14). "The *locus* is a relationship between a certain specific location and the buildings that are in it. It is at once singular and universal" (p.103); the value of the *locus* thus assumes great importance.

The hospital is included in what A. Rossi defines as the fixed activities of a city which converge in its primary elements; what unites them is their public and collective nature and 'this characteristic of a public thing, made by the community for the community, is essentially urban in nature'. Le Corbusier, when he decided to accept the commission of the Hospital of Venice in 1964, tackled the project with a much advanced awareness of the public aspect, starting with a careful analysis of the natural features of the site and its history. The project he proposed was related, from a physical and morphological point of view, to the structure of the city of Venice. Almost by osmosis it became a part of it, a continuation and organic development of its fabric and physical form, thus characterized by the natural features of the site and its civil history (Petrilli, 1999).

The hospital therefore as one of the primary elements, *res publica* of urban nature, rooted in a settlement context and capable of contributing to the construction of the city. The reference to be used as as starting point in the design of hospitals is therefore the *popolo*, namely the ensemble of people as members of the community of a certain society, which, through its architecture, constructs the city.

The concept of urban and social integration is referenced by some English guidelines for the design or redevelopment of hospital structures. To achieve urban and social integration, the guidelines suggest the topics and related issues that designers should take into account (Fig.2), such as: a sense of place; a good neighbour; a positive contribution to the community; fit with site and landscape design (BMA, 2011). In order to overcome the critical relationship between the hospital and the city three principles must be taken on board in the planning and design processes.

- The principle of urbanity. The hospital must not be foreign to the settlement context, but rather an organic part of it in a subsystem logic that must express a relationship of continuity and comparison with existing architecture, in particular when it is of great historical interest.

- The principle of sociality. Inside and outside the hospital people must rediscover the values of solidarity, a sense of belonging to the community and interdependence in daily life.
- The principle of dynamism. Cities today undergo great transformations, some of which are still only at cultural development level. The concepts of green city, eco city, smart city, and salutogenic city must be upheld at the scale of the green hospital, eco hospital, smart hospital, and salutogenic hospital. All these strategies and/or approaches to the design incorporate attention to the outdoor space, which assumes great value in the achievement of the objectives they set.

Hospital architecture, the result of undisputed interdisciplinary work, in its totality and in continuity with the consolidated urban fabric, thus helps to construct a sense of place and a sense of belonging, strengthening its social and identity function in the enhancement of diversity.

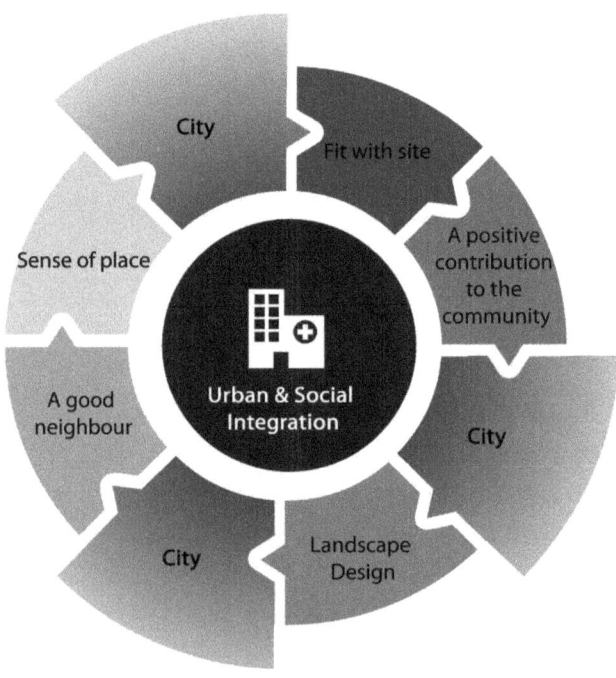

Figure 2: Achive urban & social integration in hospital structure

In *versus* out design

The outdoor spaces pertaining to a hospital and their usability are highly affected by the organizational, spatial and functional choices made in the design phase, dictated by the complexity of the activities that will be carried out within the confined space. The layout of the hospital is put together during the design process essentially based on the spatial-functional proximity relationships, deemed to be most efficient, between the activities that must be performed:
- bed-related inpatient functions
- outpatient-related functions
- diagnostic and treatment functions
- administrative functions
- service functions (food, supply)
- research and teaching functions (Fig.3).

For design purposes these functions in spatial terms are reflected in a number of sectors, which the hospital is divided into:
- bed-related inpatient sector
- outpatient-related, diagnostic and treatment sector
- general services, administrative and service functions (supply) sector
- research and teaching sector.

The sectors, in turn, are divided into functional areas and these into spatial units: for example, the healthcare services sector includes the surgery functional area, which in turn is divided into the surgical block, the day surgery block and the delivery block.

The optimization of the relationships between the different functions is closely linked to the choice of the physical configuration of the hospital building (Fig.4) in relation to the system of flows and routes of goods and people, and transport logistics. The physical configuration and the system of flows and routes influence and determine each other; indeed, when planning the expansion or reorganization of existing hospital buildings it is very difficult to find the optimal solution for the two aspects.

In recent years increasing attention has been given to the study of spaces inside the hospital building capable of making the hospitalization process less dramatic and

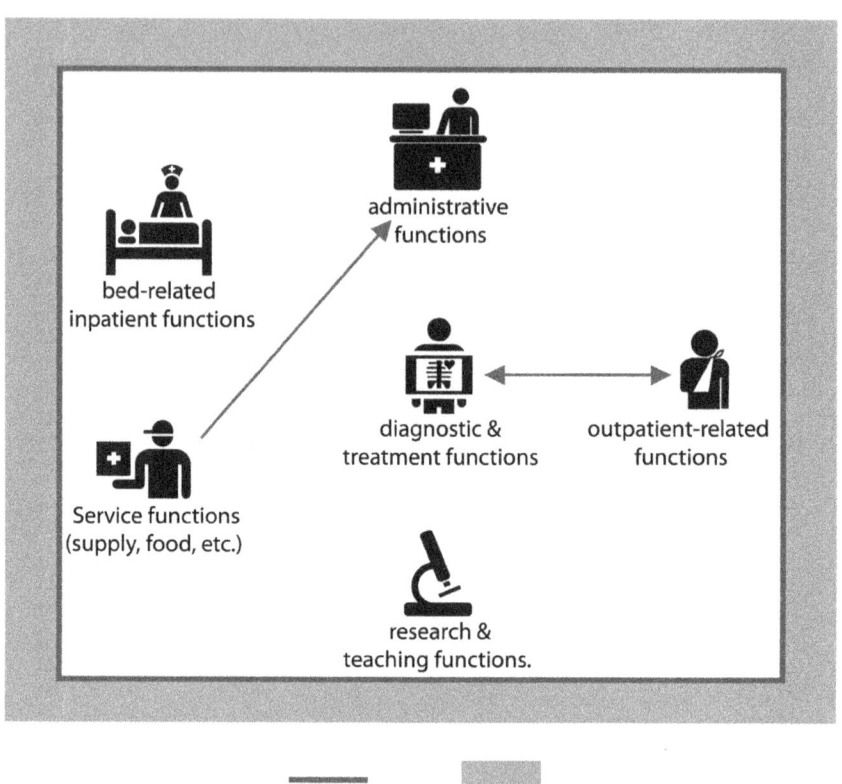

Figure 3: General hospital relationship

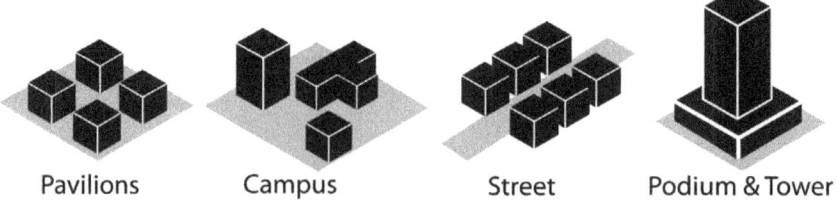

Figure 4: Hospitals typologies and outdoor spaces

stressful for the different user groups and their integration in the design programme. These spaces are defined as healthcare public spaces and serve to support and integrate the activities and functions indicated above. In this regard, the reflection made as part of the Annual Conference of the Academy of Architecture for Health on the topic of 'healthcare public space and the power of design' is of particular interest, and was presented in a video. It assumes that "both general public space and healthcare public space share the same characteristics, but healthcare public spaces also have their own special patterns." (Pangrazio, 2013).

The AAH proposes a categorization of healthcare public spaces under the following formal typologies.

- Collector spaces. These are accepting and orienting spaces with high populations. They are active and have increased noise levels.

- Introspective spaces. These are accepting but calming spaces. They also feature high populations, but are personal, quieter and highly passive.

- Purpose spaces. These are spaces with specific functions. They are service-based and feature various user volumes. Noise levels are usually moderate in these dynamic spaces.

- Mover spaces. These spaces feature constant movement as well as the ebb and flow of user volumes. These highly dynamic spaces are characterized by moderate noise levels.

- Switchboard spaces. These are orientation and wayfinding spaces with consistently high populations. These dynamic spaces feature moderate noise levels and organizational clarity.

The construction of the functional programme and of the layout of a hospital is a highly complex operation: starting from the needs of the user groups, the logistical and functional requirements must be integrated with those of the healthcare public spaces. The questions to reflect on are: «Are the external spaces pertaining to the hospital considered an integral part of the overall design of the hospital? What potential relationships can be established between the indoor and outdoor spaces of the hospital?» From the foregoing in relation to the conceptualization of the layout, it can be seen how the outdoor and open space has only residual value, just as the healthcare public spaces still have today. The outdoor space is conceived as merely functional to support the activities of the hospital: parking, pedestrian and vehicle access, orientation and routes. The technical and autonomous knowledge that generates the design of a rationally functioning and functional confined space must however now also address the renewed value that people, before scientific literature, attribute to open space. The form and spatial-functional organization of the hospital have a significant effect on the size and quality of the outdoor space. The latter must become an integral part of the overall design of the hospital, an issue to consider, equal to the other functions listed above. The outdoor related functions can thus be identified. The outdoor related functions take place in spaces that must be designed both in relation to the different levels of usability – public, semi-public, private – induced by the functional specificity of the hospital, and in relation to the requirements of the user groups. The design of these spaces is of great importance insofar as it potentially influences and alters the behaviour of the people that use it, even more so if those same people are involved in its design.

The outdoor related functions can theoretically be grouped into different types of spaces:

- Permeable spaces. These are spaces between the hospital complex and the settlement context, which place the hospital in direct dialogue with the city. They are spaces with high populations and can be designed with high identity and artistic value.

- Transitional support spaces. These spaces feature constant movement. They are support spaces for the hospital, such as parking areas (staff, visitors, suppliers, ambulances), pedestrian paths, vehicle and emergency routes, areas for storing goods and disposing of waste, and orientation and control systems.

- Interaction spaces or social spaces. These are socialization spaces for different user groups. They are close to the hospital or included as an integral part of it, again with open spaces (courtyards, liveable roofs). The different user groups are formed of medical professionals, nurses, students, researchers (staff), inpatients, outpatients and visitors.

- Introspective spaces. These are more private spaces where all users, in particular patients and visitors, can find a moment of calm and respite. These spaces are very close to the hospital or included as an integral part of it, again as open spaces (courtyards, liveable roofs, open terraces) and can be directly connected to the internal introspective spaces.

- Open healing spaces. These are spaces for long-term inpatients who spend several days in hospital and act as extensions of the healthcare activities; these spaces take on different connotations and values according to the target users (e.g. children, adolescents, adults, the elderly, etc.), the healthcare needs in relation to the treatments or interventions that the patient has received and continues to receive during the hospitalization period (e.g. following orthopaedic traumatological surgery, the treatment of cardiovascular diseases) or certain specific pathologies (e.g. Alzheimer's disease, Autism spectrum disorder).

It can be said that some outdoor related functions can potentially become an extension of and supplement to the orienting, accepting and healthcare activities that are carried out inside the hospital.

People experience their first impact with the hospital through the permeable spaces and the transitional support spaces. It is the qualities of these two categories of spaces that first help to construct a sense of place. The patient is one of the main users of the hospital. In order to understand their profile it is considered necessary to define the types of hospital stays and how much time people spend in hospital in Italy, analysing some definitions and data. Types of hospital stays can be divided into:

- Acute inpatients, who are hospitalized for a short time due to an episode of immediate and severe illness or disability and then usually have to return to the hospital for a follow-up.
- Long-term inpatients, who are hospitalized for a longer time as they require prolonged treatments before being discharged.

The package of care required after the acute phase defined with the term post-acute care is aimed at stabilizing the disease towards recovery or chronicity and is broken down into long-term hospitalization or rehabilitation.

- The patients' average length of stay in hospital is calculated based on the hospitalization typologies, which is the ratio between the number of days in hospital granted to a particular set of patients and the number of those patients. The 2014 Annual Report on Hospitalization by the Italian Ministry of Health (data from 2013, hospital discharge forms), reports the following data:
- The average length of stay for acute care is 6-8 days, it has remained almost constant around this value for some years;
- The average length of stay for rehabilitation is 25.7 days.
- The average length of a long-term stay is 27.6 days.

In Italy, as in many other European countries, the average number of hospitalization days for acute cases gradually reduced over time until it stabilized. The health statistics of the Organisation for Economic Co-operation and Development indicate for Italy an average hospitalization period of 6.8 days for acute cases (OECD, 2014). In Italy from 2009 the average hospitalization period for rehabilitation and long-term hospitalization also reduced.

In addition to the acute inpatients and the long-term inpatients the high number of outpatients must be considered, namely those who go to hospital as outpatients for diagnostics and treatments but are not hospitalized.

The types of hospital stays and the relative lengths of stay in hospital are useful information for understanding the mission of the hospital and therefore also for the potential use and characteristics of the outdoor spaces.

As stated in the introduction, the hospital that promotes health transfers some of its functions to other facilities of the network in the area, such as centres for rehabilitation and long-term hospitalization, Alzheimer's centres, houses of health, and others. The hospital becomes a facility primarily dedicated to highly technological acute cases with an average patient hospitalization period of up to 8 days. Therefore outdoor spaces first defined as permeable spaces, transitional support spaces, interaction spaces or social spaces, and introspective spaces will assume ever greater importance. For the other types of healthcare facilities it is useful, as in fact happens, to refer to the numerous studies on the characteristics of healing open spaces, which include the healing garden, dedicated and targeted for each range of users and related diseases.

A supportive design: the balance between outdoor and indoor environments

A supportive design for the hospital must consider the outdoor environment and the indoor environment with the same importance. The design language of the indoor environment is characterized by a prevalence of spaces generated by technical and scientific knowledge which must find a balance with the healthcare public spaces. The design language of the outdoor environment is totally different; it should seek to play down the hospital situation and is generated by other knowledge, always in close consideration of technical and scientific knowledge.

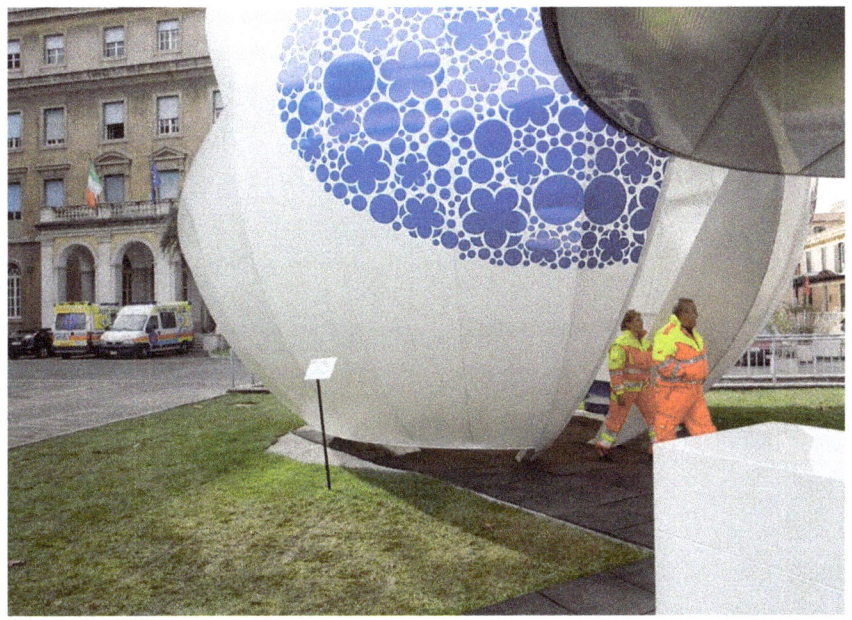

Figure 5-6: Art installation, Policlinc Umberto I, Rome, Italy (above) and visual relationship between indoor and outdoor spaces, Meyer Children Hospital, Florence, Italy (below), photo by Francesca Giofrè

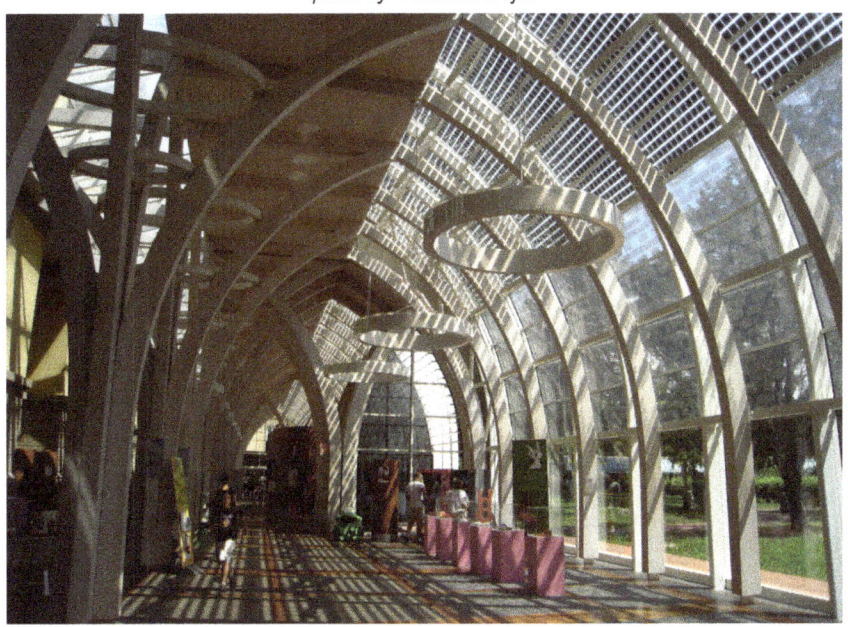

A supportive design must therefore find a balanced relationship between the outdoor and indoor environments insofar as the two environments complement each other. The identity of the hospital for the community and for user groups is established through this balanced relationship.

The outdoor related functions must be designed to achieve different objectives in relation to the needs of the user groups. Some characteristics that connote the design of the spaces where the outdoor related functions are performed are indicated below.

- Permeable spaces. The design of these spaces must relate to the settlement context of reference and at the same time identify the boundary of the lot on which the hospital stands. The boundary must have areas of discontinuity that give rise to spatial continuity and to permeability between the settlement context and that of the hospital. These spaces perform the main functions of building up the first identity of the hospital and they are transitional. In the permeable spaces different activities can be carried out, such as artistic performances and health education open to the entire community.

- Transitional support spaces. The design of these spaces is closely linked to the typological configuration of the hospital, the spatial-functional organization and the points of access to the lot of the hospital through the permeable spaces. These spaces perform the main functions of ensuring: clear and intuitive external wayfinding for all users; easy pedestrian and vehicle access to the hospital for patients, visitors and staff; a preferential and separate access to the ambulance emergency routes; a separate access for suppliers of goods and services; clear orientation, information and control points; separate areas for waste storage.

- Interaction spaces or social spaces. The design of these spaces is closely linked to the typological configuration of the hospital and the spatial-functional organization. These spaces perform the main functions of ensuring that each user group, together or separately, has places to meet and to socialize. These activities act as moments to reduce psychological distress, which has different values for the user groups as demonstrated by the numerous studies on the topic. Particular attention must be given to spaces dedicated to child patients and adolescents (Del Nord, 2006). The interaction spaces or social spaces can also host activities aimed at the entire hospital community and open to the region.

- Introspective spaces. The design of these spaces is closely linked to the

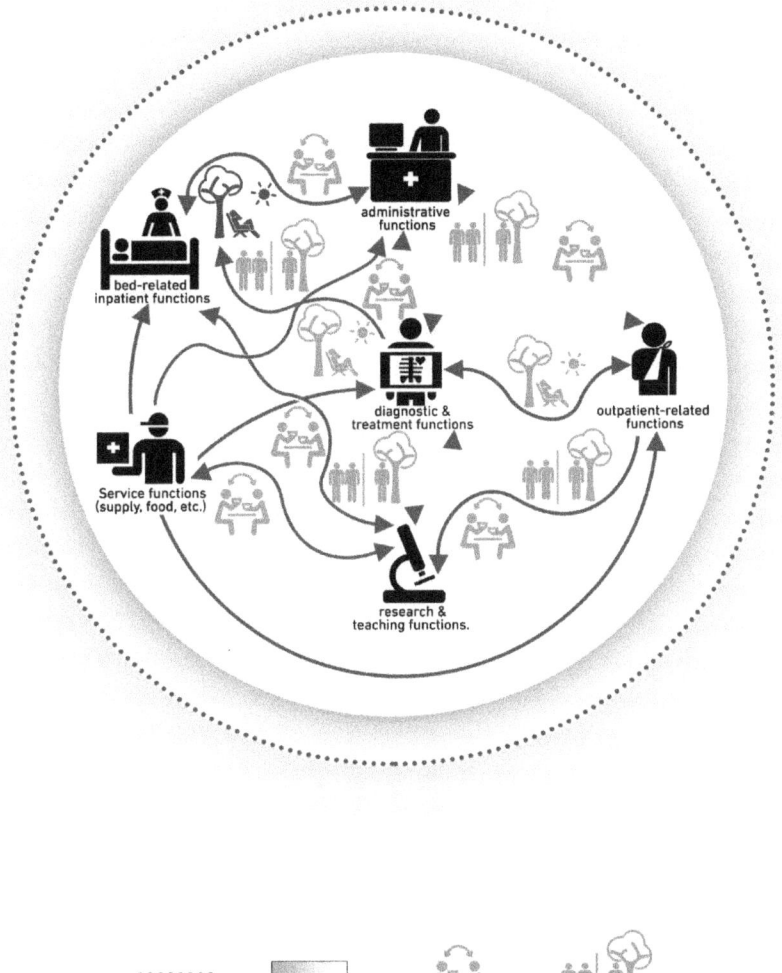

Figure 7: General hospital relationship and outdoor related functions

typological configuration of the hospital and the spatial-functional organization. These spaces perform the main functions of ensuring each user group has a place to go for an informal moment of respite and calm. They must be suitably screened from sources of noise, be secluded and have a family nature (Fig.7).

The positive values of the outdoor spaces also spill over into the inside of the hospital through the views, visual contact with the outside, natural light and green space. The inpatient rooms, connection spaces, but also functional areas, such as the operating theatre and intensive care, can benefit from views of the outside and natural light in terms of stress reduction and improving the work productivity of the staff (Giofrè, 2013). Moreover, the outdoor space experienced independently reinforces the patients' sense of autonomy.

Therefore not only 'in versus out' but also 'out versus in' design must be achieved through a multidimensional approach in order to create psychosocially supportive spaces (Dilani, 2001). A multidimensional approach is deeply entrenched with the territory and its needs and is constructed through the synergy of different knowledge bases and professionals: sociologists, psychologists, anthropologists, doctors from various disciplines, computer experts, biomedical experts, economists, engineers, architects, and among them the role of the landscape designer should not be overlooked.

Final considerations

Hospitals are the expression of the culture of a given society and must be considered an integral part of the city system and its urban fabric, namely a subsystem of the city. For these reasons hospital design must assume the guiding principles of urbanity, sociality and dynamism. In the design of a hospital it is necessary to find a balance between that which is the result of highly autonomous technical knowledge which generates the functional programme and the layout of the hospital and the outdoor spaces pertaining to it, often deemed to be residual. The characteristics of the outdoor spaces of hospitals are highly conditioned by choices concerning the functional and spatial organization decisions reached in the design phase, and this is why it is necessary to integrate the outdoor space as a design element, together with that of the building structure. The outdoor spaces of the hospital and their outdoor related functions must be designed in accordance with the needs of the user groups and with the users themselves; these spaces are an added value with respect to the functionality of the hospital itself.

It is a great challenge for the multidisciplinary design team to find a balanced relationship between the city and the hospital, and between the hospital outdoor environment and the hospital indoor environment. The identity of the hospital in the city for the entire community and for the user groups is established through a multidimensional approach that considers all the outdoor and indoor spatial components to be equally important, which become psychosocially supportive spaces.

References

British Medical Association (2011), *The psychological and social needs of patients*, London, UK, available at http://www.ahsw.org.uk (accessed 23 September 2014).

Burnett, J.,D. (1997) "Therapeutic Effects of Landscape Architecture" Marberry, Sara. O. (Ed.) Healthcare Design, John Wiley & Sons New York, USA.

Del Nord, R. (edited by) (2006), *Environmental stress prevention in children's hospital design. Technical guidelines and architectural suggestions*, Motta, Milan, IT.

Dilani, A. (2001), Psychosocially supportive design, *Scandinavian Health Care Design World Hospitals and Health Services*, 37(1), 20-4, available at http://www.designandhealth.com (accessed 23 September 2014).

Falcitelli, N.; Trabucchi, M. and Vanara, F. (2000), *Rapporto Sanità. L'ospedale del futuro*, Mulino, Milan, IT.

Foucault, M. (1976), *Sorvegliare e punire. Nascita della prigione*, Einaudi, Turin, IT.

Giofrè, F. (2002), "Innovazione nel progetto delle aree a elevata complessità tecnologica". In Baglioni A. and Tartaglia R. (edited by), *Ergonomia e Ospedale, valutazione, progettazione e gestione di ambienti, organizzazione, strumenti e servizi*. Il Sole 24 Ore, Milan, IT.

Giofrè, F. and Terranova F. (2004), *Ospedale e Territorio, Hospital & Land*, Alinea ed., Florence, IT.

Giofrè, F. and Terranova F. (2006), "Healthcare facilities from planning to design", Design & Health IV. Future Trends in Healthcare Design, IADH. Dilani A. (edited by) International Academy for Design and Health, also available at http://www.designandhealth.com (accessed 28 May 2014).

Giofrè, F. (2013), "Materiali, arredi e attrezzature",Cirialo, F.; Giofrè, F. (edited by) Sala Operatoria e Terapia Intensiva, Maggioli, IT pp.164-165.

Horsburg, C., R. (1995) "Healing by Design", The New England Journal of Medicine. 11 (333). p. 735-740.

Malkin, J. (1992), *Hospital interior architecture. Creating Healing Environments for Special Patient Populations*, Van Nostrand Reinold, New York, USA.

Marcus, C., C. and Barnes, M. (1995), *Gardens in healthcare facilities: Uses, therapeutic benefits, and design recommendations*, Center for Health Design, USA. Available at https://www.healthdesign.org (accessed 5 June 2014).

Ministry of Health (2014), Annual Report on Hospitalization, available at http://www.salute.gov.it (accessed 16 October 2014).

OECD (2014), "Average length of stay: acute care", Health: Key Tables from OECD, No. 52. DOI: 10.1787/l-o-s-acutecare-table-2014-1-en.

Pangrazio, J.,R. (2013), Planning public spaces for health care facilities, Healthcare Facilities Management, available at http://www.hfmmagazine.com (accessed 15 October 2014)

Petrilli, A.(1999), *Il testamento di Le Corbusier. Il progetto per l'Ospedale di Venezia*, Marsilio,Venice, IT, p.40.

Rossi, A. (1982), The Architecture of the City, trans. by Diane Ghirardo and Joan Ockman, MIT Press, Cambridge, USA, p. 14 and p.103.

Sack, R. D. (1986), Human territoriality. Its theory and History, Cambridge University Press, Cambridge, UK.

Ulrich R., S.; Simons R.F., Losito, B.D.; Fiorito, E.; Miles, M.,A. and Zelson, M. (1991). "Stress recovery during exposure to natural and urban environment", Journal of Environmental Psychology 11, p. 201-230.

Ulrich, R. S. (2001) "Effects of Healthcare Environmental Design on Medical Outcomes" Proceedings of the Second International Conference on Design and Health, Stockholm, SE available at http://www.capch.org/wp-content/uploads/2012/10/Roger-Ulrich-WCDH2000.pdf (accessed 15 May 2014).

Van Den Berg, A. and Wagenaar C. (2006), "Healing environments at the century mark: the quest for optimal patient experiences", in Wagenaar C. (edited by), The architecture of the hospital, NAi publishers, Rotterdam, NL, pp. 255-257.

World Health Organization (1998), Terminology of the European Conference on Health, Society and Alcohol: A glossary, Copenhagen, DK, available at http://www.who.int (accessed 15 October 2014).

06

Hospital outdoor environments on dualities and contradiction

Ružica Božović Stamenović

Abstract: Design of hospital outdoor spaces as healthful environments is a complex endeavor engaging both pragmatic and semantic design tools. The process of defining the hospital boundary tackles conceptual and functional considerations and reveals the importance of the widely understood context in the process. In this paper we raise and discuss a number of dichotomies and paradoxes intrinsic to the nature of these important hospital zones. Even the apparently well-defined topics like space, place and environment or indoor-outdoor realm are raised and questioned revealing symptoms of confusion and space for improvements. We argue that evidence based design of hospital outdoor environments needs to be put in a wider contextual frame to be effective. In this discourse the outdoor realm is put in perspective with the urban, social and personal domains. As many of the problems raised persistently endure in common practice, this discourse is directed towards their critical examination rather than solution. In conclusion, the healthfulness of the outdoor hospital environment is deeply imbedded in design's qualitative substance rather than in its formal appearance. In that sense narrative strategies and exploration of indeterminacy and multifaceted character of outdoor spaces seem more opportune for achieving the lasting positive effects on users.

Keywords: hospital outdoor, healthful architecture, wellness, social capital.

Introduction

The considerations of the characteristics of space and design in relation to health have been increasingly discussed and problematized in a number of disciplines involved in hospital design (Huisman et al., 2012; Schweitzer and Frampton, 2004; Ulrich, 1999; Dilani, 2008). The understanding of a threefold character of health as the complete physical, psychological and social wellbeing (WHO, 1948) led to comprehending the complexity of multifaceted influences involved in defining the relations of health and space (Lawson, 2010, Zimring, 2004). The salutogenic (Antonovski, 1996), rather than pathogenic approach to design is now widely accepted. However, the diverse professionals involved in the planning and design processes tend to look at the symbiosis of space and health solely from their respective professional standpoint. The stakeholders - medical staff and medical planners, architects and engineers, financial advisers and system organizers, volunteers, patients and civic representatives, also have and put forward their own views on the ideal hospital space and the outdoor areas (Mourshed and Zhao, 2012; Dijkstra, 2009; Mazuch and Stephen, 2005; Stichler, 2009). Thus, a simple and commonly shared revelation that space could improve health turns into a prolific cacophony of interpretations.

Efforts towards establishing some order into the design of hospital spaces are articulated through attempts to build diverse assessment tools for post occupancy evaluation (POE). These POE surveys are, among other objectives, investigating and justifying the effects that the design solutions for the hospital physical environments have on healthcare outcomes. If proven successful these design features are then labelled as Evidence Based Design (EBD) and recommended as guidelines for hospital design (Hamilton and Watkins, 2009). It is assumed through an increasing body of evidences (Ulrich and Zimring, et al, 2008) that EBD might raise the impact of healthcare design on health outcomes and also prevent common design mistakes. Both assumptions have been verified in practice and even more, EBD proved to have a persuasive role in situations where certain advocacy in design process was needed. Investors like the risk free enterprises and EBD seems consoling in that sense. However, the EBD trend raised criticism too. Diverse cultural and contextual circumstances in which the attempts to follow the research proven guidelines occurred, problematized the outcome of the generic EBD (Nanda et al., 2013).

Although very practical, this set of design evidences did not seem universally applicable after all. POI however, remains a useful tool but with limited effects since many of the observed problems turn to be beyond repair.

EBD research still provides valuable data in regard to design of the hospital outdoor environments. The relevance of outdoor spaces for wellbeing of all users concerned is well documented (Thwaites et al., 2005; Marcus, 2000, 2007; Joye, 2007, 2006; Leibrock, 2011). Ulrich (1991) paved the way with his seminal work on impact of views to nature on recovery of patients. Healing gardens are recognized as beneficial for stress relief and anxiety reduction (Gesler, 2003; Ulrich, 2002; Marcusand Barnes, 1999; Marcus, 2007). Sustainable design solutions are crucial for energy savings (Guenther and Vittori, 2008; Johnson and Hill, 2002). Design of outdoor space is strongly affecting public health: obesity problems and social capital are linked to certain urban characteristics and social bonding could be improved through spaces that instigate encounters (Helliwell and Putnam, 2004; Rogers, 2013). Implementation of art work in public spaces engenders numerous benefits including way finding (Hathorn & Nanda, 2008).

However, the indicative research project carried out under Module "Human ecology-health and space" at the National University of Singapore and focused on the ambitiously designed hospital outdoor spaces revealed a very interesting and intriguing discrepancy. Our survey on users' perception of these outdoor spaces discovered an inconsistency: the scores for the separately examined spaces were better than the mediocre grade given for the impression on the overall ambience. Even though this investigation was not a conclusive solid research, some valid questions arose. How come that the overall rating of the outdoor spaces is mediocre while the results for its separate constituencies are considerably higher? If the components – in this case the ideas and design- are satisfactory, what went wrong to make the overall result so blank?

The ensuing on site analysis uncovered problems and possible origins of this paradox. To cite a few: outdoor spaces were compartmentalized and not connected in a smooth and logical way, their respective image was distinct but unclearly related to the overall image of the outdoor realm-no branding attempts, lack of control and choices in space was evident and the design and art work often sent the ambivalent semantic messages. A few typical examples are worth describing.

In one of the open areas the sculpture made of shiny metal elements with sharp edges (Fig.1) was labelled in writing as 'compassion, commitment' and positioned in the middle of the small fountain. In our brainstorming exercises taking part for a decade in "Health and Space" class the word 'metal' consistently evoked 'sharpness' and 'coldness' as immediate responses. Touching metal was not reported as a pleasant tactile experience. In our example the metal sculpture labelled in words as symbolizing care, was also separated by the body of water from those in need of that care. All benches in this particular courtyard were arranged around and turned towards this sculpture, which was supporting the sense of belonging to a small community formed around it. However, there was no choice for those who might have needed to be alone and secluded from other commuters and no opportunity to form smaller social circles like family sitting together for example. The literal description, the form and the position of this particular feature were representing different notions and once put together conveyed a contradictory semantic message. Therefore, as Stigsdotter and Grahn state (2002), it may be

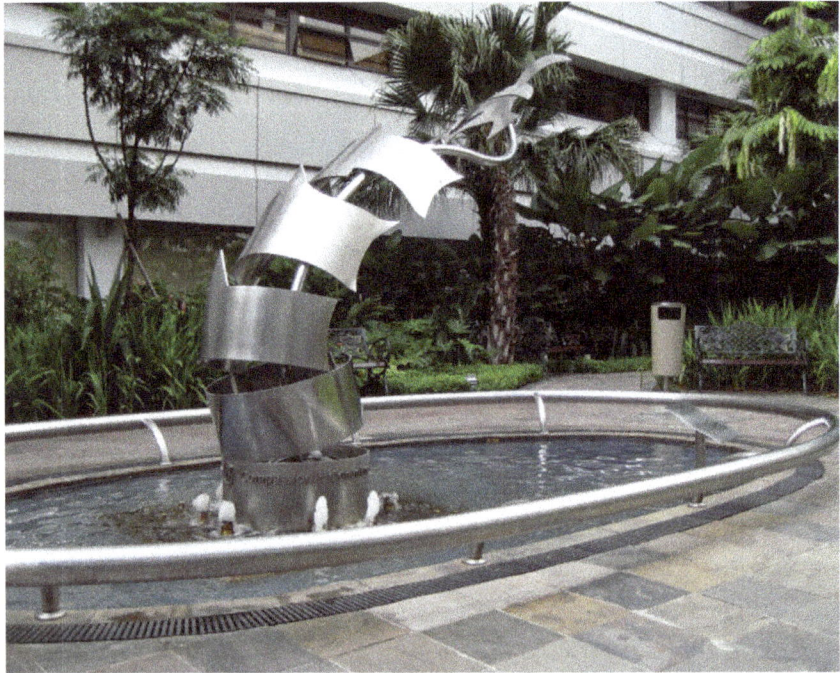

Figure 1: Sculpture named 'compassion, commitment', photo by Ružica Božović Stamenović

necessary for designers to think about a garden as a phenomenon that involves the interdependent and unspoken relations between the users and the garden.

Another spot in the same hospital was designed as a beautiful sensorial meditative courtyard. The sound of water shimmering down a tilted wall rich in tactile stimuli and the minimalist Zen design with smooth colors and refined details attracted the light and suggested calmness and meditation. Unfortunately, this courtyard was seldom used even though it was aligned with a very busy walkway connecting the two blocks of this hospital. For busy commuters on their way to, or from their destination this meditative space was not what they apparently needed. For those who might have benefited from this sophisticated supportive space this courtyard did not work either as it seemed too public and exposed to views and therefore not suitable for meditation. After some time the same courtyard changed function to become a café with tables, benches and lots of people around at all times. Interestingly, this sensory stimulating environment turned very appropriate for the café as people obviously enjoyed the ambience and the image they could connect to some resort rather than to a medical facility.

Looking at these examples, even though the implementation of art, greenery and sensorial effects are advised through research as tools for creating the healing environment, something was lacking to fulfill this objective. Why the research proven design solutions did not bring the expected outcome in these cases? What happened between planning, constructing and inhabiting these outdoor spaces? What was the cause of ineffectiveness in spite of applied concepts confirmed through evidence based design?

The biased results might have come from our comprehension and judgments regarding the outdoor spaces that too often rely on visual images only and on common, generic interpretations of the terms and issues connected to the indoor and the outdoor. With this assumption in mind our academic discourse needs to diverge from discussing the usual design outcomes and pose a few simple questions first: what is actually understood as the outdoor hospital environment, who and what defines it, who benefits from it and who is in charge of it and why do all of these questions matter for designing healthful outdoor spaces?

Space - environment

The use of the word environment already suggests that we refer to more than just the Euclidian space. It might however be anything from the semantic construct burdened with intangible and buried meanings to the phenomenological interpretations of place dependent on and articulated through personal accounts. In the core of all interpretations are the relations of men and space and implications of their interconnectedness on wellbeing (Frumkin, 2003). The Euclidian space is commonly considered healthy for its sanitary status. However, the prerequisite for impact of space on holistic health is in establishing its resonance with the human counterparts. For this, the shear presence of users in the particular space would not suffice; the relation needs to be complex in order to be meaningful and influential. Therefore, creating an environmental system with men and space as main building blocks put together in a harmonious and purposeful way is the prerequisite for good design in terms of human ecology. As much as this statement seems self-

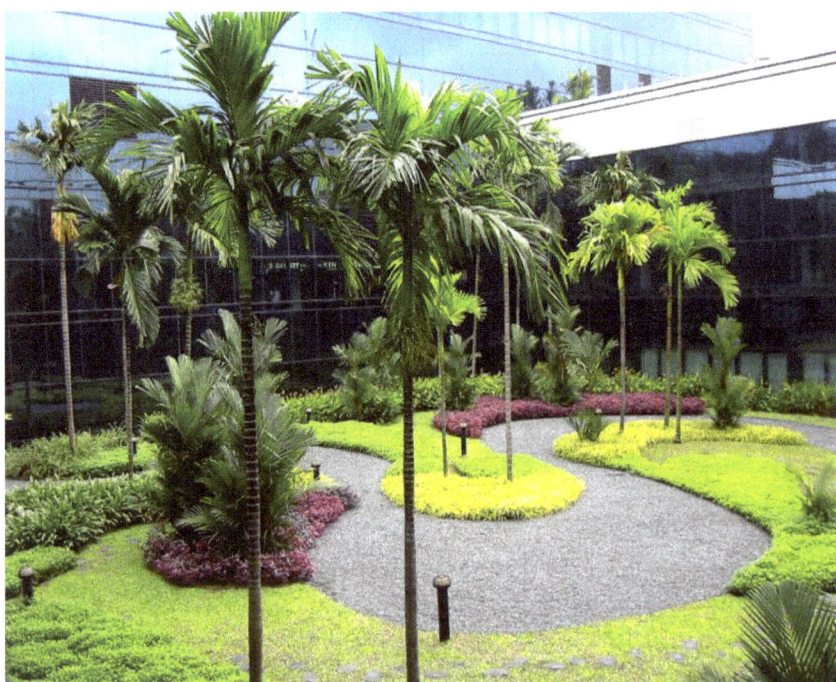

Figure 2: Green scenography for the hospital courtyard, photo by Ružica Božović Stamenović

explanatory, in many hospitals we have evidences of design failing to transcend from being just a space into an encompassing and supporting environment.

In another example of hospital green courtyards their healthful qualities proved questionable not because of the design per se but because it failed for multiple reasons to engage men to the fullest (Fig.2). The effort to make the design appealing was evident, and yet, almost at all times these courtyards seemed completely uninhabited, like a nice scenography we can look at but not touch. The courtyards are grassy with mature trees, but without much shade since the tree species are not appropriate. There are also no canopies or sheltered areas as relieve on a rainy day in the warm and wet tropical climate. The walking path is meandering, may be meant to make the experience more lasting and interesting. However, these are seldom tested since there are no railings for support or benches for rest. The paths don't begin or end in any particular point seeming to lead to nowhere. There is little to hear, taste, touch, learn or experience with senses other than the vision. And most of all, the courtyards are surrounded by facades glazed with fixed windows and shaded glass. Physical interaction between the inside and the outside seems to be literally non-existent. One can't step out or even smell and feel the air outside. Views are not encouraged since glass is tinted and changes the natural color palette of the scene. The inside space is air-conditioned and the sunny, humid and warm outside seems as an unappealing alternative from this perspective. Ultimately, except for being obviously outdoor and carved by the hospital building form, the courtyards are isolated from other hospital walkways. So, with no stimuli or reason for stepping outside and no chance of trespassing on the way to somewhere else the courtyards remain deserted most of the time. Although the design reveals good intentions it is missing the point in regard to healthfulness.

Therefore, regardless of the design scenario for the outdoor spaces, it is their habitability and connectedness with other domains that are fundamental for their relevance as healthful environments. The imminent complexity of the terms habitability and connectedness often unfortunately ends up in complicated spatial solutions providing for basic user needs and circulation. Our profession than simplifies the 'complicated' by applying sets of guidelines, EBD outputs, norms and regulations and in the process completely misses the opportunity to deal with environmental complexities. The 'complicated' may call for definite spatial solutions as relieve the 'complex' however introduces indeterminacy.

The latter is much more appropriate for hospital environments since they are perceived in distraction. Indeterminacy opens up possibilities for personal interpretations of the seen and the outdoor environment might thus become a relieving factor under the stressful hospital circumstances. Referring back to our examples, both are lacking complexity and fail to bring about what René Magritte considered essential while speaking of his self-portrait "The Son of Man": "Everything we see hides another thing; we always want to see what is hidden by what we see."

The outdoor - indoor realm

The counterparts 'outdoor-indoor' seem neither complex nor complicated to understand and yet in the hospital context the adjective 'outdoor' turns to be elusive. Every area touching all hospital facades, including the rooftop, is considered as the 'outdoor' of the hospital. In the densely nit urban matrix a hospital's outdoor space might be a public street, plaza, park, or another building's courtyard maybe. In these cases the outdoor space is skipping the authority of the hospital over its appearance since others might have the power to influence and define it both visually and in a cultural, social or some other sense. Dovey (2008) claims that in everyday life we tend to notice power 'over' while power 'to' is taken-for-granted.

Apparently, the definition of the hospital outdoor is closely connected to the empowerment, as our next example illustrates. The prominent private hospital is occupying a large part of the city block. Entrance to the hospital is at the crossroad, and the longitudinal façade is facing the street. However, except for the humble corner entry the indoor hospital spaces are neither visible nor approachable from the urban area. The hermetic façade facing the street is projecting the feel of separateness and of the purposeful ignorance of the public realm.

For the passers-by who might not be familiar with the neighborhood, this isolation of a big and architecturally prominent building raises uneasiness. The realization that the building is a hospital almost justifies the discomfort. The street becomes at that point a place to avoid or at least use in rush while probably wondering if this harsh delineation of the two entities is about protection, seclusion, exclusivity, safety or something else. And it probably is about all of these issues and more. From the private hospital management point of view, this image stands for confidentiality, distinctiveness and elitism - the brand they display for the paying clientele. Although the private hospital does not have the power over the public domain, it does in this case explicitly demonstrate the power to define it to be advantageous to them and ignore the social communal benefits. Therefore the issues of authority and control are inseparable from the discourse on 'outdoor-indoor'.

However, the mutual influence of the two domains might be very positive too (Fig. 3). It is often the case that the image of the outdoor inspires the internal design and character of the hospital ambiences. In our next example (Fig. 4) the notion of the outdoor realm deeply penetrates the inside of the green, sustainable hospital located on the fringe of the urban water reservoir. It is impossible to say where the inside ends and the outside begins. The two domains literally merge on all levels to the point that the distinction is not legible even for the trained eyes of an architect. The entrance to the hospital from the public walkway is not a point but a network of intertwined spaces, ambiences and function that attract urban commuters and hospital users alike. The synergy of the two domains creates an impression of continuity and harmony. On the ground-floor the public path and the hospital garden are inseparable and smoothly used without segregation by patients, visitors, staff and the passersby. The connectedness is established on upper levels too. The green walls, rooftop gardens, water features and natural materials are omnipresent. Distant views to the reservoir easily penetrate the interior of the hospital wards and add on to the green, supportive feel of the ambience. The distance between the realms does not jeopardize the quality of this experience since the transition is smooth and continuous due to the porous façade. From the patients' perspective the bonding experience with the outdoor space commences while still inside, with perceiving the green branded interior, touching the plants on the window edge, and then uninterruptedly observing the realistically landscaped rooftop garden followed by the distant view to the pond at the horizon.

Thus, for the patient lying on the hospital bed the sense of connectedness to the outer world is constructed due to the elusive boundary between the outside and the inside. The image of the outdoors unfolds starting right at patient's reach and ends up outside the hospital premises, connecting three different realms: the private-room, the common-rooftop hospital garden, and the urban-the public water reservoir.

The links and affiliations with the different outdoor spheres simultaneously engage men's physical, mental and cognitive mechanisms in a logical and interdependent way. In our example, viewing the pond was actually easier than noticing the rooftop gardens or other green features positioned right below the facades, unless one is standing right at the window edge and this is certainly not encouraged in hospitals. Interestingly, one particular user of this subsidized hospital ward reported in his feedback that the hospital deprived him from enjoying the rooftop garden and provided instead just the 'free view out'. The positive impact that the view out might have had on his recovery, was stained as his cognition put it in the contextual perspective – as a subsidized patient he felt stigmatized and deliberately cut off from viewing the beautiful podium rooftop garden.

Therefore, the sheer existence of the well-designed outdoor space might become irrelevant in terms of healing unless meaningfully related to the inside and the overall context.

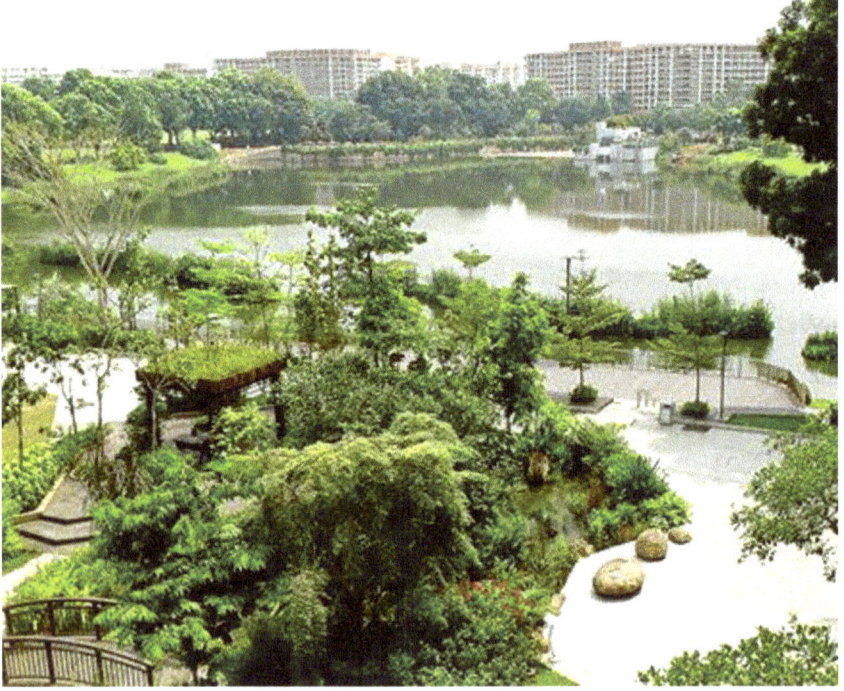

Figure 3: Rooftop garden merges with public realm, photo by Ružica Božović Stamenović

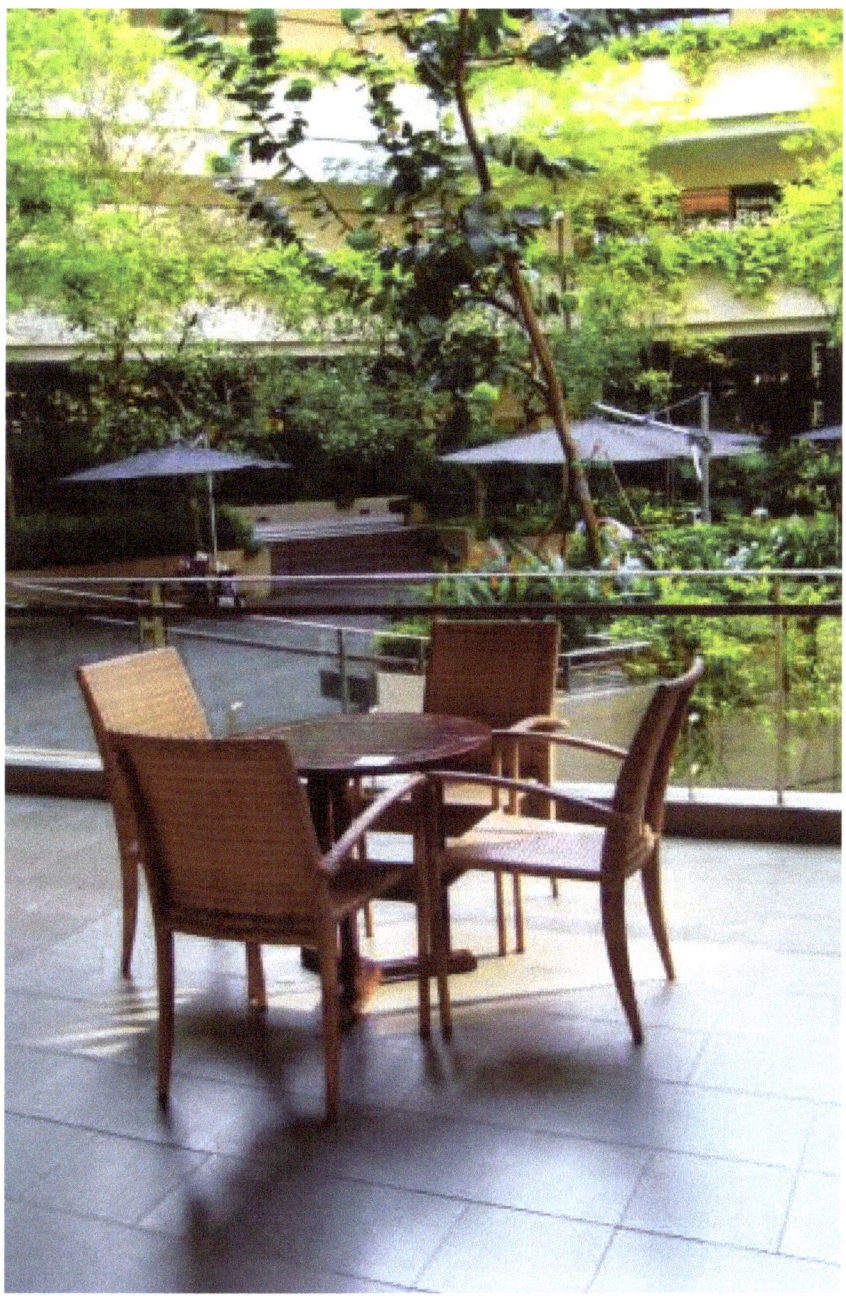

Figure 4: Image of leisure in hospital outdoor ambience, photo by Ružica Božović Stamenović

Function - semantics

The 'outdoor' and the 'indoor' are not defined through their physical position or formal features only, but also in relation to the sublime meanings assigned. Exemplary are public hospitals that often use the outdoor design to convey the messages of social care, values and support. The welcoming image is usually constructed with greenery, planters spread outside the premises, graphic symbols referring to family oriented social care, children playgrounds, resting facilities and with an air of openness and social connectedness reflected in the architecture of the building. Outdoor spaces around private hospital premises, however, often convey the same welcoming message with somewhat constrained expressiveness and distinct air of exclusivity.

The outdoor and the indoor realms merge in physical, functional and symbolic ways. The adjectives 'outdoor' and 'indoor' imply the set of corresponding functions, respective images and affiliated semantic meanings too. Our cognitive and experiential mechanisms relate the specific images to either 'indoor' or 'outdoor' based on previous experiences and common sense. However, the feel of the 'outdoor' could be and often is created indoors and vice versa. In these cases the semantic value of design features contributing to the feel of the place surpasses the relevance of their actual form or content.

In this next example, we encounter the value of paradox: if we are surrounded by the greenery, fresh air and running water we associate this image with the outdoors. The toilet, on the contrary, as a very private place is expected to be indoors. And yet, our exemplary hospital tropical toilet has this puzzling feel of both indoor and outdoor space. It is a hybrid place merging a typically indoor function with the outdoor design appeal of some tropical resort in the most unexpected place – the hospital. The overall feeling is thrilling and ostentatious – two words we hardly ever associate with healthcare environments or toilets.

The other example is the rooftop healing and activity garden of a general hospital (Fig. 5). The greenhouse atmosphere, the different species of fruits and vegetables blooming or being harvested in neatly arranged and labelled plots, gardening devices and watering pipes, the sky above and the pond on the horizon. All of these features could be a part of an accurate description of some suburban or rural yard. None of them suggest the picture of a typical hospital garden, and yet, that's exactly

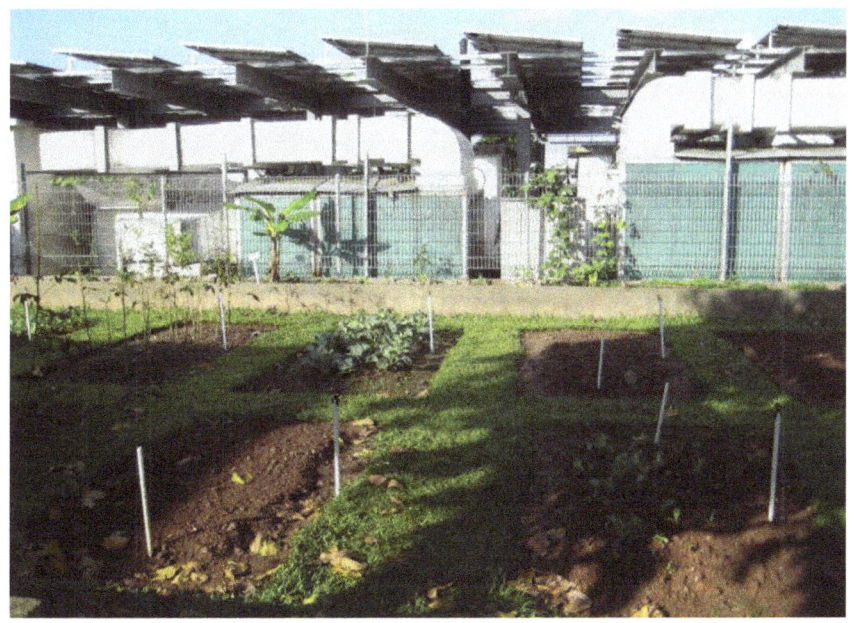

Figure 5-6: The hospital rooftop healing & activity garden, (above) and photos of nature as metaphor for healing (below), photos by Ružica Božović Stamenović

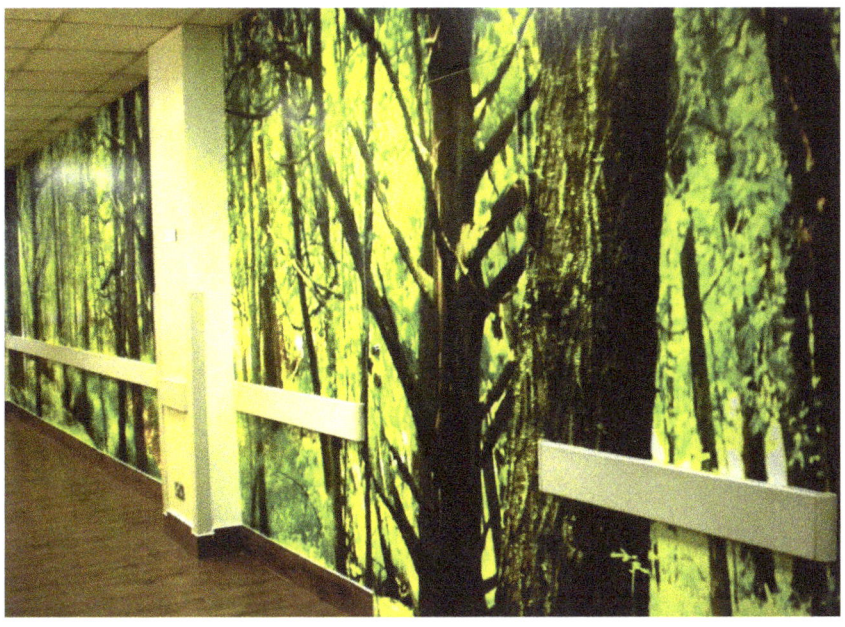

what it is: a roof top vegetable and fruit garden belonging to a big public hospital. Is the effect on users the same as if the garden was on the ground level? The semantic value of this garden is in delivering both the explicit and the implicit message. The clear enjoyment of being amongst the corn crops, mango trees and other plants is combined with the sense of surprise and astonishment due to its unexpected position and context. Furthermore, the garden is often visited and maintained by schoolchildren who otherwise would not even be in hospital premises. This garden, as realistic and functional as it is, thus becomes the surreal metaphor of healing and of returning to the 'outer' world and normalcy – the world of the healthy.

Therefore, the pragmatic function of the hospital outdoor space should not be an obstacle for creating its emblematic readings. Our examples implied a straightforward message: if the tropical outdoor toilet, the rooftop corn field, school children helping with gardening and doing their homework in hospital premises - if all of these is possible, then, just maybe, even the healing might be achievable too. In a refurbished old hospital surrounded by a beautiful garden with mature greenery, the images of plants and flowers are applied as interior decorations with confidence and enthusiasm. The images are also blown up to a size much bigger than the original plants. They are mounted to walls but also to unusual surfaces like the elevator doors, the ceiling, the food delivery containers and stations, etc. The designers were not involved into this endeavor. It was all executed by the hospital staff led by their enthusiastic CEO who issued a decree that it is only the images of nature that are appropriate to build the brand of a "hospital in the garden". Apparently, this exaggeration of the outdoor reinstalled in the interior was a great success and positively affected the patients, the staff and the visitors. The association to nature was direct while the allegory of wellness was plainly implied too (Fig. 6). The dose of surreal amplified the effect of nature as the metaphor for healing.

The real - the surreal

Metaphors, as mental concepts, are very important for human condition as they activate multiple layers of consciousness. In hospitals, however, the clear-cut messages are supposedly observed better than associations due to the omnipresent distress of all users alike. Simplicity is longed for as an escape from the uncomfortable sense of uncertainty. Nature and nature inspired art, materials, decorations and alike seem like a perfectly legible metaphor for hope and recovery.

Thus, the interiors of hospitals are often decorated with botanical motives, natural materials like timber or pebble, garden furniture and water features. Apparently, research (Wilson, 1984; Kaplan & Kaplan, 1989) confirms the preferences for very specific natural motives, like shrubs, waterfalls, deep perspective and certain height of the horizon. Apart from the obvious intent to bring the sense of the most pleasant outdoor into the institutionalized hospital ambiences, this trend is also introducing the idealistic imagery of the 'garden of Eden', a place of peace, of ultimate happiness and eternal life into the most pragmatic and functionalistic hospital environment.

In a refurbished old hospital surrounded by a beautiful garden with mature greenery, the images of plants and flowers are applied as interior decorations with confidence and enthusiasm. The images are also blown up to a size much bigger than the original plants. They are mounted to walls but also to unusual surfaces like the elevator doors, the ceiling, the food delivery containers and stations, etc. The designers were not involved into this endeavor. It was all executed by the hospital staff led by their enthusiastic CEO who issued a decree that it is only the images of nature that are appropriate to build the brand of a "hospital in the garden". Apparently, this exaggeration of the outdoor reinstalled in the interior was a great success and positively affected the patients, the staff and the visitors. The association to nature was direct while the allegory of wellness was plainly implied too (Fig. 6). The dose of surreal amplified the effect of nature as the metaphor for healing.

Neurophysiology suggests certain properties of the mirror neurons which might explain the success of semantic migration, very typical for the sensorial status of the newest outdoor spaces (Pallasmaa, 2013). In the example of the Medical Centre built as an extension to a big general hospital, the main entrance is at the same time the entry to the metro station and a medium large shopping area (Fig. 7). The lift lobby is literally immersed into the shopping mall ambience. The incoming ambulatory patients and hospital staff on short breaks mingle between the shops and intersect with metro commuters. Although spotting the elevators leading to medical facilities is challenging, the way finding seems not to be a problem. Directions to the Medical Center clinics share the same boards with popular shop brands. The surreal functional concept seems to work well and convey both descriptive and representational messages.

Apparently, certain paradigmatic visual images seem to generate the corresponding typical feelings and behavior. Park like paths and benches induce rest and relaxation while presence of children' playgrounds, vending machines, advertisements and such paraphernalia evoke the atmosphere of the quotidian. The hassle and routines of the ordinary life might be thus recalled in institutionalized hospital ambiances that are usually deprived of any connection to the life outside their premises. Creating the sense of bizarre or the nodes of surreal within the hospital outdoor premises by using the real elements of the daily life is an attempt to form these hyper-realistic strata as an effective strategy for triggering the neural mirror effect response and contending stress while boosting wellness.

Power - empowerment

Significance of the hospital outdoor environment is not only confined to its appropriate image but has its social dimension too. The effect it has on hospital users is as important as its role in boosting social capital of the wider community. However the power over this space held by the usual bureaucratic and technocratic subjects, does not exclude the possibility of empowerment over the same space by some other entities. As Dovey (2008) defines it, the capacity to imagine, construct and inhabit a better built environment is the form of empowerment too. In that sense designers' focus should be on how to inhabit the outdoor hospital space and change it with one's presence rather than on its image. In the first scenario, the design indulges the users to immerse into the outdoor realm, to use it, dream of it, change it and explore many other ways of being connected. The real image of the space and its surreal representation merge in the minds of its users to create numerous and promising positive outcomes. So, even though the arbitrary power over the outdoor hospital space usually resides in institutional bodies and specialists either inside or outside the hospital, the better outcome could be expected and achieved through the empowerment of the society and in particular the user-experts as Ostroff coined (1997).

However, this is not the usual practice. Common designers' thinking of the hospital outdoor environment is far too often about creating a seducing and pleasant image (Verderber, 2000), usually through beautifying the entrance areas by using design paradigms characteristic for hotels or home. This is a harsh simplification but

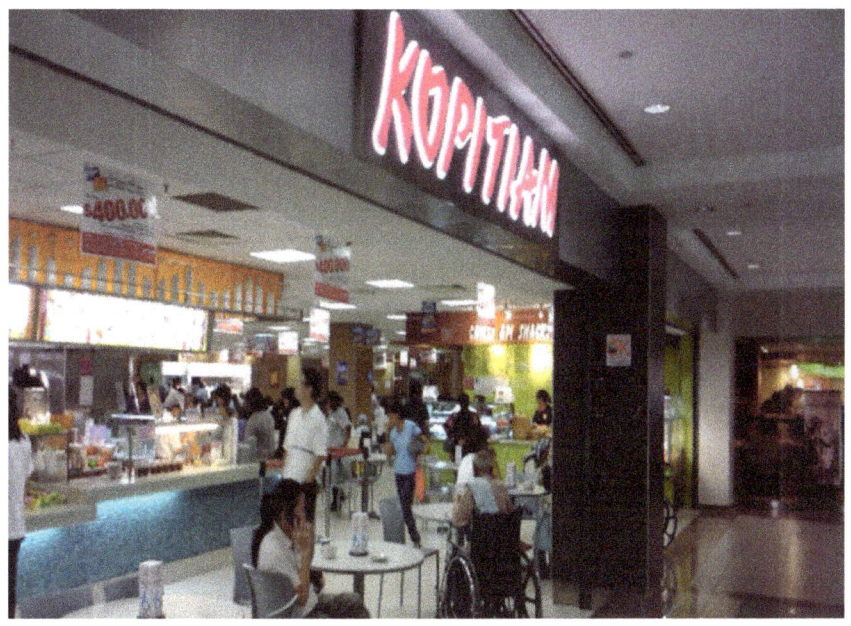

Figure 7: The mall ambience of the Medical Center, photo by Ružica Božović Stamenović

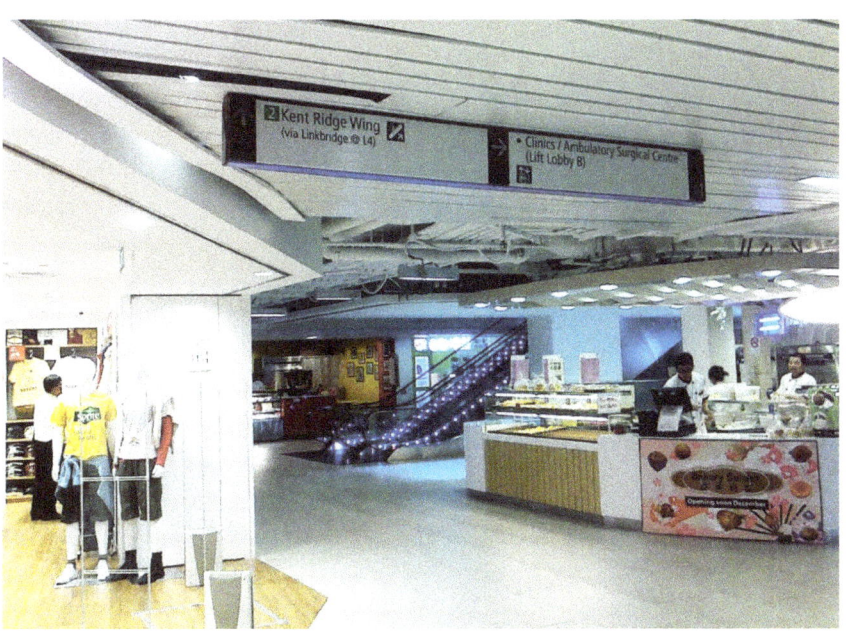

also an accurate description of many hospital examples where the open spaces resemble a scenography or a landscaped botanic arrangement not to be touched, rather than a real inhabited place. How did this happen? The criticism directed at the perceived inhumanity of the common hospital spaces and the alienation and anxiety as a result of this fallacy led to extensive work on guidelines regarding the open area design. They resemble a list of do-s and don't-s without leaving any space for alterations and inclusion of user-experts.

In connection with the empowerment as sort of transfer of power is a sense of relief and independence. Both terms are just the opposite of what the patients usually experience in hospitals where they are bound to strict procedures, expected behavior and with very little space for self-management of their actions. However, in examples of hospital spaces that diverge from the typical functionalism and its embedded prescriptiveness, the users are encouraged to form their own sense of place and to personalize the outdoor ambiences they occupy.

For example, in the design proposal for general and community hospital the entire ground floor area is landscaped and opened to commuters from the neighborhood to use for rest or as a shortcut between the two prominent streets. The entrances to general and community hospital are there too, immersed in greenery. They are visible, functional and easy to find, but still secondary in this picture of publicness and social integration. The entire community is thus empowered over the hospital outdoor space and chances of raising social bonds within this institution are high, particularly for the elderly.

The experiential approach that comes from the phenomenological discourse proves more reliable in discussing the issues of empowerment in regard to hospital outdoor spaces (Dovey, 2010). The design per se does not matter except as an entity composed of a number of segments sensed through the consecutive experiences of space. From this standpoint, the outdoor hospital environment is not any more an immobile image, but a situation, a set of circumstances that encompass many more elements than just the physical space. In connection to the empowerment are the issues of privateness and publicness of the outdoor hospital environments too.

Public - private

Although widely used to refer to spaces surrounding the hospital buildings the term outdoor is also prone to variety of diverse capacities and interpretations. Since hospitals are public institutions where one resides out of need and not choice, they might be considered as complete opposites of private homes. Yet, building the image of home in healthcare facilities has been noted throughout research literature as beneficial for wellbeing of all users. Unfortunately, the idea is often connected solely to the image and not to the concept of privateness and illustrated with iconic image of a typical western home.

Historically, the hospital outdoor space changed characters depending of the clerical, social, political, military or other authority the hospital was affiliated with. The outdoor hospital space was pragmatically used for diverse functions that served this institution, but it also resonated with the needs of the society. Looking beyond the utilitarian role it fulfilled, the outdoor hospital space was also anything from being feared of to being embraced. The range stretches from being a place of incarceration like in historic Lazaretto cases, to being a place of liberation and support in contemporary examples. In short, numerous and very diverse characters of the outdoor space developed between these two poles: the fear and the comfort. Visual symbols engaged in building the outdoor ambiences reflect the context and the era, the levels of cultural, scientific and medical developments, etc. Therefore, defining the outdoor hospital space is beyond descriptions and relies on understanding the causes that led to numerous appearances displayed over time.

The widely understood context is one of the inevitable determinants of the hospital outdoor space. The ungrounding and the fluidity of place as Dovey (2010) suggests in his discourse on place making, changes the perception of space as fixed and given once for all. The realization of the fluidity of place shifts the outdoor hospital space from being a subject with fixed qualities and prone to analysis leading to definite judgments, to a position of an object in processes that contribute to place making.

For example, in the most famous Renaissance atrium hospital the Ospedale degli Innocenti, the public civic plaza was right in front of the hospital while its inside contained atriums as very intimate outdoor spaces inserted like intarsia in the body of the building. The position that the plaza and atriums held in regard to the urban domain predetermined their character. The difference between the civic plaza and the internal private atriums and gardens was innate. Their distinct looks, levels of publicness and privateness, their meaning in regard to their social stand and medical function, their design and their usage were very clear. In the true renaissance spirit this hospital was proudly positioned in the urban matrix as a social institution celebrating the enlightened patrons and civic bodies that stood behind. Although the atriums in the interior still reflected its historic ecclesiastical affiliation, the distinct front façade with nine bay loggia symbolized this new public stand of the hospital in the society.

Even now, centuries later while visiting this historic monument and a still functional medical institution, there is this notions that nothing is to be added or subtracted to outdoor spaces, nothing seems to be missing or redone differently. Of course, the hospital is still firmly rooted into the Florentine historic urban tissue and thus any change to its outdoor spaces would not be even possible. Yet, not all historic cities remain unchanged and there are many examples where a historic hospital finds itself in a totally changed urban surroundings. The sudden inappropriateness of the outdoor space caught up between the unchanged private domain and the completely new public one is often the cause of friction and design ambivalence.

The context and authority over the hospital open spaces entails its spatial, functional, aesthetic and semantic characteristics. Context, however, is a complex system prone to changes and transformations over time. Private and public realms stand in constant opposition and flux as users transcend this sometimes invisible boundary. Thus, the urban and the cultural context in which the hospital stands should induce the fluid rather than the inflexible look of the outdoor hospital spaces to maintain their compatibility and allow for adjustments over time.

Typology - branding

Paradigmatic changes in hospital design are another significant determinant of hospital outdoor spaces. Looking down the historic line it is interesting to find the breaking point in time when even the definition of the outdoor hospital environment became a controversial issue. In the atrium hospital type the outdoor space was clearly delineated, however, in the typical nineteenth century pavilion hospital it turned elusive. The areas surrounding the hospital pavilions became bigger, filled with greenery and circulation lanes. This type of hospitals occupied larger grounds and thus required certain distance from the closely knit urban network. This, in return, loosened links with the urban hierarchical order of public spaces. The inherent clearness was lost and space required fencing to demarcate from the urban surroundings. The edge between the city and the hospital became sharp and harsh. One could be either in or out of the hospital premises and this binary character almost directly implied the fearful position of being ill or healthy.

The compact typology of a functionalistic city hospital was the opposite example, since its outdoor spaces were reduced to inner courtyards while on the outside they entirely diminished leaving the street patterns to define the hospital building and its edges. This position however, was not less harsh as the façade of the hospital facing the public domain now held the binary character and had to conform to requirements of both realms it divided.

Recent examples of green hospitals, however, escape the trap of confining their outdoor spaces to any typological requirements. The 'green' as the umbrella brand takes over the prime position in determining the design features and their connotation. The landscaped courtyards, the rooftop gardens and green walls of the hospital merge and relate to similar features in the nearby urban neighborhood. The outdoor hospital space thus establishes connections between the domains due to its brand and not necessarily its type. The 'green' as branding theme is appropriate for supportive environments and easy to recognize. However, in examples of smaller medical facilities inserted in shopping centers or university campuses for example, other branding themes are adopted too. Waiting rooms resembling a café, a library or an IT studio with corresponding outdoor terraces are some of the attempts to brand the space differently and shift it out of the expected hospital typology.

Links – boundaries

The utilitarian role of the hospital outdoor space still defines its boundaries. Circulation and traffic, public transportation link points, pedestrian lines and service accesses allow for people and goods to reach their destination within the hospital building. The spatial characteristic and position of the entrances determines if the approach is smooth and efficient, or confusing and obstructive. With established principles of universal design we expect the outdoor to be accessible to all users regardless of their capabilities and under all imaginable conditions. From the functional point of view the efficient transition from outside to the inside and vice versa is the main role of the outside hospital space.

However, the links with the urban infrastructure pattern, even though important, still can't define any exact character of the outdoor hospital space. The elusive description of an apparently very simple attribute–the outdoor, suggests that further dissection of the term is needed before its meaning is taken for granted.

Outdoors is also the opposite of indoors. This opposition conceives numerous dichotomies characteristic for the outdoor hospital environment. To name a few: separation and connectedness, clashes and bonds, contradictions and harmonies. The healthful qualities of the outdoor hospital environment depend on links, semantic bonds and harmonious transitions between these opposing pairs and in particular from the inside to the outside and back. The importance of links is easy to understand - if the outdoor space is not well connected and easily reachable from the inside then it would not be frequently visited. If it is not visually present and revealed from different indoor spaces then it would not be considered relevant for healing processes. If its appeal is negative looking from the street, than the institution will be stigmatized and avoided.

However, the links are not physical only; they might be indirect and metaphorical too. If the view to outside is not provided, than the shear existence of the healing garden will not benefit all patients in the wards but only those who can step out and visit it. Even they might not succeed in doing so as they might not be informed on the existence of the garden or not feel strong enough to visit or simply might not feel tempted to overcome these and other obstacles and go to a healing garden. In response to these common circumstances the indoor space often adopts some or all of the symbols and qualities of the outdoor and presents itself as a reminiscence of the real, the copy of the unreachable original. The nostalgic icons of the outdoor, like potted greenery or veranda furniture are elements often found in the interiors of the hospital waiting areas or corridors for example. The inside and the outside change sides and thus create the elusive boundary between the two, always in move and striving for balance and harmony.

The edge - the threshold

Speaking of the physical boundaries that shape the outdoor hospital environment we actually refer to the urban edge, the zone between the hospital and the city, but also to the edge delineating the inside and the outside, the private and the public, the opened and the secluded, the social and the intimate, etc. We can easily discuss the outdoor space from singular standpoints as a functional edge, protective edge, beautifying edge, demarcating edge or even the disappearing edge. The issue of threshold is however more complex.

From the geometric perspective two planes are defining the outdoor environment: the horizontal and the vertical one constituting the basic demarcation of three-dimensionality. The ground floor areas surrounding the hospital building, but also the sunken courtyards, rooftops and terraces are the horizontals, while the verticals are the facades of the hospital buildings and vertical communication connecting the horizontals. Why discussing the obvious? Because far too often only the most evident out-door spaces like ground floor gardens and atriums are considered and specifically designed to contribute to healing and the rest of the possibilities is neglected.

However, if we consider the edge with reference to the sides it delineates than the pragmatic, descriptive approach seems inadequate. The edge in that sense needs to be treated as a threshold. Although both terms might be mistaken as synonyms, the thresholds are constructs that are both mentally and materially present, as Stavrides (2007) states. This subtle difference is based on the human ability to delineate the act of passage from its representation. The design of the outdoor hospital realm thus always has a twofold role – to allow for the passage and to induce its meaning. Yet, in both cases the literal and the symbolical control over this important point makes a big difference. Who is setting the symbolic clues that turn the edge into the threshold? Who insures the synergy of both? With participatory, flexible and intuitive design of the outdoor areas some of these questions might be answered. For example, the edge of a hospital surrounded by a lush tropical garden is fenced. The threshold, however, is recognized in other details: the pattern of leaves imprinted on the concrete walkway, the butterfly garden, the nature inspired logo of the institution, typical park-like benches and other details that users discover and read thus constructing their own symbolic hospital threshold.

Sympathy - empathy

The affective response to space is in the core of healthful architecture. If a place is perceived as pleasing it is more likely that one would feel good about it. Imaging results suggest that brain activity related to the formation of the affective response depends on the processing dynamics, or the time needed to comprehend the seen and to generate the reaction to it (Bechtel and Abrahamsen, 2002; Reber et al., 2004).The faster we comprehend the seen, the better we apparently react to it. While designing the hospital outdoor realm we are actually setting the stage for formation of an affective reaction to the aesthetics of the environment (Cold, 2001).

However, our example of the outdoor space of the hospice medical facility shows that not all the clues, no matter how carefully conceived, trigger the desired emotional response. The wish to create supportive outdoor environment for all users resulted in creation of a specific sympathetic scene in front of the hospice entrance. The theme of the spatial arrangement seems religious probably symbolizing the hospice patrons. Statues of Holy Mother and Child in baroque posture and saints' face expressions ghostly emerging from the rocks were interwoven with flower arrangements, koi fish pond and lights, almost suggesting an image of heaven. The intention based on sympathy is clear although the emphatic messages are questionable considering that hospice users are terminally ill patients and that the emotionally shaken visitors need not be reminded on this outcome each time they enter.

The contextual determinant of sympathetic and empathetic response is recognized in research (De Vignemont and Singer, 2006; Harris et al, 2002). The empathic brain response is strongly connected to environmental properties and determines the most effective social behavior under the respective circumstances. However, although the environmental characteristics and notions of sympathy are connected on the drawing board we seldom tackle the issues of empathy and anticipated behavior triggered by design.

End notes

The development of the hospital urban edge transgressed from being detrimental to becoming vital for hospital function and beyond. Its design characteristics are now recognized as valuable for the healing processes and wellness but also as a prominent social and mercantile asset tapping on the various urban resources. The outdoor hospital space still preserves its functional role and efficiently coordinates hospital operations with urban infrastructure systems and at the same time boosts levels of social capital in the neighborhood.

However, the true value of the outdoor hospital design is in its capacity to adapt in reaction to the ongoing contextual changes. This recently gained sense of the importance of vitality and ability to continuously transform over time is genuinely new and unprecedented in the history of hospital development. We might not need to have specific plans for hospital outdoor spaces in the future. Instead, they might be considered as public spaces that the commuters occupy for recreation, the young for ad hoc events, families for visits, entertainment or even shopping, patients and medical staff for relaxations, support and for immersing in the atmosphere of the quotidian where stigma disappears, etc. At the same time, it should be the space that hospital systems easily take over and use for emergency containment as both functional and protective zones.

To design the outdoor hospital spaces as open frame calls for new and evolutive design processes where only principles and clues are set in advance and the rest left to evolve over time. In this scenario the continual engagement of user-experts and society as a whole is essential. Design-wise the open frame model offers opportunities for engagement of new technologies as they appear and for flexible and far more effective usage of space in times of major medical crises.

References

Antonovski, A. (1996), "The salutogenic model as a theory to guide health promotion", *Health Promotion International, vol. 11*(1).Oxford University Press, Oxford, GB, pp.11-18.

Bechtel, W. and Abrahamsen, A. (2002), *Connectionism and the mind: Parallel processing, dynamics, and evolution in networks*, Blackwell Publishing. Oxford, UK.

Cold, B. (2001), "Aesthetics, well-being and health", In Cold, B. (Ed) *Essays within architecture and environmental Aesthetics*, Ashgate,Aldershot.

De Vignemont, F. and Singer, T. (2006), "The empathic brain: how, when and why?",*Trends in cognitive sciences, 10*(10), pp.435-441.

Dijkstra, K. (2009), *Understanding healing environments: Effects of physical environmental stimuli on patients' health and well-being*. University of Twente, Netherlands.

Dilani, A. (2008), "Psychosocially supportive design: A salutogenic approach to the design of the physical environment", *Design and Health Scientific Review, 1*(2), pp.47-55.

Dovey, K. (2010), *Becoming Places: Urbanism/Architecture/Identity/Power*, Routledge, New York; London.

Dovey, K. (2008), *Framing places: mediating power in built form*, Routledge, London.

Frumkin, H. (2003), "Healthy places: exploring the evidence", *American journal of public health, 93*(9), pp.1451-1456.

Gesler, W., M. (2003), *Healing places*. Rowman & Littlefield Publishers, Washington DC.

Guenther, R., & Vittori, G. (2008), *Sustainable healthcare architecture*, John Wiley & Sons.

Hamilton, D., K. and Watkins, D., H. (2009), *Evidence-based design for multiple building types*. John Wiley & Sons.

Harris, P. B., McBride, G., Ross, C., & Curtis, L. (2002), "A Place to Heal: Environmental Sources of Satisfaction Among Hospital Patients ", *Journal of Applied Social Psychology, 32*(6), pp.1276-1299.

Hathorn, K., Nanda, U. (2008),"A guide to evidence-based art", *The Center for Health Design*,1, available at http://artshealthnetwork.ca/ahnc/guide_to_evidenced_based_art_.pdf (accessed 28.11.2014).

Helliwell, J., F. and Putnam, R. (2004), "The Social Context of Well-Being", *Philosophical Transactions of the Royal Society London*, 359, pp.1435-1446.

Huisman, E. R. C. M., Morales, E., van Hoof, J., &Kort, H. S. M. (2012), "Healing environment: A review of the impact of physical environmental factors on users", *Building and Environment*, 58, pp.70-80.

Johnson, B. and Hill, K. (Eds) (2002), *Ecology and design: frameworks for learning* (Vol. 1). Island Press, Washington, D.C.

Joye, Y. (2007),"Architectural lessons from environmental psychology: The case of biophilic architecture", *Review of General Psychology*, 11(4), p.305.

Joye, Y. (2006), "Cognitive and evolutionary speculations for biomorphic architecture", *Leonardo*, 39(2), pp.145-152.

Kaplan, R. and Kaplan, S. (1989),*The experience of nature: A psychological perspective*, Cambridge University Press, New York, NY.

Lawson, B. (2010), "Healing architecture". *Arts & Health*, 2(2), pp.95-108.

Leibrock, C., A. and Harris, D., D. (2011), *Design Details for Health: Making the Most of Design's Healing Potential* (Vol. 9). John Wiley & Sons Inc.

Marcus, C.,C. and Barnes, M. (Eds) (1999), *Healing gardens: Therapeutic benefits and design recommendations*, John Wiley & Sons Inc.

Marcus, C., C. (2000), "Gardens and health", *Design and health: the therapeutic benefits of design*, International Academy for Design and Health, pp.61-71, available at http://www.designandhealth.com/uploaded/documents/Publications/Papers/Clare-Cooper-Marcus-WCDH2000.pdf (accessed 22 November 2014).

Marcus, C. C. (2007), "Healing gardens in hospitals", *Interdisciplinary Design and Research e-Journal, 1*(1), available at http://www.intogreen.nl/en/topics/care/research/if-nature-has-healing-properties-why-is-there-so-little-green-in-hospitals/cooper_marcus.pdf (accessed 22 November 2014).

Mourshed, M. and Zhao, Y. (2012), "Healthcare providers' perception of design factors related to physical environments in hospitals", *Journal of Environmental Psychology, 32*(4), pp.362-370.

Mazuch, R., & Stephen, R. (2005), "Creating healing environments: humanistic architecture and therapeutic design". *Journal of Public Mental Health, 4*(4), pp.48-52.

Nanda, U., Bajema, R., Ortega-Andeane, P., Solovyova, I., and Bozovic-Stamenovic, R. (2013), "Investigating the impact of culture and education on students' art preferences", *Journal of architectural and planning research, 30*(4), pp. 291-310.

Ostroff, E. (1997), "Mining Our Natural Resources: The User as Expert", *Innovation*, the Quarterly Journal of the Industrial Designers Society of America, 16(1).

Pallasmaa, J. (2013), *The eyes of the skin: Architecture and the senses*, John Wiley & Sons, USA.

Preamble to the Constitution of the World Health Organization, Official Records of the World Health Organization, no. 2, p. 100, available at http://www.who.int/about/definition/en/print.html (accessed 28th November 2014).

Reber, R., Schwarz, N., Winkielman, P. (2004), "Processing fluency and aesthetic pleasure: is beauty in the perceiver's processing experience?", *Personality and Social Psychology Review*, Vol. 8, No. 4, pp.364-382.

Rogers, SH., Gardner, K.H., Carlson, C.H. (2013), "Social capital and walkability as social aspects of sustainability", *Sustainability*, 2013, 5, pp.3473-3483, available at http://scholars.unh.edu/cgi/viewcontent.cgi?article=1083&context=civeng_facpub (accessed 20.03.2014).

Schweitzer, M., Gilpin, L., Frampton, S. (2004),"Healing spaces: elements of environmental design that make an impact on health", *Journal of Alternative & Complementary Medicine*, 10Supplement 1, pp.71-83.

Stavrides, S. (2007), "Heterotopias and the experience of porous urban space", in Franck, K., Stevens, Q. (Eds), *Loose Space: Possibility and Diversity in Urban Life*, Routledge, New York, London, pp.174-192.

Stichler, J., F. (2009), "Healthy, healthful, and healing environments: A nursing imperative", *Critical care nursing quarterly, 32*(3), pp.176-188.

Stigsdotter, U., & Grahn, P. (2002), "What makes a garden a healing garden", *Journal of therapeutic Horticulture,13*(2), pp. 60-69, available at http://www.protac.dk/Files/Filer/What_makes_a_garden_a_healing_garden_Stigsdotter_U__Grahn_P.pdf (accessed 22 November 2014).

Thwaites, K., Helleur, E., Simkins, I., M. (2005), "Restorative urban open space: Exploring the spatial configuration of human emotional fulfilment in urban open space". *Landscape Research, 30*(4), pp.525-547.

Ulrich, R., S., Zimring, C. M., Zhu, X., DuBose, J., Seo, H., Choi, Y., et al. (2008), "A review of the research literature on evidence-based healthcare design", *Health Environments Research & Design, 1*(3), pp.61-125.

Ulrich, R. S. (1999), "Effects of gardens on health outcomes: Theory and Research", In Marcus, C., C., and Barnes, M. (Eds) *Healing gardens: Therapeutic benefits and design recommendations*, John Wiley & Sons Inc. chapter 2, pp.27-86.

Ulrich, R., S. (2002),"Health benefits of gardens in hospitals", In *Paper for conference, Plants for People International Exhibition Floriade* (Vol. 17, No. 5, p.2010).

Ulrich, R., S., Simons, R. F., Losito, B. D., Fiorito, E., Miles, M. A., &Zelson, M. (1991),"Stress recovery during exposure to natural and urban environments", *Journal of environmental psychology, 11*(3), pp.201-230.

Verderber, S., Fine, D. (Eds) (2000), *Healthcare Architecture in an Era of Radical Transformation*, Yale University Press, New Haven, CT.

Wilson, E., O. (1984), *Biophilia*, Harvard University Press, Cambridge, MA.

Zimring, C., Joseph, A. and Choudhary, R. (2004), "The role of the physical environment in the hospital of the 21st century: a once-in-a-lifetime opportunity", *Concord, CA: The Center for Health Design*, available at http://www.herg.gatech.edu/Files/ulrich_role_physical.pdf (accessed 22 November 2014).

Ružica Božović Stamenović

07

**Health facilities and open spaces:
Integrated policies at the landscape and territorial level**

Rosalba D'Onofrio and Elio Trusiani

Abstract: The paper examines the relationship between health facilities and open spaces from a landscape and territorial point of view, considering not just the hospital closest surroundings, but also more distant areas. Such an approach might appear not in line with the present book, but it can suggest nonetheless new possibilities and ideas in a global review of the current planning policies and practices, as far as the enjoyment and usage of common goods and public services are concerned. As a matter of fact, the open spaces' network is a connection system of different green areas and natural amenities, inside and outside the city, comprising a variety of functions at different levels. Therefore, it has to be carefully planned in a strategic and multi-scalar way, in order to preserve the highest possible degree of biodiversity, as a primary element for our environmental comfort, health and wellbeing. By some national and international examples, we want to show how a different use of natural parks and other protected areas could represent a precious opportunity, still unexplored, for human health and social wellbeing. Sometimes hospitals, especially if located within the city boundaries, are quite far away from the largest natural areas, nevertheless a new possible connection between each other could foster innovative planning policies and give back vitality. This would imply to overcome the old and boring quarrel about passive or active nature conservancy, in favour of a dynamic and comprehensive management of landscape as a common good, involving various private or public bodies, institutions and social-health service providers, which are not sharing plans and policies yet. In many cases, however, hospital facilities are close indeed to highly valuable open spaces. Thus, from a territorial perspective, they could establish fruitful and innovative relations in many respects: functionally, therapeutically, formally and perceptually. Moreover, the economic crisis we are still passing through, might even convince someone that the protection of nature in the parks is a luxury we cannot afford anymore. But the scientific research of the last decades has highlighted how a loss in biodiversity can undermine human health and comfort, whereas living in close contact with nature has very good effects on our physical and mental wellbeing. People today have an increasing need to restore a balance with the natural environment, in order to improve the quality of their own life. Worldwide, some experimental projects in forest-therapy and eco-therapy, in parks and natural areas, are very interesting not only for obvious positive outcomes in terms of mental and physical health, but also for very good social, ethic and economic prospects. These new experiences can relaunch strongly the key role of natural parks and protected areas, supporting both their primary goals' achievement and their further contribution to the cultural, social and economic development of contemporary world.

Keywords: natural park, healthy, integrated policy, planning, quality of life.

Introduction

A Chinese saying reads: "...Pleasure for one hour, a bottle of wine. Pleasure for one year, a marriage; but pleasure for a lifetime, a garden". This saying representswell our common sense about the natural environment, which can obviously help people maintain a physical and psychological wellbeing and therefore a good quality of life. In Europe, during the Middle Age, monastic hospitals encompassed gardens and orchards for the purpose of contributing to the physical and spiritual healing of patients(Gerlach-Spriggs et al. 1998). In the second half of 19th century Florence Nightingale, who is considered the pioneer of modern nursing, wrote in her Notes about the importance of providing visual connection with nature to sick people, in order to speed up and ease their physical recovery. Notwithstanding this common sense, which is present in the eastern as well as in the western countries, it is just since few decades that researchers are trying to give scientific evidence of the relationship between natural environment and human health and wellbeing. A lot of various disciplines and fields are involved in these studies: environmental psychology, psychiatry, medicine, but also environmental science, ecology, urban planning and landscape architecture. Some scholars have highlighted, in fact, how human beings depend on nature not only for their materialnecessities (food, water, livelihoods in general, etc.), but even more, perhaps, for their psychological, emotional and spiritual needs. According to researchers, gardens, parks and natural areas would decrease the levels of anxiety and stress, while enhancing our concentration ability (Kaplan, 1995; Kaplan & Kaplan, 1989; Ulrich, 1984; Ulrich, Simons, Losito, Fiorito, Miles & Zelson, 1991). In this sense, they speak about *remedial effects*, capable of recovering from mental exhaustion caused by modern lifestyles (Kaplan & Kaplan, 1989; Ulrich, 1999). A resting period spent in a refreshing natural environment, even if for only few minutes, could help people regain their mental and physical balance (Pretty, J. and Barton, J., 2010). Other scholars have also demonstrated that those living inside large green areas are more protected from cardiovascular disease, diabetes and obesity (Mitchell & Popham, 2008; Björk, Albin, Grahn, Jacobsson, Ardo, Wadbro, Östergren & Skärbäck, 2008).

Recently, studies on the relationship between human health/wellbeing, biodiversity and climate change have attracted increasing attention. In particular, the preservation of biodiversity and ecosystem services, according to some authors

(Niemelä, Tyrväinen& Schulman, 2009), can be considered as a way to protect humankind's health from catastrophic impacts of climate change. This linkage has been the subject of the UN Millennium Ecosystem Assessment in 2005 and of the Global Environmental Change and Human Health project 2014 (GEC&HH). These reports have focused on the threats to human health caused by global environmental changes and on the adaptive strategies to be hence implemented. The European Union, by the COST Action E39 Program "Forests, Trees and Human Health and Wellbeing", aims to enhance the awareness that natural places have a positive influence on Europeans' health and wellbeing. By exploring the relations between health, natural environments in general, and forests in particular, this research has gathered experiences of scholars from 25 countries, who work in the fields of forestry, health, environmental and social sciences (Nilsson, K., Sangster, M., Gallis, C., Hartig, T., de Vries, S., Seeland, K., Schipperijn, J. , 2011).

All of the above mentioned researches, as well as others, have relevance not only from a sanitary perspective, but are intended to renovate the national policies in the sector of parks and natural areas, in the hope of an upcoming strategic and integrated territorial planning. This paper aims to examine these new possibilities, by referring specifically to some ongoing experiences.

Parks, nature and health: what is the link?

Although scientific research has proved since decadesthe health benefits of natural areas, there is still a general undervaluing of the important implications that might influence from this point of view the policies of each country as far as the management and planning of natural parks and green areas are concerned. That is instead what already happens in the case of sports and recreation activities (Rohde and Kendle, 1997). However, some national and international organizations, governments and parks can be considered pioneers in this new field. One of the first non-profit organizations to pay much attention to the relationship parks/public health was the Canadian Parks/recreation Association (CPRA ACPL), which in "The Benefits Catalogue" of 1997, updated in 2009, determined tight liaisons between parks' objectives and people's health. In the catalogue, some basic functions of parks were defined: parks help people live longer; they extend the active life of elderly people; help in decreasing the number of heart diseases and strokes (major causes of death in Canada); fight women's osteoporosis; fight diabetes; contribute to cut down the risk of contracting particular tumours (colon, breast and lung cancer); help in preventing and rehabilitating from back trouble; enhance mental health; reduce stress; etc. The catalogue aimed to provide instructions for a global reorganization of parks, namely, to enable parks to supply better services and to share these new possibilities of development with local stakeholders. As for the national governments, then, we cannot but mention the Scottish experience. In 2008 the Scottish Government launched the "Good Places Better Health", which theorized a close connection between health policy and environmental policy, between people's health and wellbeing and the quality of the environment they are living in. The programme consists of various strategies and is intended also to reduce social inequalities and national health costs. One of the strategies put in place from 2009 and updated in 2015 is the "Woods for Health strategy". The Government has in fact supported the national health care by promoting a wider and more frequent use of outdoor spaces, in particular woods and natural areas, for therapeutic purposes. According to the researches brought in support of the programme, woods would be able to decrease: risk of heart disease, obesity, diabetes, cancer, osteoporosis and other life-threatening. Furthermore, woods would enhance people's mental wellness; would improve their sense of belonging to the neighbourhood they are living in; would favour social integration; would help hence in reducing cases of social isolation. By this strategy, the Government is committed to:

- provide everybody accessibility to forests and woods;
- enable health-care providers to use much more woods and natural areas;
- maximize the potential of green networks in urban regions;
- promote and increase the opportunities to enjoy woods and natural areas.

This strategy has generated various initiatives, a lot of which are now in progress, such as: the supply of services in close relation with hospitals to people with different kinds of health troubles; precautionary measures, for instance in the form of 'walks in the woods by medical prescription'; rehabilitation programmes such as 'green gyms'. All of this has implied a great involvement of the health care services, the local institutions, the voluntary associations, etc. These activities have been arranged through an Action Plan, which is periodically updated and defines: the objectives to achieve, the indicators to be checked for monitoring their fulfilment, the specific actions and who is responsible for each of these. Some of the goals of the 2013-2015 Action Plan are: to live longer and healthier; to live in pleasant areas where services are easily accessible; to help children live their lives in the best way; etc. The planned actions include: a network of pathways for various disabilities; projects in the schools to train pupils in outdoor games and physical activities in the woods; medical prescription of open-air activities; etc. The growing interest and willingness to improve people's health by means of parks and natural areas has been promoted through increasing activism by parks themselves. An international congress titled "Healthy Parks, Healthy People" took place in Melbourne (Australia) in 2010 and 37 nations participated. At the end of the proceedings, the "Healthy Parks Healthy People" document was approved and subscribed, in order to encourage a rediscovery of the relationship between healthy environment and healthy society. This report calls everybody to build up healthier communities and to face our planet's troubles starting from the recovery of a good and balanced relationship with nature. It has highlighted in fact the key role of parks to better cope with problems such as pollution, global warming, biodiversity loss, deforestation, but also obesity, cardiovascular disease, diabetes, stress, anxiety, etc. Besides, the Melbourne document has underlined that the implementation of policies and actions, which hold together nature conservancy and people's health and wellbeing, can boost tourism and create new job opportunities for local inhabitants. It really suggests a "modus operandi" to governments and humanitarian/environmental organizations, making them able to adopt the concept "Healthy Parks Healthy People" within their programmes and institutional activities.

In line with that, the international campaign "No Child Left Inside" wants to fight the 'deficit of nature' in the young generations. Its principles have been adopted, as a motion, from the World Conservation Congress IUCN (Barcelona 2008). This campaign aims to recover the relationship between nature and children for their own benefit. In Italy, the project is called "Equilibri Naturali" ("Natural Balances") and is promoted by the Sibillini Mountains National Park.It has the primary object of fostering children's wellbeing through the development of more opportunities to get in contact with natural environments (1). The campaign begins by noting that, gradually, children (and their families) are losing acquaintance with the "True Nature", as they spend an average of 36 hours per week in front of a TV screen, play-station, computer. The increase in children's diseases such as obesity (Italian children are the most affected in Europe!), would result just from this 'departure from nature'.

The "park-therapy" and the "repositioning" of the Park Authorities in some ongoing experiences

Since the 2003 Durban World Parks Congress in South Africa, reveailingly entitled "Benefits Beyond Boundaries", a firm belief has begun to circulate internationally: parks cannot simply keep on dealing with nature conservancy, fostering tourism or attesting indirectly the quality of local products. There is widespread opinion that parks should play as activators of positive models of land management and leadto new kinds of proactive policies and development. In this regard, the most interesting experiences are right dealing with new development processes, based on creative formulas which combine environmental protection with local micro-economies. Thus, the possibility of a repositioning of the Park Authorities,by redefining and relaunching their functions and role, is just in line with the above. In this perspective, the possible offer of new services for people's physical and mental wellbeing, is still utterly to be explored. Although most of us is aware of the health benefits brought about by sports and recreation activities, the range of all other benefits resulting from contact with nature is very much unknown. On this subject, a shared international purpose is to further enhance the key role of parks in promoting and maintaining human health and environmental quality. Actually, few meaningful experiences have been undertaken so far, but there is growing interest nonetheless. The trend towards more comfortable lifestyles could find in protected areas a favourable terrain. Our impression is that the future of parks points very much in this direction. Below, two of the most significant experiences now in progress: the Japanese *"Shinrin Therapy Stations"* and the Italian *"Parchi Terapeutici"* (*"Therapeutic Parks"*) of Umbria Region.

Japan: the Blueprint for shinrin therapy stations

According to a 2000 survey by the Ministry of Health, Labour and Welfare of Japan, 54.2% of respondents (32,000 Japanese individuals older than 12 years) evaluated their stress level as 'very high' or 'relatively high'. Moreover, nearly half of respondents self-perceived their health condition as 'mediocre', in a range from 'poor' to 'good'. These data state clearly that modern society is a 'high-stress' one and that many people, even if not affected by any particular disease, perceive themselves as sick. Doubtless, Japanese people consider nature therapeutic since ancient times, but the Shinrin-yoku invention, which can be defined as "taking in the forest atmosphere or forest bathing", is quite recent; one of the most interesting experiences of forest-therapy is right linked to it and is completely changing the services and functions provided by Japanese parks. The project has begun as a marketing campaign, strongly wanted by the Japanese Forestry Agency since the 80s of the last century. The Shinrin-yoku strategy was entirely based on the people's deeply-rooted perception that spending time in nature, especially in the lush forest trails of Japan, would have benefit mind and body. This argument has been supported by the "National Land Afforestation Promotion Organization in Japan", which has fostered a field research in 24 forests all over the country. Afterwards, the number has increased and the research activities have shown that a walk in the forest reduces blood pressure and heart rate and improves the immune system. Experiments have also proved that even the mere display of a picture of a forest for 20 minutes, is able to cut down the stress hormone, cortisol, by 13 percent, thus reducing depression, fatigue and emotional confusion. Since 2005, the Japanese Government has allocated 4 million dollars for Shinrin-yoku researches, aimed at providing scientific evidence of the physiological effects caused by the forest environment on the central nervous activity (e.g. smell of wood, sound of springing water, landscape). From 2005 to 2009, studies have been conducted in several parks and forests in order to prove the beneficial effects on human health. A system of forest certification has originated from these studies and the certificate can be requested by prefectures, cities, towns, villages and farms. These various parties can in fact candidate places and forests they belong to. The award is issued on the basis of three criteria. The most important considers the physiological study which is carried out for each applying area. The study is to compare the physiological effects of similar activities in different environments, such as walking or resting in a forest with old trees, listening to the natural sounds and enjoying the landscape, with their analogue in urban areas. Measured parameters are: the hormone stress level in saliva, the blood pressure, etc. The second criterion looks at the distinctive features of the place, such as: the presence of hot-water springs; the local food, history and culture; the cost of living; etc. The third is linked finally to the quality of the natural environment and of the provided services (hospitals, health facilities in general, etc.). The primary objectives of the strategy are: the economic development of cities, towns and communities; the revival of popular interest and care for Japanese forests; the activation and improvement of the Community Forests; a reduction of the national health-care expenditure by launching a kind of preventive medicine. From 2005 to 2010, 42 sites have been awarded: Japanese people visiting these forests are estimated between 2.5 and 5 million each year. The "Walking Forest Therapy Roads ® with a Doctor" are among the activities developed within the Shinrin Therapy Stations. In these occasions, participants take a walk in the forest, take a sit or just lie down on the ground, enjoy the landscape, relax and benefit from the forest's healing power. The specific venues for these events are several trails (nearly 50) selected all around the country on the basis of experiments which measured the forest's positive impact on the hormone stress levels. The Shinrin therapy approach has proved so convincing that other countries have followed the Japanese example, as for instance Finland and South Korea, which is investing huge resources on its national forest-therapy project.

Italy: The Therapeutic Parks of Umbria Region

Umbria Region is commonly named the green heart of Italy, due to its 7 natural parks: the Sibillini MountainsNational Park, the Regional Parks of Monte Cucco, Monte Subasio, Trasimeno Lake, Colfiorito and the River Parks of Tevere and Nera. Besides landscape and natural beauty, this territory is deeply influenced by the figure of San Francesco d'Assisi, who is inextricably linked to the image of this land, suspended between nature and spirituality. The idea of the Therapeutic Park originates from an intuition of the Environmental and Health departments of Umbria Region in collaboration with the Mountain Community of Martani, Serano e Subasio. They were able to envisage the social, health and tourism potential of some places and facilities within the boundaries of the Regional Parks. In line with the original concept, a study committee has been established by gathering experts in the fields of health care, architecture and society, in order to draw up a feasibility study and a pilot project. The latter was financed through the "POR FESR 2007-2013" funds and generated, as a first outcome, a massive information campaign aimed at promoting the project idea by means of a widespread distribution of highly eye-catching posters about nature.

The principal goal of Therapeutic Parks is to combine the promotion of the major landscape beauties of Umbria Region with eco-therapy, a special kind of caring of physical and mental disease. The project is designed to achieve several targets in the social, economic, tourist and environmental spheres. Its innovative drive is to be found in the great effort of integrating, around the inclusive idea of the Therapeutic Parks, policies and plans carried out separately by different bodies and departments of Umbria Region Authority, that in fact do not communicate at all between each other. In particular, the project aims to:

- foster concrete measures in favour of people's wellbeing, with special regard to the most disadvantaged social groups, by means of a sensorial therapeutic approach able to overcome physical, neurological and psychological disabilities;
- equip spaces and places with proper facilities for people's welcome and social-health recovery of the weakest;
- set up a centre of excellence fortherapy and rehabilitation, which provide pilot experiences to be repeated in other regions;
- strengthen the collaboration, integration and social dialogue between institutions and other organizations operating in the social, cultural and environmental sectors.

These targets' accomplishment will benefit also the economic activities and social integration of people with disabilities, by:

- increasing the job opportunities for most disadvantaged people;
- training specialized staff in non-conventional therapeutic activities;
- engaging those with the great difficulties in the management of their own therapeutic and rehabilitating programmes;
- reusing existing structures and thus saving resources and money for health care.

In addition to the above, further goals are: promotion of sustainable tourism in Regional Parks, by setting up a network of therapeutic places which could generate related income and jobs; implementation of a fullyopen network of park users, from the local to the national and European level; establishment of institutional links between the Parks' Administrative Bodies and the local health & social service-providers.

The Therapeutic Parks project, in this early experimental stage, has involved the Regional Parks of Monte Subasio and Monte Cucco, which are becoming places really qualified to take care of diseases such as cardiovascular pathologies, diabetes, Alzheimer, etc. In a second step, the project will involve as well the other regional protected areas.

The Park of Monte Subasio is a unique environment with a strongly naturalistic character and a deeply spiritual meaning. The Therapeutic Parks project (Fig.1) sets up a series of therapeutic, recreational and sports activities, which ensure people to get specific benefits from the surrounding nature. In particular, the programme is devoted to:
- Alzheimer-suffering people and their families;
- people with Down's syndrome;
- autistic children and teenagers;
- people undergoing social reintegration;
- disabled people;
- people with various kinds of psychiatric pathologies.

There are three venues for these either outdoor or indoor activities:
- in Assisi, in Torgiovannetti neighbourhood, there is the Day Centre;
- in Spello, in Madonna di Colpernieri district, a group of facilities named the Therapeutic Farm;
- in Trevi, Villa Fabri, a building of remarkable historical interest, which is a multi-functional centre and the reference point for the entire Therapeutic Park (Fig.2). The project recommends a number of therapeutic activities, which are carried out basically outdoor, either in the very Park or in the gardens around each facility.

In particular, an area for garden-therapy has been localized in close proximity to the Day Centre and a green house is there located as well, equipped with both raised and ground-level flower beds. In the remaining open space, it is possible to undertake other activities, such as pet-therapy, physiotherapy, music therapy, art therapy, etc.

The Therapeutic Farm in Spello will host an info-point serving as promotional centre of the Therapeutic Park, a riding school with a particular rehabilitation centre, a covered structure for exhibitions, open spaces for outdoor therapy and receptive premises to give support to all activities.

In its turn, Villa Fabri in Trevi will promote, manage and monitor the therapeutic activities carried out in each of the park facilities. In particular, training courses for the personnel will take place inside the building, as for instance:
- garden-therapy courses;

- art therapy courses;
- aromatherapy courses.

Special regard has been directed to the project management and promotion, but also to its financial and monitoring issues.

A thorough assessment of the territory has identified possible users of the park facilities and have also detected several associations already working in the Region at guardianship of disabled and weak people's rights. The project is in fact designed to involve as well these social cooperatives, especially in the management and training of professional figures in possession of the needed skills and competences for the mentioned activities.

The monitoring of the project through time has also great importance. Some regional offices are right in charge of caring about that. The monitoring indicators are related to:
- the project goals achievement;
- the compliance with the regulatory standards;
- theacknowledged therapeutic benefits;
- the social and health consequences.

Additionally, the monitoring will consider:
- economic benefits;
- brand and image benefits;
- comfort and wellness benefits.

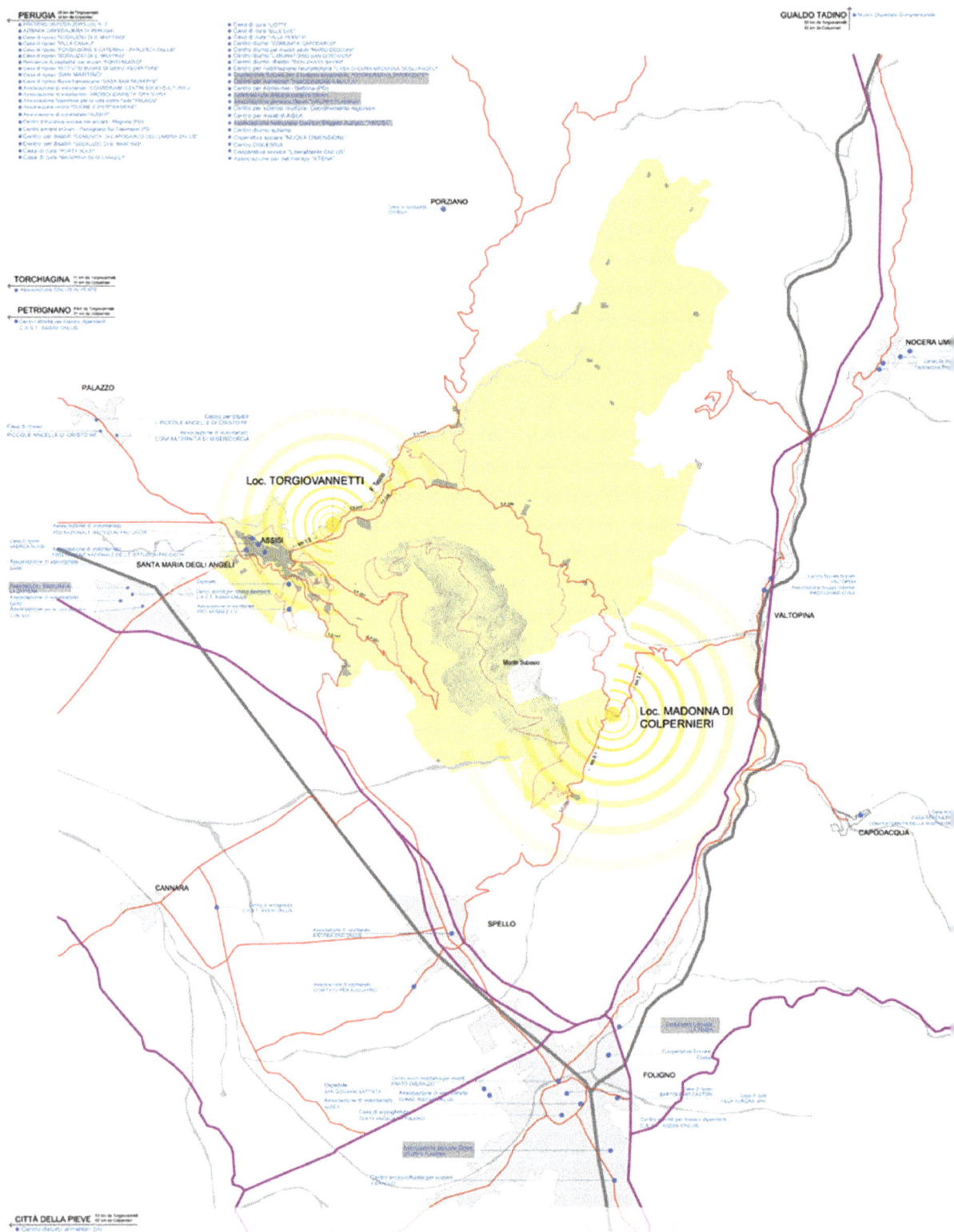

Figure 1: Therapeutic Park Monte Subasio. Territorial analysis, source: Umbria Region. Therapeutic Park Project.

PARCO TERAPEUTICO

ANALISI TERRITORIALE DEL PARCO DEL MONTE SUBASIO
Sistemi sanitario, culturale e sportivo

REGIONE UMBRIA
DIREZIONE REGIONALE RISORSA UMBRIA, FEDERALISMO, RISORSE FINANZIARIE, UMANE E STRUMENTALI.
SERVIZIO AREE PROTETTE, VALORIZZAZIONE SISTEMI NATURALISTICI E PAESAGGISTICI.
COMUNITÀ MONTANA DEI MONTI MARTANI, SERANO E SUBASIO
PARCO DEL MONTE SUBASIO

PROGETTISTI
ARCH. MONICA BOTTA
DOTT. ROBERTO BENOTTI

COLLABORATORE
ELISABETTA NUCERA

DATA: DICEMBRE 2011   SCALA 1:40.000   TAV. 1

LEGENDA

- Parco Regionale del Monte Subasio
- Centri abitati
- Autostrada
- Strade provinciali e statali
- Strade secondarie
- Linea ferroviaria
- Fiumi e torrenti
- Percorsi ciclistici
- Ippovie
- Sentieri trekking/nordic walking
- Strutture del Parco Terapeutico
- Strutture di interesse socio-sanitario
- Punti di interesse culturale/naturalistico
- Edifici religiosi
- Maneggi
- Atterraggio/decollo volo libero

Mappa Sentieri Monte Subasio

- Sentiero dei Mortari (Assisi - Spello sentiero n. 50)
- Sentiero Francescano (Assisi - Nocera Umbra sentiero n. 51)
- Collepino - Monte Subasio (sentiero n. 52)
- Sentiero dei fossi (S. Giovanni - Mortarone sentiero n. 53)
- Tre Fontane - Forca Bregno (sentiero n. 54)
- Armenzano - Monte Subasio (sentiero n. 55)
- Abbazia di S. Benedetto - Il Lago (sentiero n. 56)
- Monte Civitelle - Vallegina (sentiero n. 57)
- S. Giovanni - Madonna della Spella (sentiero n. 58)
- Armenzano - Mulino di Valentino (sentiero n. 59)
- Eremo delle Carceri - Pontecentesimo (sentiero n. 60)
- Costa di Trex - Monte Subasio (sentiero n. 61)
- Ponte S. Vittorino - Armenzano (sentiero n. 62)

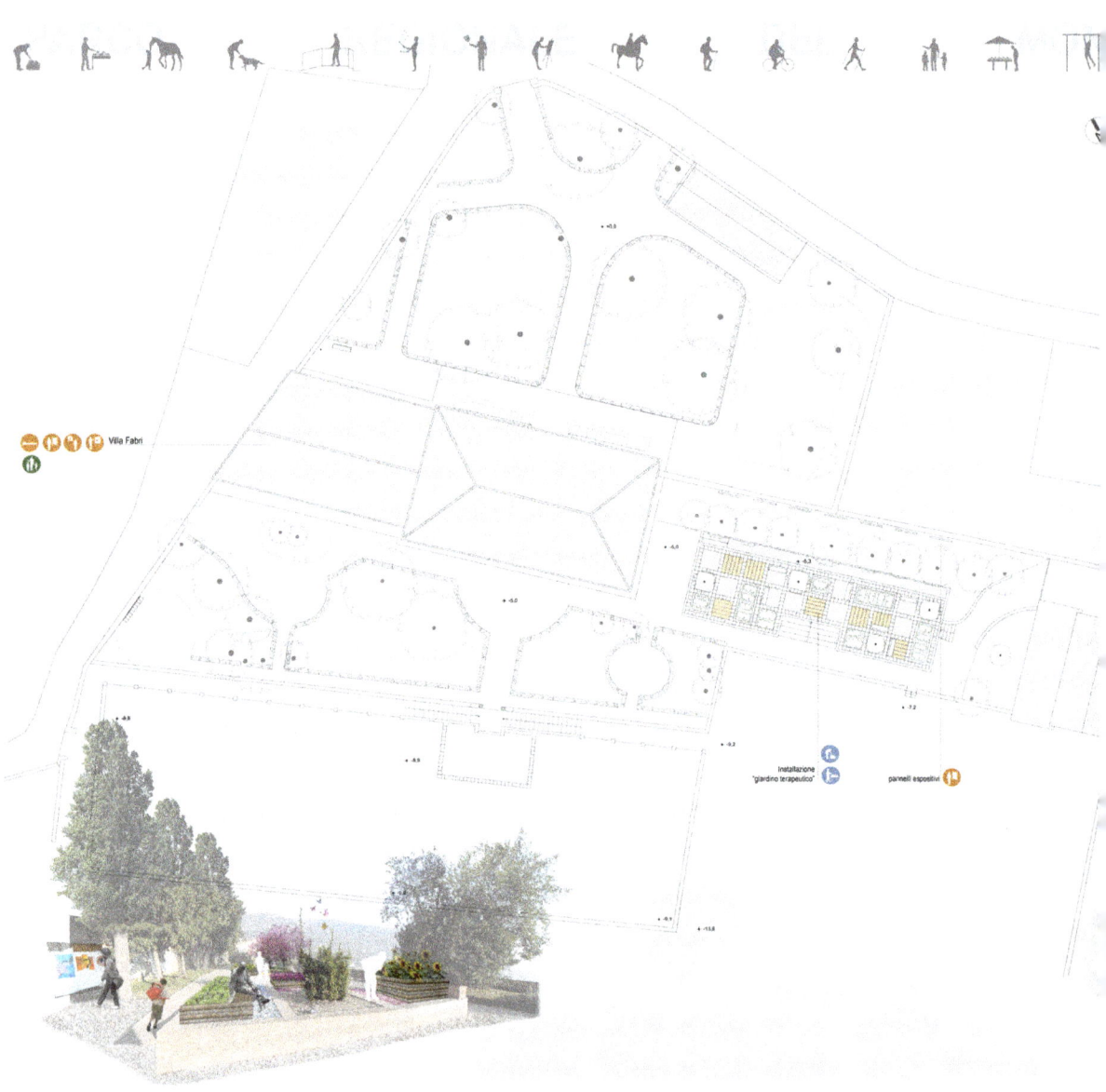

Figure 2: Activities and facilities of the Therapeutic Park. Villa Fabri Center, source: Umbria Region. Therapeutic Park Project.

Conclusions

The contemporary man has an increasing need of restoring a balance with the natural environment, in order to improve the quality of his own life. Therefore, some ongoing experiences undertaken recently in Europe and worldwide, are giving rise to much interest and attention owing to their social, etic and economic implications, besides their undoubted benefits for mental and physical health. These new projects of forest-therapy/eco-therapy can bring an important contribution to relaunch the key role of open spaces, urban vegetation and parks, from a completely new perspective related to the health/wellness factor. Such a combination could foster integrated policies, with new programmes and goals, reviving the pivotal roleof parks and other protected areas that are to become strategic in the overall picture of the economic, social and cultural dynamics of present-day world. These new experiences reflect new sensibilities of our changing society, but preserve at the same time the original mission of parks, that is nature conservancy. They could lead parks to a profound renewal, pushing them forward, beyond the mere activities of preservation. Parks in fact should become places where man could find again his good relationship with nature, by promoting a range of activities aimed at caring of health and preserving physical and mental wellbeing. Such an evolution, in compliance with the Parks' core mission and principles, would require anyway:

- a much intense communication and education campaign. In other words, it is necessary to make institutions, communities and stakeholders understand that the binomial Health/Parks has a momentous potential, which can be used to improve and maintain people's health and wellbeing; that in so doing Parks would have a chance to reduce the health-care expenditure; that Parks can foster a holistic/ecological approach in relation to health and wellness, which is useful (and essential) for each individual, for the society and for the environment;

- the activation of administrative management processes, keeping together health care, tourism, safeguard of protected natural areas, sports, cultural heritage recovery, job promotion, welfare in support of people with physical disabilities and thus most disadvantaged. This would be really innovative, since any sector tends traditionally to work isolated, notwithstanding the opportunities of working and planning together. Promoting a comprehensive management would reflect a modern perspective also in termsof health;

- the integration of different use practices of the natural environment, as already implemented through the development of sports, cultural and artistic disciplines, able to catalyse different users (from students to elderly people, from athletes to the most disadvantaged, including disabled, etc.);

- the practical contribution of local communities, by experiencing new forms of health-care services' management, both for them and for tourists, in order to fulfil an optimal balance between conservation and development needs;

- the conceiving and planning of open spaces from the most recent perspective: namely, the open space as a continuous system with different uses and functions, which can thus accomplish several goals and host various activities, at very different scales (from the building to the neighbourhood, city, territory). Ecological networks and biodiversity are essential components of the picture, as they keep a territorycohesiveand functional, leading us in fact to the final three key-words of a contemporary landscape project, which are biodiversity, multi-scalarity and geo-urbanity.

Notes

(1) Taking the role of "promoters", the following have joined the call of the Sibillini Mountains National Park: Parco Nazionale del Circeo; Parco Nazionale Dolomiti Bellunesi; Agenzia Regionale Parchi del Lazio; Parco Regionale del Po Torinese; Area Marina Protetta del Plemmirio; Associazione Ambientalista Mare Vivo; Istituto Pangea Onlus (Labnet-Lazio); Parco Regionale del Fiume Irno; Parco Nazionale del Gran Sasso, Monti della Laga; Parco Nazionale d'Abruzzo, Lazio e Molise; Parco Regionale dei Castelli Romani; Parco Regionale dei Monti Lucretili; Parco Regionale Marturanum; Parco Regionale dei Monti Aurunci; Ente Regionale RomaNatura; Agenzia Regionale per la Protezione dell'Ambiente-Sicilia; Ente Foreste Sardegna; Parco Nazionale della Sila; Parco Nazionale del Pollino; Parco Nazionale dell'Appennino Lucano-Val d'Agri-Lagonegrese; Area Marina Protetta di Punta Campanella; Direzione Regionale Ambiente-Regione Lazio; Amministrazione Provinciale di Roma-Ente gestore dei parchi provinciali.

(2) Ministry of Health, Labour and Welfare, Japan. Trend survey on health and welfare in Japan; 2000.

References

Barton J. and Pretty J. (2010), "What is the best dose of nature and green exercise for mental health? A meta-study analysis",*Environmental Science & Technology*, p.44.

Björk J, Albin M, Grahn P, Jacobsson H, Ardö J, Wadbro J, Ostergren PO. (2008), "Recreational values of the natural environment in relation to neighbourhood satisfaction, physical activity, obesity and wellbeing", J*Epidemiol Community Health*. 2008 Apr; 62(4).

Gerlach-Spriggs, N., Kaufman, R., & Warner, Jr., S. (1998), *Restorative Gardens: The Healing Landscape*. New Haven, CT and London: Yale University Press.

Kaplan, R., & Kaplan, S. (1989), *The experience of nature: A psychological perspective*, Cambridge University Press, New York.

Kaplan, S. (1995), "The urban forest as a source of psychological well-being",in G. A. Bradley, Ed., *Urban Forest Landscapes: Integrating multidisciplinary perspectives*, University of Washington Press, Seattle.

Lee J., Park B.J., TsunetsuguY. and Miyazaki Y. (2011), "Forests and human health - recent trends in Japan", in: *Forest Medicine*. Ed by Q. Li. Nova science publishers.

Maller C., Townsend M., Anita Pryor A., Brown P. and Leger L.e St (2006), "Healthy nature healthy people: 'contact with nature' as an upstream health promotion intervention for populations", *Health Promotional International*, Oxford University Press.

Maniglio Calcagno A. (2012), "Per ilBenesserenelPaesaggio". In Anguillari E., Ferrario, V., Gissi E., Lancerini E., *Paesaggio e Benessere*,FrancoAngeli, Milano.

Mitchell, R. and Popham, F. (2008), "Effect of exposure to natural environment on health inequalities: an observational population study". The Lancet 372(9650).

Miyazaki Y., Park B.J., Lee J. (2011),"Nature therapy",in *Designing our future: Perspectives on bioproduction, ecosystems and humanity (Sustainability Science*, Vol. 4. Eds.by M. Osaki, A. Braimoh and K. Nakagami. United Nations University Press.

Niemelä, J., Tyrväinen, L. & Schulman, H. (2009), inM. Faehnle, P. Bäcklund& M. Laine. eds. (2009), *Kaupunkiluontoa kaikille - Ekologinen ja kokemuksellinen tieto kaupungin suunnittelussa*. Edita Prima Oy, Helsinki.

Nilsson, K., Sangster, M., Gallis, C., Hartig, T., de Vries, S., Seeland, K., Schipperijn, J. (Eds.) (2011), *Forests, Trees and Human Health*, Springer.

Rohde, C. L. E. and Kendle, A. D. (1997)," Nature for people", in Kendle, A. D. and Forbes, S. (eds) *Urban Nature Conservation—Landscape Management in the Urban Countryside*. E. and F. N. Spon, London.

Urlich, R.S. (1984), "View through a window may influence recovery from survey".In:*Science*, 224.

Ulrich, R. S., Simons, R. F., Losito, B. D., Fiorito, E., Miles, M. A., & Zelson, M. (1991). "Stress recovery during exposure to natural and urban environments", in *Journal of Environmental Psychology*.

Ulrich, R. S. (1999). "Effects of gardens on health outcomes: theory and research", in: Cooper Marcus B.,Barnes M. (Eds.), *Healing Gardens: Therapeutic Benefits and Design Recommendations*, John Wiley, New York.

Vries, S. (2010). "Nearby Nature and human health: looking at mechanisms and their implications", in Ward Thompson C., Aspinall P., & Bell S. (Eds.), *Innovative approaches to researching landscape and health. Open space: People space 2*, Routledge, New York.

Williams, A. (ed) (1999),*Therapeutic Landscapes: The Dynamic between Place and Wellness*, University Press of America, Lanham MD, USA.

Williams, A. (ed.), (2007),*Therapeutic Landscapes*,Ashgate Publishing Ltd., London.

Canadian Parks/Recreation Association (1997), "The Benefits Catalogue", available at http: //lin.ca /sites/default/files/attachments/Complete1997Benefits%20Catalogue.pdf (accessed 20 August 2015).

Forestry Commission Scotland (2009), "Woods for Health", available at http://www.forestry.gov.uk/ pdf/fcfc011.pdf/$FILE/fcfc011.pdf (accessed 20 August 2015).

Healthy Parks Healthy People Congress (2010),"Proceedings 2010", available at http://www.hph pcentral.com/congress, (accessed 20 August 2015).

The Scottish Government (2008), "Good Places, Better Health is about responding to the challenges we face in creating safe and positive environments which nurture better and more equal health and wellbeing", available at http://www.gov.scot/Publications/2008/ 12/11090318/0 (accessed 20 August 2015).

Regione Umbria, (2011), "Il Parco Terapeutico", available at http://www.parchi.regione.umbria.it/ mediacenter/FE/articoli/il-parco-terapeutico-001.html, (accessed 20 August 2015).

Regione Umbria, (2012), "ParchiAttivi", available at www.parchiattivi.it. (accessed 20 August 2015).

08

A Master Plan for regeneration:
Piacenza Hospital complex, Italy

Anna Maria Giovenale

Abstract: The paper illustrates the "Piacenza Hospital Complex Master Plan" tool, the result of the synergy of different skills and different specialisms, and highlights the originality of this tool.

Starting with a frequently asked scientific question, I will examine the design of a hospital building, in particular the prevalence of functionality rather than architecture, highlighting how the Master Plan in question represents a possible solution which is 'outside the box.'

To be more specific, a first response is explained by the cognitive framework, from having placed the planning criteria of the spaces within the hospital system and the functional reorganization in the overall macro-areas as the basis for the elaboration of the strategic choices for the new organizational structure.

Another response is determined by having substantially followed the concept of a user-centered facility, paying particular attention to: reception, orientation, and the needs of minority groups.

One of the most original elements (also by way of an answer to the aforementioned question) is represented by having reinterpreted the hospital in Piacenza (made up of different buildings from different eras, that have been constructed over time, without an overall strategic plan) as a place where citizens should be able to meet. Thus the issue of program choices arises, which should be developed to recover the sense of the hospital being an "urban site".

In conclusion I emphasise, as one of the fundamental factors for the Plan's success, the orientation towards operational status and to boosting, through planning, all of the conditions for the implementation of the works; with reference to the monitoring systems, structured through processes which have been specifically developed to make the programming tool feasible

Keywords: hospital, strategic planning, regeneration, monitoring.

A repeatedly asked question

In the history of hospital building, in the Italian national context, for the last thirty years there has been a frequent preference for a functionalist approach: the organisation of functional areas and spaces needed as a priority element in the design project of a new hospital or when restructuring an existing hospital.

For several years, in the light of the known functional, technological, economic, organizational and managerial complexity inherent in a 'hospital system', the new priority is given to planning (and meta-planning) definition of the access system, the system of internal relations: the hospital like a machine, with all its gears, possibly well informed in terms of the needs of clients and users.

All this is done with an aim in mind, from a methodological point of view, to plan upstream and to define the project guidelines, and in particular to prefigure a functional and working system that is above all flexible in light of the change to the specific requirements that had motivated it.

The best results achieved: those represented by works created and used, within a reasonable time, responsive as much as possible to projects developed with the quality objectives and social, economic and environmental sustainability. There are few examples within the Italian context. Examples which, in some cases, are not identified by an element which strongly contributes to the overall quality obtainable from a new hospital construction or renovation project: the awareness of the hospital as an 'urban site' with its complexity of relations between the buildings enclosed in the sector and between the sector itself and the city.

These areas, differing from the traditional programming tools and for the purposes of an in-depth study carried out during the preparation, express themselves in the opposite way, and fit into the Piacenza Master Plan according to two different meanings.

The first is that the Master Plan represents a possible 'outside of the box' answer to a question already formulated almost ten years ago, in a book. A question that, in turn, made references to an article published years ago: "Three years ago, an article entitled "The Hospital: Architecture and Technology" proposed a provocative question, asking an architect: why are Italian hospitals so 'ugly'?" (Palumbo and Giovenale, 2006).

The second meaning relates to the fact that here we are talking about a Plan that, as such, constitutes an instrument which addresses the later stages (design and construction) while, in reality, it possesses a specific orientation towards 'operational status' of the works, and is characterised as a strategic tool and, at the same time, a highly operational one. From here, along with other essential and very concrete aspects, which will be highlighted in the course of this work, the overall success of the Plan, in terms of implementation of the works and the deadlines set (construction sites and construction sites planned in 2003/2004 and funded for the next three years).

Regarding the first meaning, it appears that the Master Plan of Piacenza Hospital (published in October 2004) was a decisive moment of clarity within the long history of the Piacenza hospital. The overall objective of the Plan was, in fact, to combine the strategic vision of the local healthcare authority, as part of the city and the province of Piacenza, with concrete solutions towards critical issues and problems.

The introduction of "Conceptual References and an Operational Plan", relating to 'structural interventions as an essential condition for the development project of the hospital', included: "The design of a new hospital poses a dilemma every time: 'what shall prevail, architecture or functionality? ' It is a sensitive issue because in both cases the risk is a hospital devoid of all the qualities that should be specific. Only a truly multidisciplinary approach through a process of successive refinements to reach an excellent result is a compromise between the two requirements."

The answer: the cognitive framework, the planning criteria of the spaces and the overall functional reorganisation

The first answer (for the planning of a new hospital or the requalification of an existing one) to the dilemma whether architecture or functionality ought to prevail is certainly represented, in this case (and others) by the cognitive framework and the programming criteria regarding the outcome of the spaces, as a guide for the overall reorganisation of the functions.

The approach to the development of the Piacenza Hospital Plan was systemic in nature and is materialised, starting with the Strategic Plan and the Plan of Organisation (which allowed to determine the relationship between the principals and the territory) in the structural and organisational redevelopment of areas of the hospital, through the logic of the redefinition of the spaces into functional subsystems.

The entire complex was analysed through an in-depth study of the state of affairs of individual buildings, in particular, from the moment that we are dealing with a hospital that consists of different buildings that have appeared over time and have been gradually added to, losing sight of the overall design. The total design is immediately added to with certain individual functions and, above all, the adequacy or inadequacy of the buildings themselves in the performance of certain functions and the provision of certain services; in view of an overall plan that would guarantee maximum functionality.

To understand how the Piacenza hospital complex of is composed of a set of buildings, of different ages, and with functions that do not always relate to each other in an efficient way, with different vocations, dictated by the very structure of the buildings, as is what happens in many large hospital complexes (especially university hospitals); we must briefly retrace the evolution of the buildings, and of the city, since its origins.

The construction of Piacenza Hospital began in 1471 (foundation year) in which the first centre was constructed in the shape of a 'Greek cross', which is difficult to make out in the hospital's current state. Over time many changes have taken place, including the annexation, in 1818, of the former Olivetan Monastery of St. Sepulchre, improvements implemented within the urban development of the seventeenth - eighteenth century, the hospital complex of the Psychiatric Hospital etc.

Subsequently (XIX - XX century), major changes were made including the Pavilion former surgical hospital, the children's hospice, orthopedics pavilion, and the building of the Laboratory.

The most significant and noticeable transformation, which occurred over time is, probably, due to the construction of the poly surgeries building (1994). Later, a series of measures were also implemented, dictated primarily by the state of emergency, the urgent need for restructuring and adjustment, as frequently occurs in the history of hospitals.

One decisive aspect has been the awareness that together all of buildings demand a single area with two complexes divided by the road Canton del Cristo and that such an aspect was particularly significant not only in the reorganisation of the overall design, but also regarding the functionality of spaces, the system accesses and paths.

Within this complex and detailed framework, criteria for the strategic planning of the spaces were:
- the centrality of the user;
- the productive concept of space: functionality and functionalisation;
- the rationalisation of the distributive function;
- the accessibility of services;
- qualification of the assets.

These criteria have guided the entire development of the Plan and, above all, were the keys to the reorganisation of the entire hospital system in macro areas (Fig.1).

The need to identify these subsystems in the overall reorganisation was dictated by the need to make the entire complex clear and readable.

The rationalisation of the distribution scheme, through the articulation into seven main areas (medical; surgical and emergency; outpatient clinical activities; mental health; clinical pathology; training) was revised in parallel with the reorganisation of the system of accessibility and traffic in order to differentiate concrete paths for groups of users and facilitate travel within the complex.

Specifically, with regard to the medical area, the renovation of historical pavilions and the creation of a new square (which we will return to later), the transfer of medical functions from the polysurgical building made it possible to create a hospital within a hospital, consisting of the inpatient unit, day hospital, outpatient services and endoscopy departments of medicine, geriatrics, nephrology, pulmonology and gastroenterology, along with dedicated reception points.

In parallel, regarding the surgical and emergency areas, all surgery activities and the entire emergency area (previously located in two different locations) have been moved together to the polysurgical building.

Regarding the macro-area of outpatient clinical activities, in an attempt to overcome the high existing fragmentation, the diagnostic and therapeutic outpatient ambulatory external activities were previously concentrated in a renovated and refurbished pavilion historically used for inpatients. This is now considered to be unsuitable to adequately accommodate the functionality of a hospital stay.

As for the macro area of mental health, which territorially has a great tradition in terms of answers to specific needs, it is expected that this unit will find home in a building called 'Villa Speranza'. This will contain patient beds and the psychiatric residency for intensive treatments, as well as a single pole for emergency psychiatric, while the outpatient functions will be located in the building overlooking Via Campagna. Obviously, in a framework which includes restructuring already in place and others planned for the following years, to be carried out in due course, it also provides quality spaces devoted to mental health, with different levels of performance.

Regarding the macro-area of training, the plan is to adapt the Saint Sepulchre building, an Olivetan cloister (where training took place during the plan processes). These two buildings will be adapted to the modern training needs. This will include adapting the existing ones and creating brand new spaces specially dedicated to training, assuming that such activities would grow over time.

One of the highly strategic guiding criteria, which certainly has been crucial to the success of the reorganisation of inpatient stay, was to give priority to patient management and interdisciplinary collaboration for service management.

In this sense, starting with the cognitive framework of detail, the allocation of space was made taking into account functional particularities; from hypothesised flexible standard solutions that would promote the best conditions of comfort and, at the same time, facilitate the efficiency and the productivity of the service.

In this sense, the main objective was to overcome the concept of space aggregation in a personalised way (as often happens in the reorganisation of functional areas of the hospital or in the design from scratch), assuming a functional and productive space concept, congruent with current organisational needs and the use of instrumental resources.

An answer: hospitality, orientation, minority groups' needs

One of the fundamental guidelines for the strategic planning of the spaces - the centrality of the user - has been converted into specific areas: the subsystem of hospitality; orientation; concentration on minority groups' needs.

In particular, the attention to hospitality and reception was reflected in the overall reorganisation, creating services including:

- the one-stop shop system aiming to unify the functions of the Local Healthcare Authority for the citizens;
- reception points, both to fulfil the tasks of information, acceptance of outpatient booking, medical bills payment etc., and the general tasks of information and booking of all the various services provided in other places by the Healthcare Authority;
- the waiting areas and refreshment points; informal areas closely integrated and relating to healthcare functions; these are increasingly important elements in contemporary reality in order to provide quality services;
- hotel services, a strong focus on comfort, and patient and visitor confidentiality. These services have been created, in particular, through the organisation of recovery areas endowing them with hotel standards, which nowadays are indispensable.

Regarding orientation, major attention was dedicated to the functional complexity and the different categories of users in terms of modes of use, outlining clear and recognisable routes, as well as spaces of where different functions integrate with each other through unifying elements.

Regarding focusing on the most vulnerable groups, we must emphasise how specific categories of citizens were identified and recognised as the users whose needs must inspire the design, to determine specific choices both in terms of redefining the intended use and reworking the distribution patterns. An emblematic example in this sector, is the creation of the 'Women's Health Center'.

It is a building situated within the general area of the Piacenza Hospital of, in the north-west of the city, a building built in the early thirties. The organisational-functional configuration lent itself to allow clear identification of distinct paths, with separate expectations, with different information points, to ensure targeted responses to the actual needs of different nature, closely related to distinct phases of women's health.

The best answer is: the hospital as a place where citizens should be able to meet

One of the key elements of the Piacenza Master Plan, regarding the actions on the scale of a hospital complex, was the conceptual guideline (anticipated at the beginning) of the hospital as an 'urban site' that can foster a sense of belonging to the community and represent perceptions, and feelings related to the site being part of the city.

Very often, the hospitals made up of so-called 'pavilions' are presented as separate sites throughout the city. Typically, they are formed of isolated blocks or sectors that have lost all the connotations of urban sites and sense of identity with respect to the territory.

The Piacenza Hospital was also configured as an isolated facility, with further elements of separation and fracture inside: between the older and the newer parts.

Unlike other projects of preliminary design and reorganisation of a hospital complex, in the Piacenza Master Plan particular attention was paid to outdoor spaces, the reorganisation of the system in terms of its viability and liveability as a place of citizenship, taking due account of the profound changes that have occurred in the understanding of the management and development of land and therefore of hospital premises.

This included, to some extent, a task of recognising the importance of shared vision of the hospital, in the broadest, contemporary sense, focusing on the lives of citizens, the identity of the place in the urban context. Another inherent aspect was overcoming the approach according to which a hospital, due to its major function, is often considered as a 'bad', 'ugly' place (as we have mentioned in the question posed at the start), not liveable, especially regarding its outdoor spaces.

The overall effort was to reconstruct a process of reappropriation, focused on outdoor areas of the hospital sector, outside of the formal rules and institutional codes.

In fact, the prevailed consideration was that of a hospital as an opportunity for the local community to meet.

Basic elements of intervention under the Plan which led to a major transformation in this sense were: the reorganisation of the vehicle and pedestrian traffic system within the complex; the return of the green spaces; the creation or reconstruction, in terms of recovery, of equipped outdoor areas and aggregation points.

In particular, a key point in the reorganisation of access paths and internal roads was to regulate access, in order to reduce the inconvenience to users, visitors, staff,

by the following means:
- the placement of Cantone del Cristo road (which, as mentioned earlier, divides the Hospital into two complexs) and the construction of a new access system with guards and supervision services;
- the reorganisation of the parking system;
- the reorganisation of vehicle and pedestrian circulation system, including planning of a protected walkway;
- the rationalisation of internal routes (both overground for general public and underground designed to ensure internal flows and logistics support (transport of food, medicines, linen).

Regarding the reorganisation of the system of movement and paths, the redevelopment has been particularly focused on the restoration of pedestrian walkways in the various routes, with attention to identify different types of flooring, with great attention to the particular surrounding buildings, thus also trying to exploit the routes that form a part of historic building heritage inside the hospital complex (Fig.2).

Regarding the 'protected' walkway, it was planned as a route starting from authorised access areas and crossing the entire complex. In this sense, the goal was to recreate an internal path between the two cloisters (St. Sepulchre and S. Maria della Campagna), while also providing the redevelopment of the green areas and walkways among them. It's a route that, in its prefiguration, is intended to cross the entire complex and that continue beyond it. The attempt, in this sense, was to re-integrate the facility in the surrounding urban fabric, giving a sense of identity to the hospital site and, simultaneously, to the city: the historical and architectural values in the hospital complex.

Regarding the recovery of the identity of the green spaces, I must say that over the years, mainly due to the succession of the buildings inside the complex, the designers have increasingly failed to give due attention and consideration to the outdoor areas and to make them sufficiently green.

In this regard, the work started from an analysis of the planimetric the hospital complex of the 1930s, which still showed an obvious and clear layout of the green areas. We looked at their design, especially in terms to the gardens and flower beds present, and the turf with trees and shrubs.

Based on this analysis the mapping of areas was redefined, restoring lawns and flower beds and creating new green areas.

The decisive aspect was the study and the subsequent realisation of equipped outdoor areas (Fig.3) and aggregation points within the hospital complex, starting from the identification of three subsystems used for these purposes.

The first subsystem has been identified as the 'square' to be created as the linking element between the old hospital and the newest one, near the polysurgical building.

The second subsystem has been located in the open space in which the ramp was placed, leading to the underground link.

The third subsystem was the green area enclosed (absolutely not valued) between parts of the Medicine building. This area was planned to be restored as a green space, with attention to the pre-existing plantings.

The Plan also defined an element of originality regarding the creation and reconstruction of equipped outdoor areas: 'The water element as the Ariadne's thread': placement of fountains and pathways between different areas of the complex, using the element of water as a way to trace the linking routes. The water element, in addition, was also used as a symbolic element pointing to the notion of an exchange between 'life' and 'health'. In this sense, were also provided with elements of street furniture for the stop, integrated with the new system of relationships created.

A further objective was to create places that facilitated the meeting and communion of people, promoting a positive sharing in the hospital as a place where all users, but also in general the users of the public spaces in between the buildings, could share emotions, thoughts, experiences, in a historic part of town.

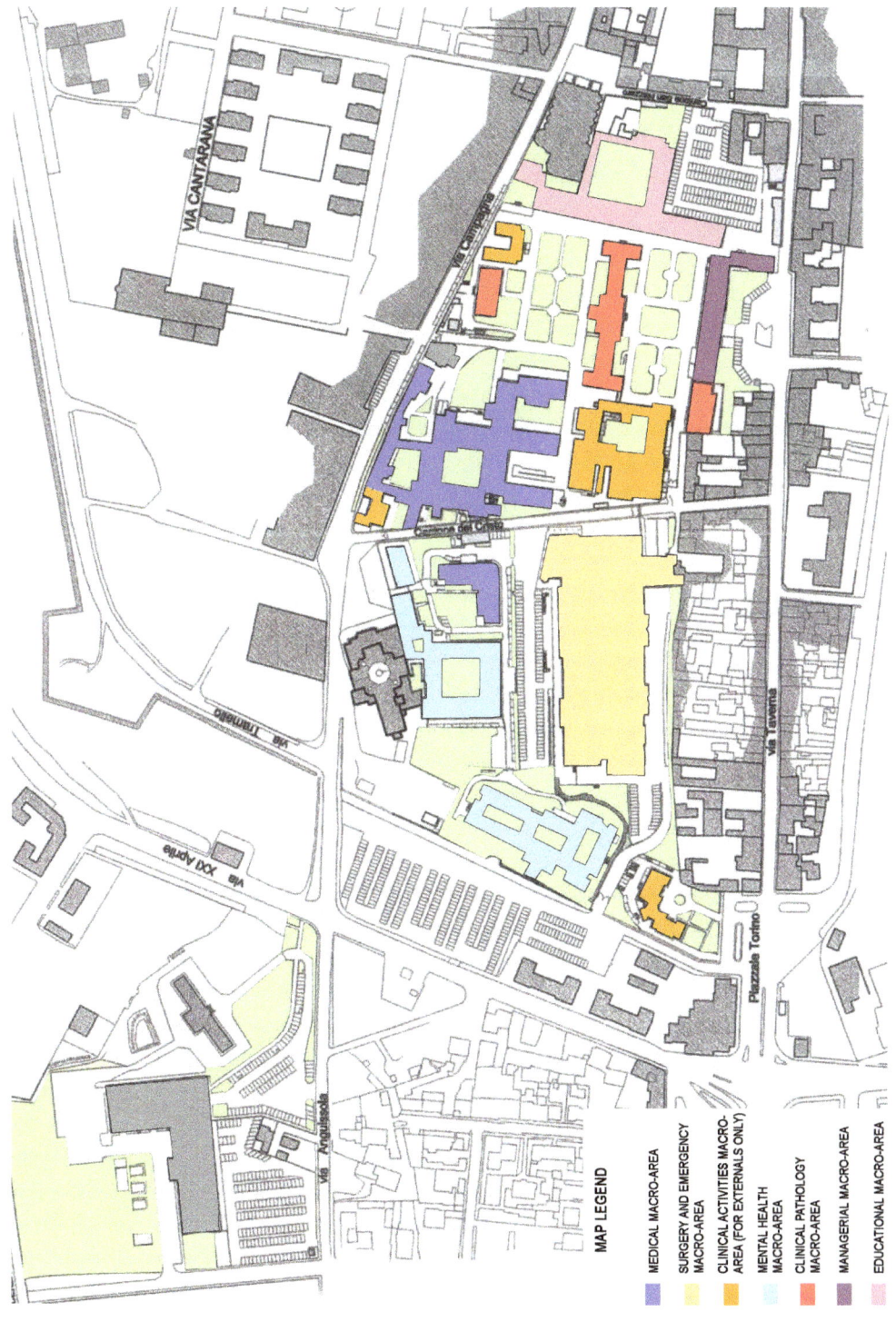

Figure 1: Hospital system: the macro areas

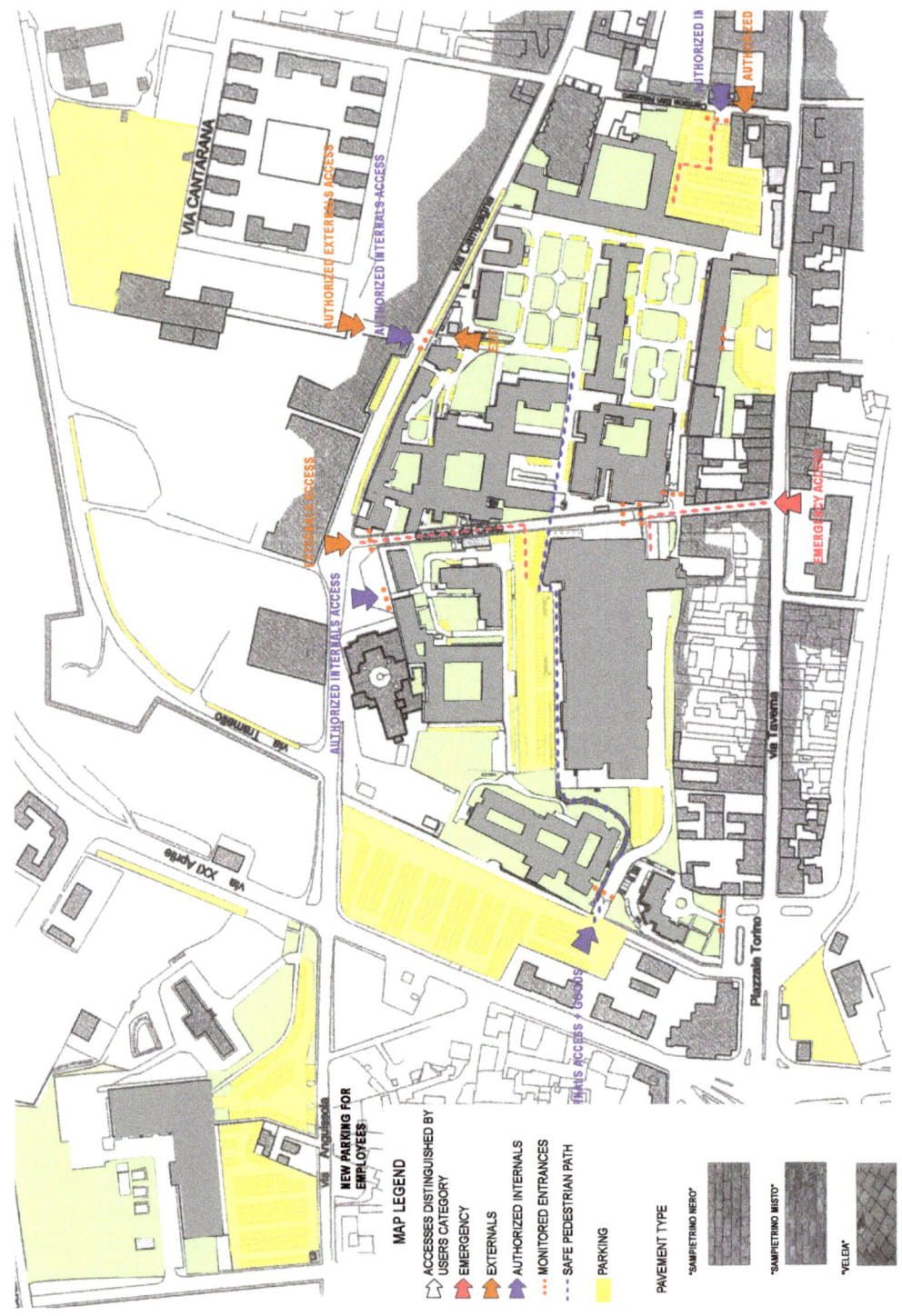

Figure 2: Restoration of pedestrian walkways

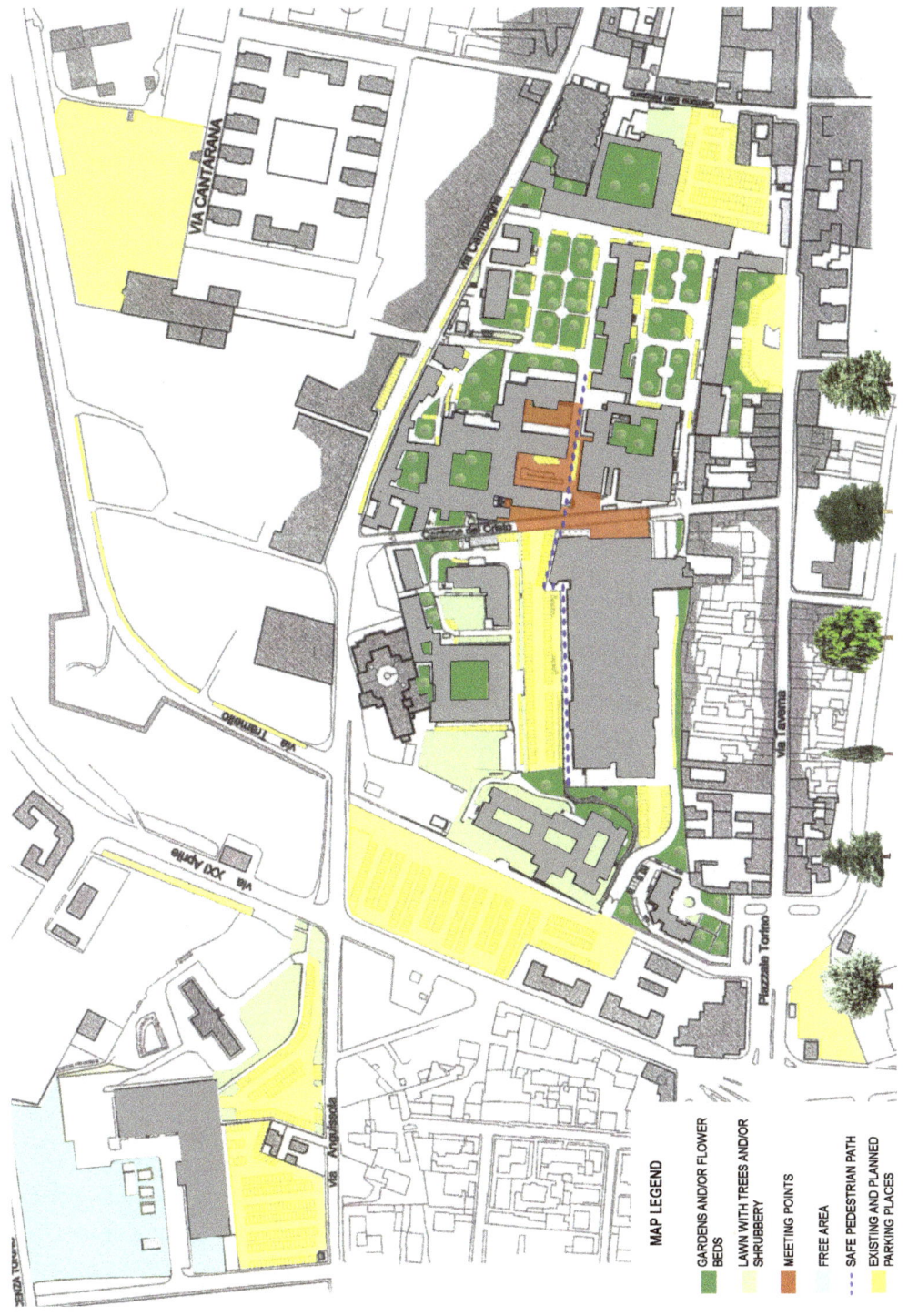

Figure 3: Equipped outdoor areas

A Plan aimed at feasibility

The Master Plan of the Piacenza Hospital of consists of 19 operations, with different levels of complexity.

As mentioned in the introduction, a key feature was that the Master Plan had been, from the beginning, strongly oriented to operational status and in this sense it obviously dedicated a great amount of attention to all the conditions, during the development and implementation phases, to assure that all building operations were implemented.

The fact that a programming tool, since the formulation of the criteria for reorganisation of space, sets itself a goal of the construction and use of the works, with precise schedules and costs, gives singularity to the instrument and shall give reasons for the success in terms of implementation.

In particular, in the organisation of the Master Plan itself, the second part was divided into dealing with the outstanding issues in 2003/2004, and that relating to construction sites planned and funded for the next three years.

For each work stage, regardless of the level of complexity, data sheets were organised which reported: the location of the operation, the time frame for completion, the problems that the intervention would solve, the expected results.

Regarding the planning of the times and costs, whereas all planned works have been realised, some with small margins of deviation from what was expected, it should be reported that all the critical moments and elements of internal consistency have been considered as much as possible in the scope of every single intervention and in the general scope of work, taking into account the highly critical aspects due to the period of construction site alongside the need to not interrupt the hospital service.

I would also like to point out that the work stages were supported by strict funding frameworks that were constantly monitored.

Regarding this last point, it should be noted that to implement the Plan, a monitoring system was developed, articulated for each process step, such as to constitute a dynamic database shared by different operating units of the Company, updated on a quarterly basis.

With regard to the monitoring system, the part relating to the programming phase has taken into consideration: objectives, functions, program budget, chief officer of the procedure, the estimated time for completion; the part relating to the design stage: the state of design, approval dates for the next stage, the estimated time for completion of the design, procurement procedures, professionals responsible for specialisations, opinions and approvals; the part relating to the implementation: procedures for contracting work, contracted companies, dates (planned and actual) related to procedures and, above all, dates for the actual construction.

At the completion of each data sheet a summary was issued containing: the priority level of each work stage, the improvement in terms of security, the impact on credit, tasks identified for the next steps, updates.

In conclusion, I can say that it was an integrated and comprehensive plan, a collaboration of all the professionals involved and the necessary specialisations, and this was crucial to building the synergy needed to make feasible a programming tool.

References

Giovenale A.M. (2006), "Quando la centralità dell'utente non è solo un assunto teorico", in Il Sole 24 ore, Aziende/territorio, 5-11 dicembre 2006, Rome, IT.

Palumbo R. e Giovenale A.M. (2006), "I criteri di progettazione: un futuro che viene dal passato", in Serarcangeli, C. (Ed.), Il Policlinico Umberto I. Un secolo di storia, Casa Editrice Università degli Studi di Roma "La Sapienza", Roma, pp. 27-36.

Scarpelli F. e Romano A. (edited by) (2011), Voci della città. L'interpretazione dei territori urbani, Carocci, Roma.

Anna Maria Giovenale

09

**Barriers between hospital and city:
Seven Italian case studies**

Francesca Giofrè

Abstract: This paper discusses the relationship between the city and big university hospitals in the Italian context. Using the data provided by the national statistics system of the Italian Ministry of Health, seven Italian university hospital complexes with more than 950 beds were selected. Drawing on the analysis of seven Italian hospital complexes using the computer software Google Earth Pro, the paper offers insights on the city context, the types of barriers separating the hospital from the city and other relevant data such as the percentage of open and built surfaces, systems of access to the hospital and the number of employees. The aim of the analysis is to offer a reading, also photographic, of the current situation of hospital complexes and their relationships with the city and to analyse the data collected in order to understand the redevelopment potential of the external spaces of the hospital complexes.

Keywords: hospital complex, university hospital, city, quantitative data.

Introduction

In Italy, around a quarter of hospitals are housed in historical buildings built before 1900 (Inail, 2012). The hospitals, once built outside populated areas for hygiene reasons, over time have become fully integrated into the urban contexts, becoming an integral part of them. Of the different types of hospitals, large hospital complexes, such as university hospitals, qualify as cities within cities insofar as they occupy large areas of land. A high flow of people, goods and services cross the boundaries of the hospital complex on a daily basis generating an osmotic process between the outside, the city and the inside, the hospital and its surroundings.

These hospital complexes on account of their year of construction, location and typology, often have architectural, structural and plant restrictions that affect how they operate and the availability of spaces and services. The necessary adaptation and expansion of the hospital complexes in order to meet new demands linked to the health needs of the reference population and the advancement of innovations in the various fields of medicine, as well as innovations in management and sustainability innovations, are very costly and difficult.

In Italy the possibility of using some of these hospital complexes for other functions and creating new ones in more accessible areas of the city with fewer restrictions – the Policlinico Umberto I in Rome is a case in point – has been debated several times, but today these hospitals in any case represent an almost unavoidable point of reference for the citizens. These hospitals are an integral part of the evolutionary history of the urban fabric in the city, and, through their typology, they tell the story of the development of medical practice and form part of the collective memory of citizens.

The analysis presented has two objectives.

1. Firstly, to analyse the relationship existing between the lot of the hospital complex and the surrounding constructed fabric by identifying the form of its border, namely the type of barriers that separate the hospital from the urban fabric.

2. Secondly, to photograph the situation of big Italian hospitals incorporated into urban contexts in terms of typologies and dimensions in order to understand the quantity and quality of the open spaces and their potential.

Seven case studies of public hospitals with different legal statuses under Italian law were selected: Hospital, University Hospital, General Hospital, and Scientific Institute for Research, Hospitalization and Health Care. Inside the hospitals, insofar as general hospitals, in addition to diagnosis and treatment functions research and training activities are also carried out. The catchment area is the health authority of reference up to regional level, but the hospitals also accept patients from all over Italy. (*)

Methodology

The type of research used in this study is quantitative research. The following methodology is used.

Choice of hospitals. Hospital complexes with more than 950 beds were selected using the latest data provided by the National Statistics System of the Italian Ministry of Health (2011). Through the computer system, data useful for the purposes of the investigation was collected on: the number of personnel, employed by both the national health service and the university, the number of admissions and the average number of days spent in hospital. It is necessary to point out that the number of employees indicated does not include those employed by cooperatives or other organizations, visitors, etc., as this data is difficult to obtain. For the number of outpatient admissions reference was made, where possible, to the data indicated on the website of the facilities being studied.

The data on the regional population and the cities was obtained through the GeoDemo system of the National Institute of Statistics (2013, ISTAT).

The data on the redevelopment works or new constructions started in the last 15 years was collected from information obtained on the websites of the hospitals or other sources mentioned.

Typologies and dimensions. Using the computer software Google Earth Pro, which allows the use of advanced measurements tools, each hospital selected was identified and photographed (1) by a satellite at a height of 1.55 km from the ground, with north in the same position. Using Google Earth Pro a reconstruction was made of all the profiles of the lots and individual buildings and the following data and information was calculated and obtained.

- Access systems: emergency department, pedestrians and vehicles.
- Types of barriers on the perimeter of the lot, classified as: high wall (max. height 2.50 m.), high wall with railings, high wall with sound barriers; building front; low wall (max. height 1.80 m.), low wall with railings and mesh, low wall with mesh, low wall with handrail; mesh; guard rail; sound barriers; concrete bollards.
- Dimensional data of the lot: covered and uncovered areas; park areas; areas used for uncovered parking; construction site areas on the surface.
- Where deemed necessary, some information was taken from a reading of the municipal master plans.

For each case study, in order of geographical location from the north to the south of Italy, the obtained and processed data and information are given.

Case Studies: University Hospitals

Seven Italian cases:
- Santa Maria della Misericordia Hospital in Udine (Region: Friuli Venezia Giulia) University Hospital;
- Niguarda Ca'Granda Hospital, Milan (Region: Lombardy), Hospital;
- San Martino Hospital in Genoa (Region: Liguria). Scientific Institute for Research, Hospitalization and Health Care. University Hospital. National Institute for Cancer Research;
- Sant'Orsola Malpighi Hospital in Bologna (Region: Emilia Romagna). University Hospital;
- Careggi Hospital, Florence (Region: Tuscany). University Hospital;
- Sant'Orsola Malpighi Hospital in Bologna (Region: Emilia Romagna). University Hospital;
- Umberto I Hospital, Rome (Region: Lazio). General Hospital;
- Bari Hospital (Region: Puglia). General Teaching Hospital.

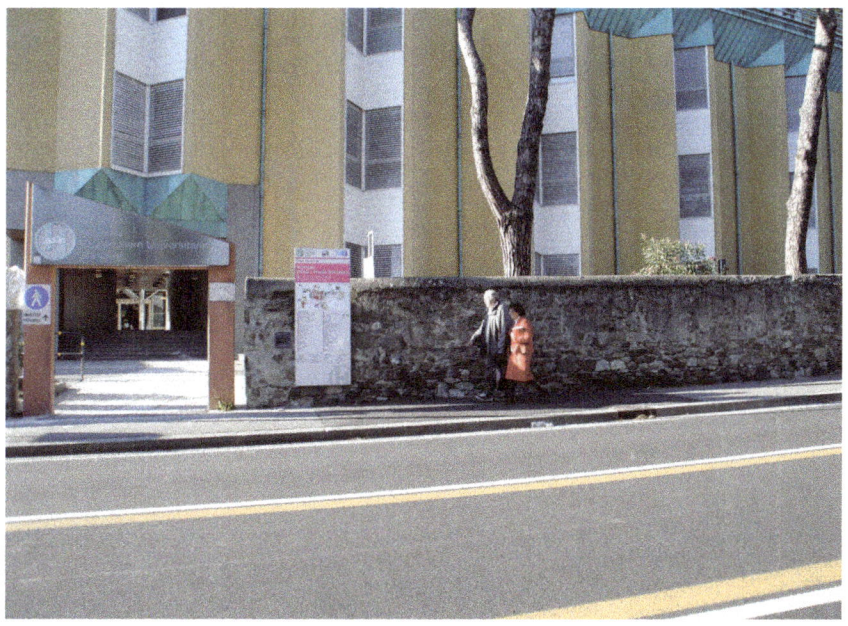

Figure 1-2: Barriers/entrances Careggi Hospital, Florence, Italy (above) and barriers/entrances Umberto I, Hospital, Rome Italy (below)

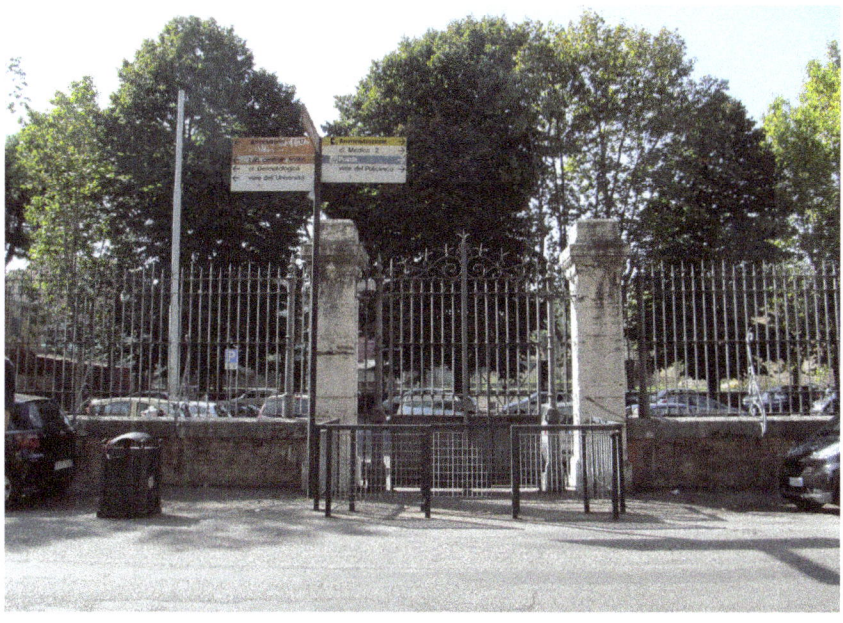

Santa Maria della Misericordia Hospital in Udine (Region: Friuli Venezia Giulia) University Hospital

Region: 1,221,860 inhabitants.

City of Udine: 98,780 inhabitants.

The start of construction of the hospital complex on the current lot dates to the first half of the 1920s, with a separate buildings (pavilions) typology.

The hospital complex is located just outside the edge of this historical centre, in the northern part of the city. The hospital lot borders on all sides with predominantly semi-intensive residential areas. To the north there is a large green area pertaining to the hospital lot; there are four parking areas in strategic positions with respect to the entrances.

The types of barriers detected are: high wall, low wall with railing or handrail, mesh and guard rail.

The total area of the lot is 37,2560 sq m, of which 28,200 sq m are construction site areas and 51,400 sq m are park land. Excluding the construction site areas, 21% is occupied by built areas and 79% by open areas.

The municipal master plan indicates a building of great architectural interest and one of typological interest within the lot.

The hospital currently has 937 beds and 3,696 employees. The hospital handles 30,312 admissions per year and the annual average ordinary hospitalization period is 9.2 days.

Redevelopment works on the hospital complex have been underway since 2002. The works affect different areas within the lot and a total of 900 beds will be reallocated to the new facilities (http://www.ospedaleudine.it/). The main building was opened in January 2013 and has a capacity of 300 beds. The process of upgrading the entire complex also includes turning a large surface area into spaces with greenery.

Figure 3: Santa Maria della Misericordia Hospital in Udine
The acquisition date: 01/05/2012. Position: 46°04'42.85"N 13°13'41.99"E.

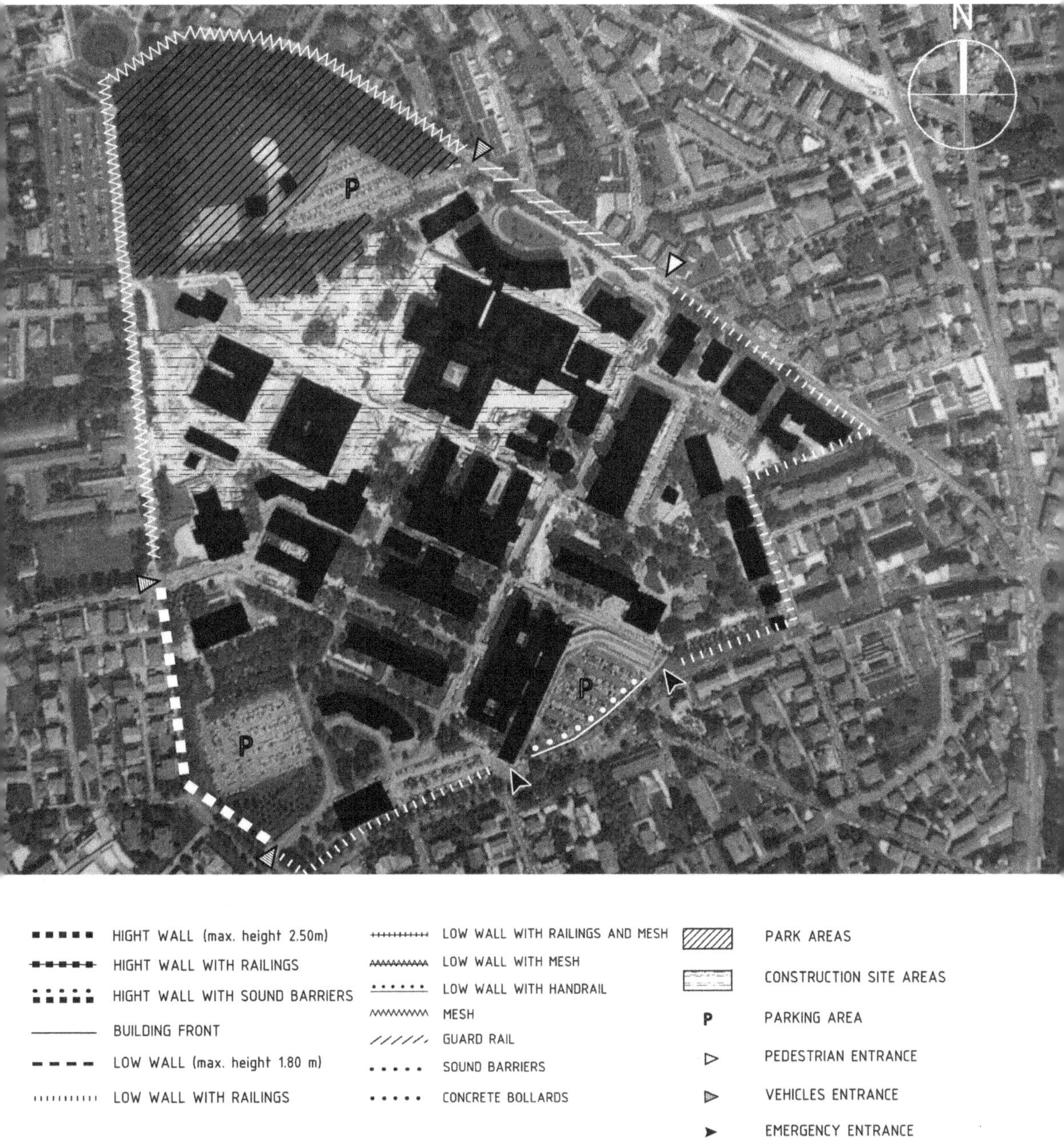

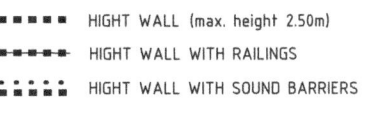

Niguarda Ca'Granda Hospital, Milan (Region: Lombardy), Hospital

Region: 9,794,525 inhabitants.

City of Milan (regional capital): 1,262,101 inhabitants.

The start of construction of the hospital complex on the current lot dates to the early 1930s, with a multi-block typology.

The hospital is located beyond the Milan ring road, in the area defined as the North Park. The lot is on the eastern side and located in a semi-intensive residential area with services. There are parking areas pertaining to the lot.

There are two types of barriers surrounding the hospital lot: a high wall with sound barriers in some stretches and a low wall with railing, and cement bollards. The total area of the lot is 334,712 sq m of which 33% of the surface is built on and 67% is open.

The hospital has 1,052 beds and 3,895 employees. The hospital handles 31,582 admissions per year and the annual average ordinary hospitalization period is 10.4 days. There is an estimated daily flow of 9,000 people including workers, patients, relatives, suppliers, representatives and others (http://www.ospedaleniguarda.it/).

The hospital complex has undergone and is subject to redevelopment works through the demolition of some historical buildings and the renovation of those that have restrictions placed on them by the Sovrintendenza per i Beni Architettonici (Architectural Heritage Office). Works on the South Block were completed in 2010. The South Block is dedicated to high care, namely emergency medicine, highly specialized medicine and the treatment of patients in intensive care, and has 469 beds (ordinary inpatient wards, specialized inpatient wards, Day Hospital and Day Surgery). The last big project was started in 2011 for the construction of the North Block, dedicated to average intensity of care, basic specializations and the maternal and child health area. The North Block has 450 beds. The works were completed in 2013 and transfers from the other buildings are scheduled for the early months of 2015 (http://www.ospedaleniguarda.it/).

Figure 4: Niguarda Ca'Granda Hospital, Milan.
The acquisition date: 04/05/2014. Position: 45°30'34.42"N 9°11'16.44" E.

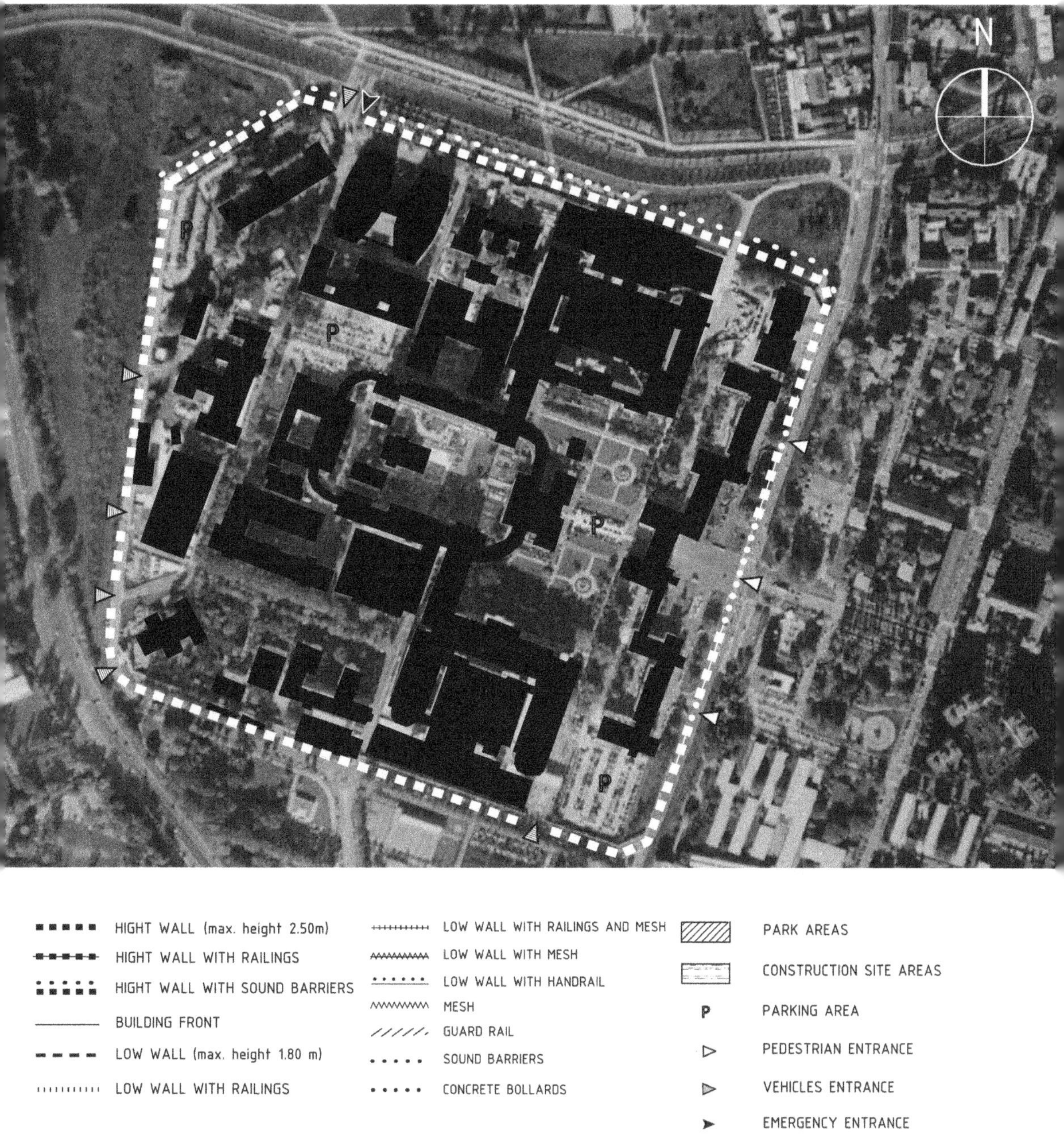

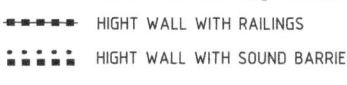

San Martino Hospital in Genoa (Region: Liguria).
Scientific Institute for Research, Hospitalization and Health Care.
University Hospital. National Institute for Cancer Research

Region: 1,565,127 inhabitants.

City (regional capital): 582,320 inhabitants.

The start of construction of the hospital complex on the current lot dates to the early 1900s, with a separate buildings (pavilions) typology.

The hospital is located in the central area of the city of Genoa, in the homonymous district of San Martino.

The area pertaining to the hospital complex (lots A, B, C) is incorporated within an intensive residential area.

The types of barriers surrounding the three hospital lots are: high wall also with mesh or railing; low wall with mesh and railing, and sound barriers.

The total area pertaining to the hospital is 374,103 sq m – lot A, 343,124 sq m; lot B, 14,032 sq m and lot C, 16,947 sq m – of which 21% of the surface is built on and 79% is open. It should be noted that the large green area to the north within the hospital area is on a slope and therefore cannot be used as a park.

The hospital has 1,345 beds and 4,803 employees. The hospital handles 41,171 admissions per year and the annual average ordinary hospitalization period is 10.2 days.

In 2004 the hospital announced a competition of ideas for the creation of a new hospital through the transformation of the facilities and the arrangement of the areas. The competition also provided for an increase in the number of beds to 1,500. The new functional reorganization of the settlement structure had to take into account the current configuration and the significance of the architectural, historical and environmental heritage of the hospital complex (http://www.hsanmartino.it/).

Figure 5: San Martino Hospital in Genoa.
The acquisition date: 04/05/2014. Position: 45°30'34.42"N 9°11'16.44" E.

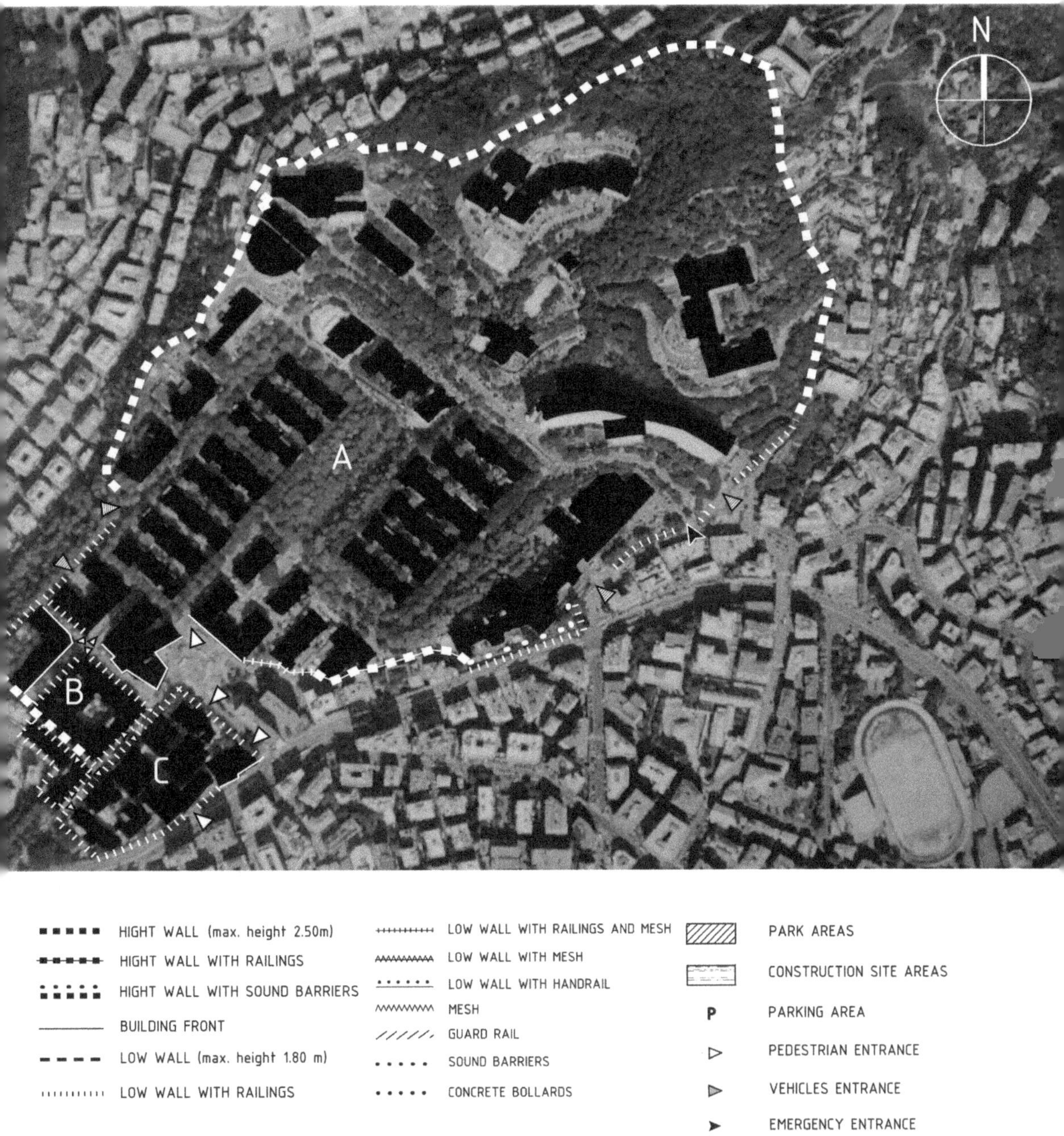

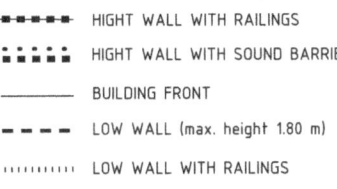

■ ■ ■ ■ ■ HIGHT WALL (max. height 2.50m)	++++++++ LOW WALL WITH RAILINGS AND MESH	▨ PARK AREAS
■●■●■● HIGHT WALL WITH RAILINGS	⋀⋀⋀⋀⋀ LOW WALL WITH MESH	▨ CONSTRUCTION SITE AREAS
⁞⁞⁞⁞⁞ HIGHT WALL WITH SOUND BARRIERS	⋯⋯⋯ LOW WALL WITH HANDRAIL	**P** PARKING AREA
─── BUILDING FRONT	⋀⋀⋀⋀⋀ MESH	▷ PEDESTRIAN ENTRANCE
─ ─ ─ LOW WALL (max. height 1.80 m)	////// GUARD RAIL	▷ VEHICLES ENTRANCE
⋅⋅⋅⋅⋅⋅⋅ LOW WALL WITH RAILINGS	• • • • SOUND BARRIERS	▶ EMERGENCY ENTRANCE
	• • • • CONCRETE BOLLARDS	

Sant'Orsola Malpighi Hospital in Bologna (Region: Emilia Romagna). University Hospital

Region: 4,377,487 inhabitants.

City (regional capital): 380,635 inhabitants.

The start of construction of the hospital complex on the current lot dates to the first half of the 1600s.

The hospital is located in the central area of the city of Bologna, immediately outside the ring road.

The area pertaining to the hospital (lots A, B, C) is incorporated within a residential area, mainly comprised of garden neighbourhoods. The types of barriers surrounding the three hospital lots are: high wall, building front, low wall also with railing or mesh, mesh.

The total area of the lots is 237,479 sq m – lot A, 193,553 sq m; lot B, 14,320 sq m and lot C, 29,606 sq m – of which 34% of the surface is built on and 65% is open.

Lot A, where most of the buildings are concentrated, is crossed by a cycle path and is marked by the presence of some buildings of historical and architectural interest (Municipal Structural Plan).

The hospital has a total of 1,651 beds and 5,429 employees.

The hospital handles 53,776 admissions per year and the annual ordinary average hospitalization period is around 7.9 days.

There is an estimated daily flow of 20,000 people including employees, university students and professors, patients, visitors and suppliers, etc., and over 3,000,000 specialist services for outpatients.

An underground car park was opened in 2002. From a reading of the 2010-2012 three-year streamlining plan of the hospital, there are various retrofitting and renovation works that affect various buildings of the hospital complex (http://www.aosp.bo.it).

Figure 6: Sant'Orsola Malpighi Hospital in Bologna.
The acquisition date: 01/06/2014. Position: 44°29'26.66"N 11°21'54.08" E.

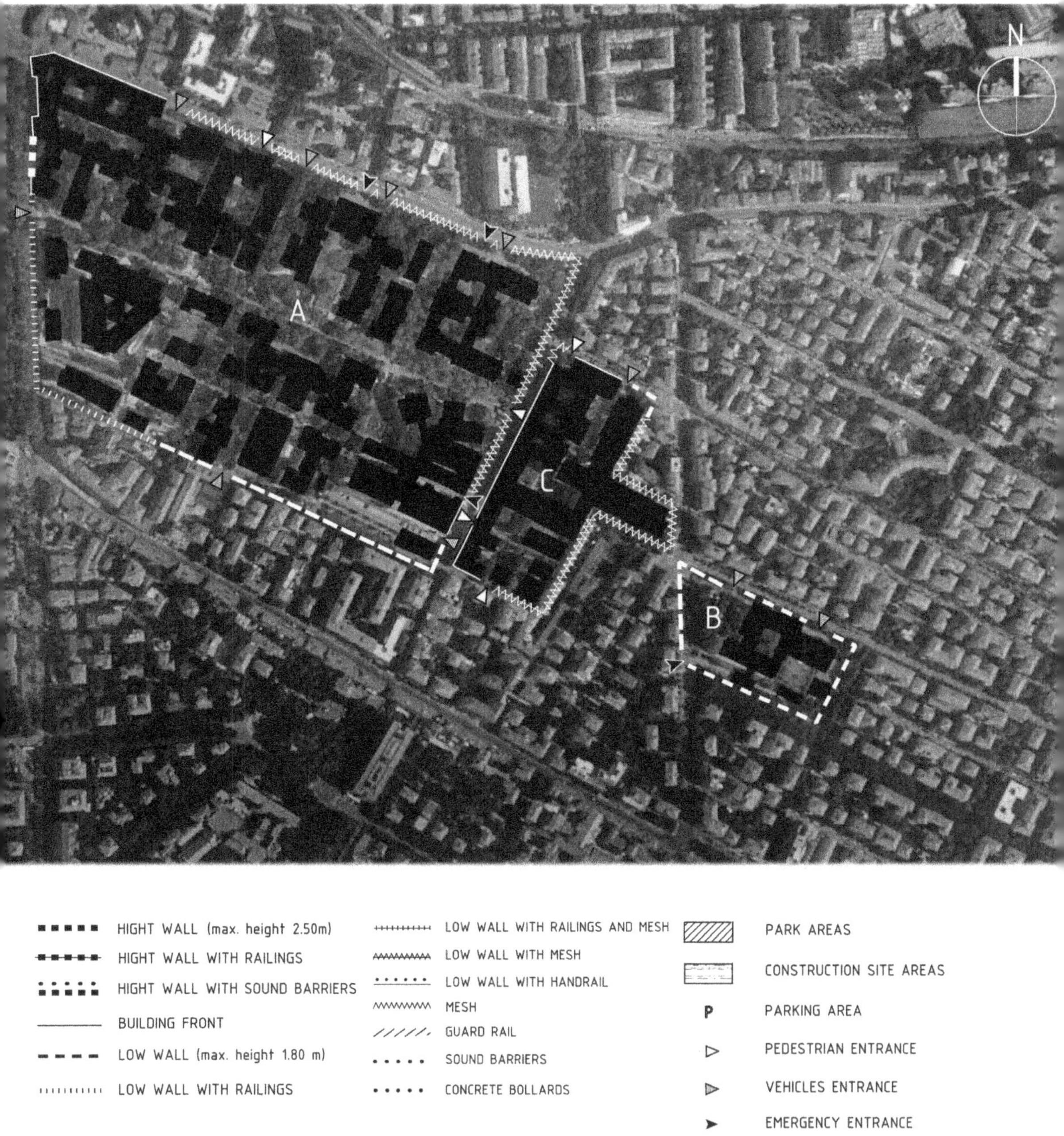

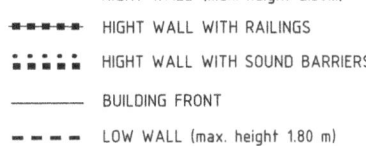

▪▪▪▪▪ HIGHT WALL (max. height 2.50m)	┼┼┼┼┼ LOW WALL WITH RAILINGS AND MESH	▨ PARK AREAS
▪●▪●▪● HIGHT WALL WITH RAILINGS	ᴧᴧᴧᴧᴧ LOW WALL WITH MESH	▭ CONSTRUCTION SITE AREAS
⁞⁞⁞⁞⁞ HIGHT WALL WITH SOUND BARRIERS	⋯⋯⋯ LOW WALL WITH HANDRAIL	
─── BUILDING FRONT	ᴡᴡᴡ MESH	P PARKING AREA
─ ─ ─ LOW WALL (max. height 1.80 m)	///// GUARD RAIL	▷ PEDESTRIAN ENTRANCE
⁞⁞⁞⁞⁞⁞⁞⁞ LOW WALL WITH RAILINGS	⋯⋯ SOUND BARRIERS	▷ VEHICLES ENTRANCE
	•••• CONCRETE BOLLARDS	▶ EMERGENCY ENTRANCE

Careggi Hospital, Florence (Region: Tuscany).
University Hospital

Region: 3,692,828 inhabitants.

City (regional capital): 366,039 inhabitants.

The start of construction of the hospital complex on the current lot dates to the first two decades of the twentieth century.

The hospital is located in a periphery area to the north of the city of Florence.

The area pertaining to the hospital complex (lots A, B, C) is incorporated on three sides within an intensive residential area and to the northeast there is a large green area where the Medici villa of Careggi is located.

There are parking areas pertaining to the lots.

The types of barriers surrounding the hospital lots are: high wall, building front, low wall, mesh.

The total area of the lots is 425,335 sq m – lot A, 336,284 sq m; lot B, 32,381 sq m and lot C, 56,670 sq m – 34% of the surface is built on and 66% is open.

The hospital has 1,329 beds and 5,744 employees.

The hospital handles 53,745 admissions per year and the annual average ordinary hospitalization period is 7.2 days. In 2012 there were an estimated 10,611,854 outpatient services for both inpatients and outpatients (http://www.aou-careggi.toscana.it/).

A variety of modernization works are underway which involve parts of the hospital complex.

Figure 7: Careggi Hospital, Florence.
The acquisition date: 01/10/2014. Position: 43°48'26.60"N 11°14'50.70" E

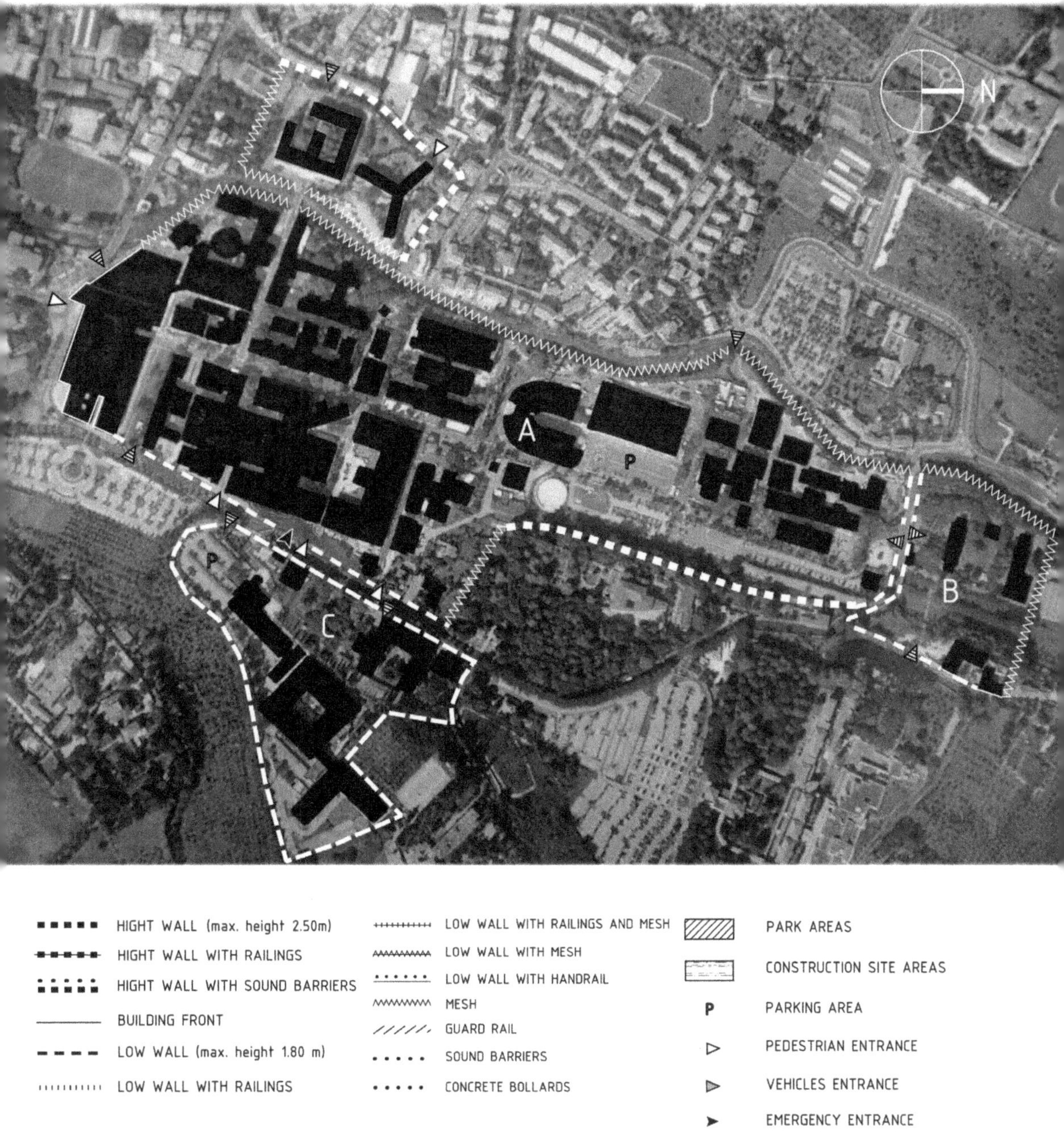

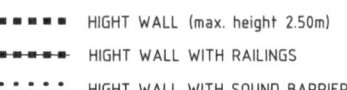

Umberto I Hospital, Rome (Region: Lazio). General Hospital

Region: 5,557,276 inhabitants.

City (regional and national capital): 2,638,842 inhabitants.

The start of construction of the hospital complex on the current lot dates to the end of the 1800s, with a separate buildings (pavilions) typology.

The hospital is located in the central part of the city of Rome, in the northeast area.

The lot is incorporated on four sides within a residential area with a predominance of services.

The types of barriers surrounding the hospital lot are: high wall also with railing, low wall also with railing.

The total area of the lot is 148,864 sq m, 45% of the surface is built on and 55% is open.

The hospital has 1,196 beds and 4,823 employees. The hospital handles 38,535 admissions per year and the annual average ordinary hospitalization period is 9.8 days.

There are an estimated two million outpatient services per year. A variety of modernization works are underway which involve parts of the hospital complex (http://www.policlinicoumberto1.it/).

Figure 8: Umberto I Hospital, Rome.
The acquisition date: 01/10/2014. Position: 41°54'24.15"N 12°30'53.06" E.

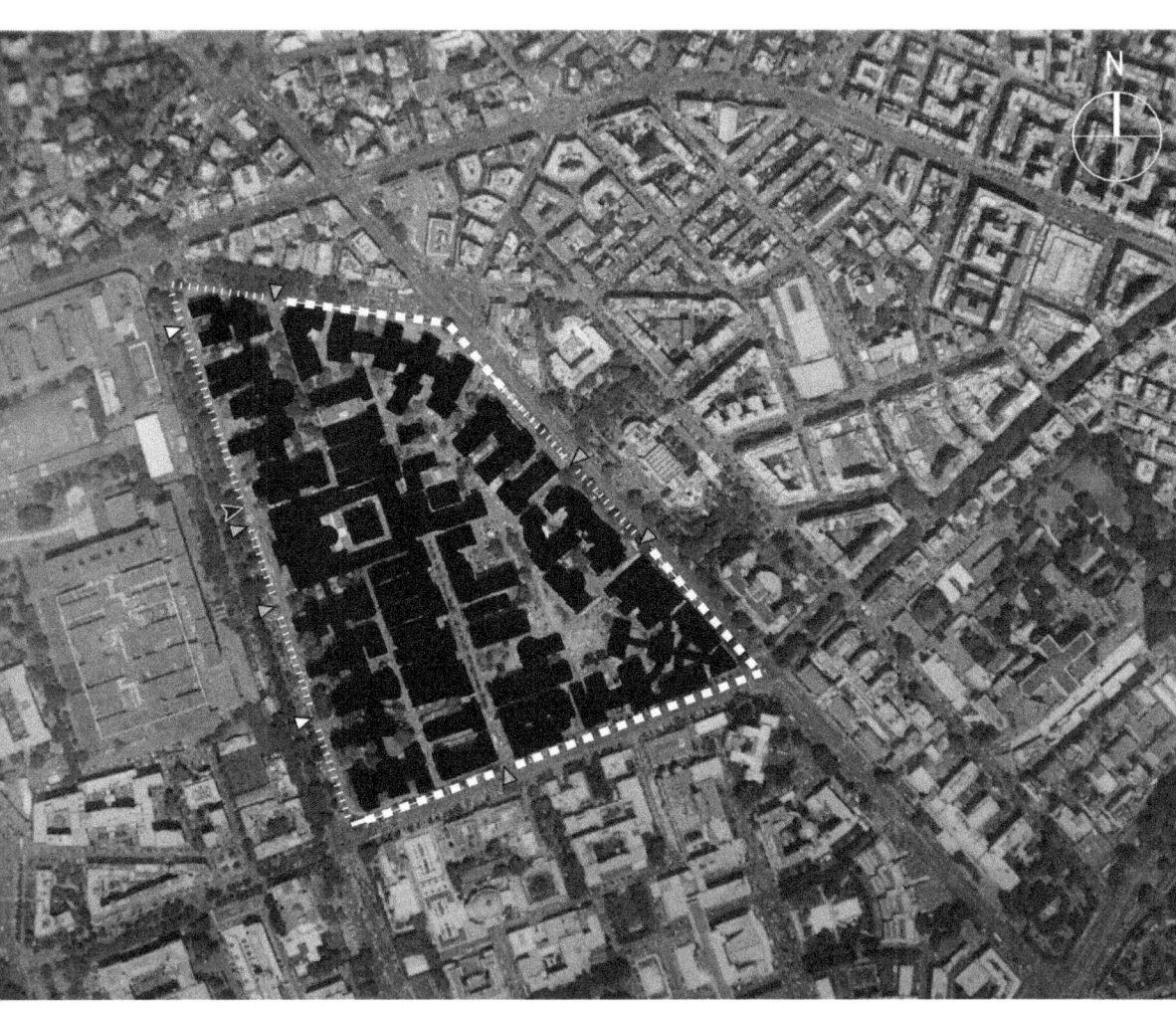

Bari Hospital (Region: Puglia). General Teaching Hospital

Region: 4,050,803 inhabitants.

City (regional capital): 313,213 inhabitants.

The start of construction of the hospital complex dates to the second half of the 1930s, with a multi-block typology.

The hospital is located in the central zone of the city of Bari, in the south area.

The lot is incorporated on four sides within a predominantly residential area with services.

The main entrance faces onto a large square.

The types of barriers surrounding the hospital lot are: high wall also with railing, low wall also with railing.

The total area of the lot is 2.1921 sq m, 32% of the surface is built on and 68% is open.

The hospital has 1,286 beds and 4,409 employees.

The hospital handles 48,888 admissions per year and the annual average ordinary hospitalization period is 7.4 days.

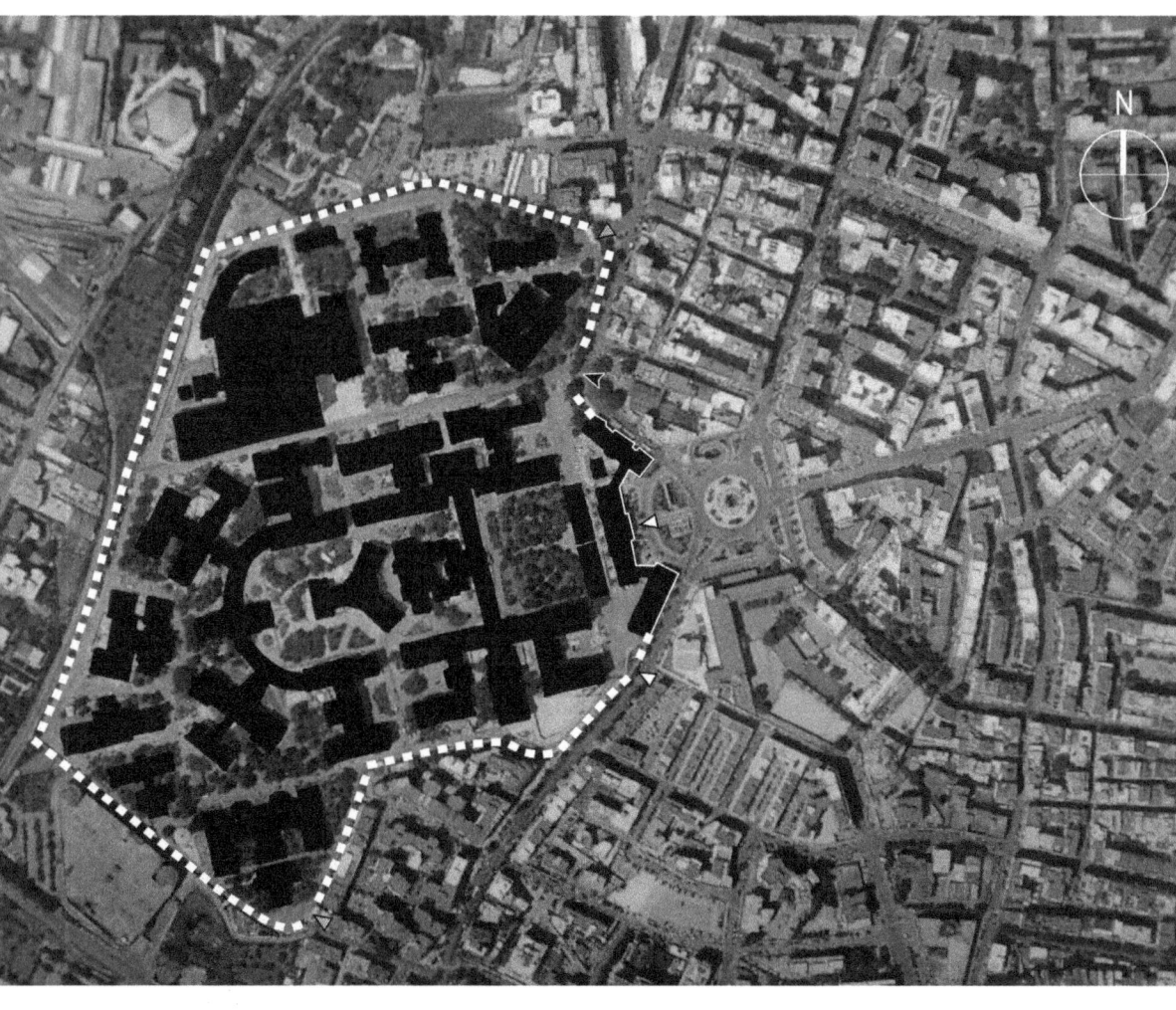

Figure 9: Bari Hospital.
The acquisition date: 01/10/2014. Position: 41°06'41.78"N 16°51'43.26" E

Final notes

From an analysis of the seven hospitals it is possible to draw the following conclusions.

- Location. The hospitals are currently situated in central or semi-central areas of the city, within building contexts that have consolidated over time.
- Typology. The initial architectural typology of the hospital complexes can still be partly recognized today in the distribution of the buildings. The architectural typology of the past is not always suitable for accommodating healthcare activities.
- Barriers. The hospital lots are all delimited by different types of barriers, which are disparate to each other. In some cases the problem of noise from the surrounding environment is resolved through sound barriers. Some barriers are permeable and allow the facility to be seen from the outside, creating a visual relationship with the city.
- Open spaces. The open spaces are treated as insignificant and are not integrated with the building structures or their activities. The hospitals, however, have great potential in terms of open spaces to be used as roads, pedestrian areas and green spaces.
- Users. The daily flow of people inside the hospitals is impressive (outpatients, visitors, suppliers, etc.), as is the number of healthcare workers employed. The average hospitalization period for inpatients varies from 10 to 7 days.
- Refunctionalization. The hospitals are all subject to constant redevelopment and expansion works.

Three aspects should be highlighted and reflected on: recovering dialogue with the city, the potential in terms of outdoor spaces pertaining to the hospital complexes, and the constant need for redevelopment and expansion works in the buildings.

The continuous redevelopment and expansion works denote the inherent difficulties of adapting such imposing hospital complexes to the new requirements of plants, equipment, security, hygiene, logistics, etc. The hospital complexes in fact become permanent construction sites within the city, with all the inconveniences that a construction site involves.

There are two ways forward that can be envisaged at theoretical level:
- seizing the opportunity of an important challenge, namely that of taking the three aspects highlighted above into consideration, simultaneously and with equal

importance, in order to construct a new identity for the hospital in the city and for the city over the long term;

- rethinking a new use for the hospital complexes, preserving their architectural qualities and transferring the ensemble of healthcare and research activities to other parts of the city.

The two alternatives are closely linked to healthcare policy decisions at national and regional level, a careful cost-benefit analysis, and town planning regulations. From a reading of what has occurred in Italy up until now, the flow of funding provided to the hospitals by different state bodies has not made it possible to implement long-term redevelopment strategies, but rather the carrying out of spot interventions on the individual buildings of the hospital complexes in the absence of an overall design strategy.

Notes

(*) Paper published in 2end International Multidisciplinary Scientific Conference on Social Sciences & Arts, SGEM 2015. 26 Aug - 01 Sept 2015, Albena, Bulgaria. Conference Proceedings Book n.4, pp.581-592.

(1) The image data varies in relation to the latest data acquired by satellite.

References

National Institute for Insurance against Accidents in the Workplace and Occupational Diseases (2012), Safety in the hospital, Inail: IT, available at http://www.inail.it/internet_web/wcm/idc/groups/internet/documents/document/ucm_portstg_114876.pdf (accessed 14 October 2014).

Italian Ministry of Health (2011), National Health Service Database, available at http://www.salute.gov.it/portale/documentazione/usldb/reguslDB.jsp (accessed 14 October 2014).

National Institute of Statistics (2013), Demographics in figures, Istat: IT, available at http://demo.istat.it/ (accessed 15 October 2014).

Santa Maria della Misericordia Hospital in Udine, http://www.ospedaleudine.it/

Niguarda Ca'Granda Hospital, Milan, http://www.ospedaleniguarda.it/

San Martino Hospital in Genoa, http://www.hsanmartino.it/

Sant'Orsola Malpighi Hospital in Bologna, http://www.aosp.bo.it/

Umberto I Hospital, Rome, http://www.policlinicoumberto1.it/

Francesca Giofrè

10

Image of a hospital city: Clinical center of Serbia

Ivana Miletić

"Technology must not dictate choices to us in our cities. We must learn to select modes of action from among the possibilities technology presents in physical planning" Maki, 2008, p.48

Abstract: The study presents the Clinical Center of Serbia, university hospital complex that spreads over more than 40 hectares on a prime city land of a capital city. Taking in consideration the particular historical background of the context as well as very actual theme of re-urbanizing hospitals and need to reinvent their relation to the city, open spaces within the Clinical Center are observed in terms of the urban environment, its structure and the public image they create. Identifying and structuring of the environment is carried out following basic elements of city form (Lynch, 1990): enclosure and permeability in relation to the city and its inner structure- districts, paths, anchor points and landmarks. The result is a very varied and confusing conglomeration that passed through different social systems and therefore constantly changes its organization, methods of management and urban planning with significant repercussions on physical layout.

Keywords: city, hospital, permability-enclosure, identity, environment.

Introduction

ID of Clinical Center of Serbia

The Clinical Center of Serbia (CCS) is the major of four clinical centers in republic of Serbia (1). It is located in capital city of Belgrade and as a referent medical institution of tertiary (2) level provides highly specialized diagnosis and treatment with the catchment area that includes the whole state. The CCS is also a medical research center and teaching base of the Faculty of Medicine, University of Belgrade providing undergraduate and post-graduate medical education and development.

The University Hospital complex of CCS in the central city core presents a city within a city: with its own population and working rhythm it has great implications both in the immediate and in the wider environment. Its permanent inhabitants are the employees - about 7000 staff of which 4700 is medical, and students of medicine with 500 enrolled every year. The temporary inhabitants are presented through 880 000 ambulance patients and more than 90 000 admissions (almost 50% of all admissions in Belgrade).

The CCS with 3600 hospital beds is one of the biggest in Europe, covering about 43 % of city capacity (10% of state capacity) (Miletić, 2008). Within the hospital 50 000 surgeries and 7000 births are carried out each year, while in Day Hospitals annually are treated 25000 patients and more than 5000 surgeries (Klinički centar Srbije, 2013).

Currently consists of 41 organizational units: 23 clinics, 9 centers, 1 Polyclinic and 9 facilities for service activities. The CCS complex is a pavilion type with scattered villas distributed over an area of about 44 hectares and compromising of more than 60 buildings with total gross area of 280 000 sqm (idem).

This form of fragmented hospital organization with numerous scattered departments provokes a substantial increasing of costs on the running of the hospital system. As a result, there is the wasteful duplication of expensive services and equipment, duplicating work force and the area itself is twice as large compared to a modern teaching hospital center of this type (Euro Health Group Denmark, 2004).

Barely more than a quarter is actually built area. Green spaces occupy almost 40% of the area, while for vehicular roads is reserved 20%, parking areas about 7% , only

10% remained in total for pedestrians, their sidewalks, lanes, access areas, squares ext. (Miletić, 2008) (Fig. 1).

The hospital buildings inside the CCS have undergone various changes over time thanks to organizational changes of the Center, often change of destination of use, as well as need to adapt to technological requirements that are in constant mutation. Modification of facilities and their accesses affected users and goods flux, which consequently made a great impact to the open space and its use.

The role of open space in extensive end functionally complex urban environments as the CCS is multiple. For the center itself, open spaces are actually inner connections of the hospital organism unimaginable for successful daily functioning. However, open spaces are also a sort of public space that contribute in creating an overall pattern of the center that relates also to the rest of the city of Belgrade.

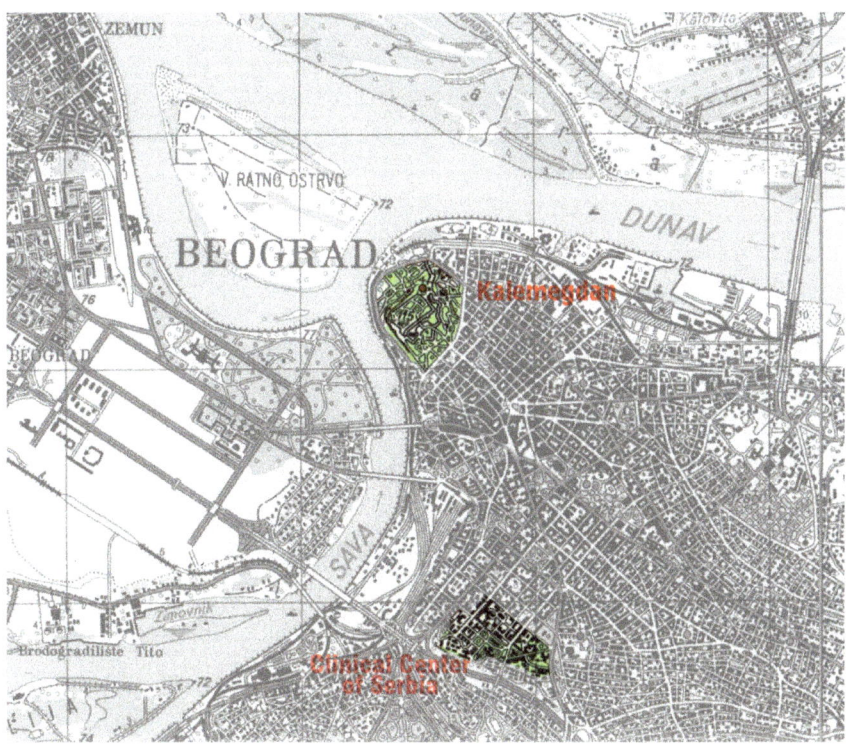

Figure 1a: Position

Initial considerations

Framing the problem - relation to the city

In general, a development of hospitals depends on economic and social frame, different public authorities and is closely linked to technological progress and continuous improvement of treatment and diagnostic methods. Over the time, the role of the open spaces changed along with the evolution of the hospital typology.

Looking at the timeline the first important moment was during the enlightenment with contextualizing hospitals into the greenery, glorifying the power of nature. Direct contact with the environment and the access to the fresh air were essential for healing process. In mid-twentieth century, along with modernism and development of new technologies and new construction methods, rationality in functional organization took the priority. Hospital became healing machine, often mega-structure. They grew physically due the complexity of functions and new technologies they needed to accommodate but without proper planning and organization. Finally, they became the complex labyrinths; often mix of different buildings from different periods without the clear form as whole. The hospitals lost their «spatial frame of reference» because of weak integration and interaction with urban tissue and low flexibility to keep up with the dynamic development of the urban context (Schaefer, 2006).

The Globalization era brought new tendencies: the need for re-urbanizing hospitals or to make open space an active participant in the healing process but also to integrate better hospitals within the city. Thereby large hospital structures would cease to sterilize urban areas and at the same time would respond to the urgent need for humanizing the hospital space.

Framing the identity – look backwards

The tension between the space and socio-political forces according to Lefebvre (1990) is realized spatially as «contradictions of space». Harvey (1996) finds «spatial permanence» as a reflection of political-economic, social and cultural processes and problems where «spatial powers created in the course of urbanization are in persistent tension with the fluidity of social processes» (p.419).

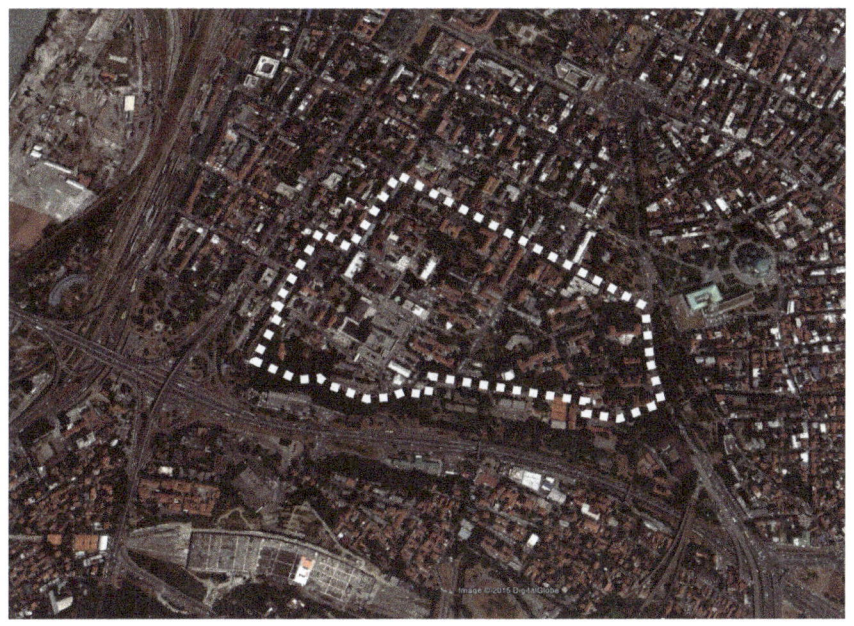

Figure 1b: Klinički centar Srbije, Belgrade, (above) and Policlinico Umberto I, Rome, (below)

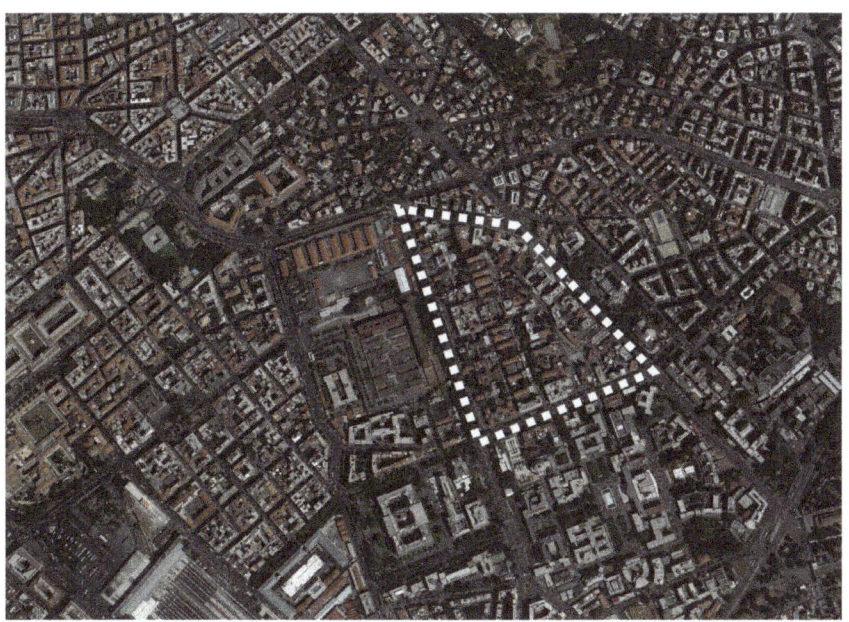

Considering the political turmoil that Serbia underwent in twentieth century, the case of CCS offers opportunity to see what kind of imprints different historical periods left in healthcare space. It was formed gradually for more than 100 years, passing through different social systems therefore constant changes of its organization, methods of management as well as its relationship to the city, depending on the social occasions. The result is a very varied and confusing conglomeration that was continuously spreading within the central urban tissue.

Framing the image – structuring

The perception of this complex mechanism as a whole is difficult and open spaces play a decisive role in creating the first general picture of it. Lynch (1960) defines an environmental image as a generalized mental picture of the exterior physical world held by individuals that becomes public if it is common for large number of inhabitants. He retains that legibility or clarity are the visual qualities of the special importance in particular when considering environments at the urban scale of size, time and complexity. Spaces «where the parts can be easily recognized and organized into the coherent pattern» give good environmental image with a sense of emotional security and intensify the human experience of the space. For Lynch in creating the environmental image basic components are identity, structure and meaning. While the last one depends of the individual, structuring and identifying of the environment can reveal the physical qualities of the space that provoke the strong image or in other words give the "imageability" of the place.

Given the importance of interrelation with the surroundings, for understanding the CCS and its open spaces the focus is on a center as a whole, as a hospital city, with reference on different historical periods. The complex is presented in terms of urban neighborhood following the five basic elements of a city form defined by Lynch as "empirical categories" (idem): edges (borders), regions (districts), paths (connections), nodes (anchor points that connect paths) and landmarks (orientation points, focus).

Historic Overview

The development of the site with the healthcare purpose begins in the second half of the 19th century at the time of the Principality of Serbia (the period before gaining total independence of Ottoman Empire) and Duke Mihailo, when in 1861 opened a

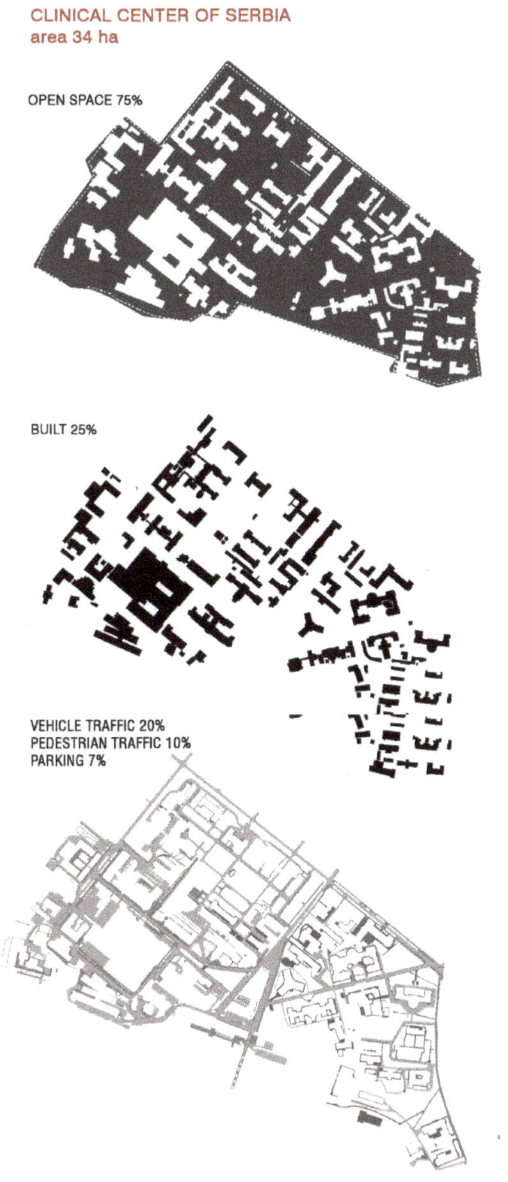

CLINICAL CENTER OF SERBIA
area 34 ha

OPEN SPACE 75%

BUILT 25%

VEHICLE TRAFFIC 20%
PEDESTRIAN TRAFFIC 10%
PARKING 7%

Figure 1c: General data

home for the mentally ill in the Doctor Tower (Fig. 2) which is now a monument of culture. It was built in 1824 as a family house for Italian doctor Dr. Vita Romito (RTS, 2011); one of the first medical doctors in the renewed Serbia and is one of the first houses built in Serbia after the Second Uprising (3). This 'home' eventually grew into a psychiatric clinic that is now part of the Clinical Center of Serbia.

Afterwards, the decisive moment in further developing of this location was the building of the Main Military Hospital (Fig. 2) in 1904-1909. It was a pavilion type complex with a system of individual buildings immersed in greenery. It was considered as the most modern hospital in the Balkans for that time comparable with similar institutions in the world, with advanced concept of architectural end town planning solutions. Today it occupies the larger part of the subject area and consequently its position, organization and inner interrelations to some extent conditioned the overall morphology of today's clinical center. The Military Hospital complex was built as a whole, in uniform style, in the spirit of romanticism with well-defined borders and accesses and traffic patterns in correspondence for the sanitary and social needs of that period. This complex has a manifold historic significance not only for its architectonic values but also as a referent medical institution that had a decisive role in developing the medical services on both the city and the country level. Further, it was major educational centre, the nucleus of the present day Medical School of Belgrade University (Cultural Properties in Belgrade, 2010).

After liberation from the Ottoman Empire, the newly created Kingdom of Serbia (since 1921 Kingdom of Yugoslavia) continued to build its institutions, which included the development of the medical school and medical practice in general. The bases of different branches of medicine are set up which was followed by the establishment of specialist hospitals. The subject area consolidated its healthcare identity with new building interventions. In proximity to the Military Hospital, an area which was still on the outskirts of the city at that time, on a hill, surrounded by greenery, a series of different hospitals and clinics were erected, mostly in the 1920's (gynecology and maternity ward, first intern clinic, first surgical clinic, first pediatric clinic, faculty buildings, different institutes ext.).

The final form, both physical and organizational, the Clinical Center gained after the Second World War. In the new Yugoslavia, now socialist republic, the area retained its primary purpose. The few new facilities were erected, such as gynecological and obstetric clinics and clinics for Neurosurgery. However, a decisive factor was delivering the first detailed Master plan in the 70's for the clinical center as a whole that introduced radical organizational and spatial changes. The Master plan predicted a series of demolitions and relocations of existing clinics as well as new traffic patterns and accesses in order to stratify movements by purpose and type of user. A key element was the construction of the central building of the clinical center with intention to concentrate the diagnosis and therapy in coherence with the spirit of that period and new trends in the healthcare architecture. The pavilion type has long been abandoned as ineffective and in its place took a hospital as an efficient machine for treatment and care with a rational approach in planning and organization.

The central Polyclinic (Fig. 2) building designed by arch. Dragoš Balzareno was built in 1974 but never completed. The design predicted two towers with patient wards positioned on a *podium* block where intention was to concentrate the diagnostics and treatment. That implied also numerous relocations of some surrounding clinics closer to central one. The idea was to form an efficient Clinical center complex as whole that included also the area of Military hospital. In 1983, the military hospital transferred to a distant location into a newly built hospital complex that provided space for other clinics to move in and to concentrate other distant civil hospital institutions on a single area.

The Master plan was never completely realized. Without new traffic network routes and accesses, it was not possible to obtain ambitious plans. The central building itself remained unfinished, without second tower and unfortunately, about 62% of built area is still out of use. The spaces enabled for utilization are used as receiving centers and Polyclinics with day activities. Still the central building dominates the site and panoramic view of that part of the city. This old (new) organization gave the spatial and visual core to the site but not the functional one.

However, the Clinical center of Serbia in present form and organization was founded in 1983 as a unique medical institution, created by joining clinics and Institutes of Medical Faculty in Belgrade: the Clinical Center of the Faculty of Medicine.

The Clinical center remained a referent healthcare institution but after dissolution of Former Yugoslavia in the 90s its coverage was drastically re-dimensioned (4). The country already in 1990 started the long process of transition from socialist to market system. The transition implied changes in urban planning and land use in general as well as conception of property (5). Unresolved questions regarding the right to dispose the urban land between the central government and cities slowed urban development.

All these aspects had their repercussions on the healthcare system and in particular to the Clinical Center both layout and management (6). It is still unclear the levels of authority regarding the open space inside of the Clinical center, the City or the center itself.

In 2009 the government started ambitious investment plan to reorganize the present clinical center. The new Master plan predicts finally enabling the central building and bringing originally envisioned purpose in coherence to the present needs and trends in healthcare.

The Look from Outside. Enclosure and Transparency of the Center

The CCS is located in the central zone of Belgrade, municipality of Savski venac and surrounded by the primary city traffic routes: highway on south-west and the Boulevard of Prince Milos on the north-west, the Boulevard of the Liberation on the east (Fig.2).

The perimeter of CCS is variable and its permeability is conditioned by a physical and architectural frame as well as by the terrain morphology. Looking from the outside it can be observed that the center has not emerged as a unified whole, but eventually grew and encompassed the surrounding areas since the border itself is non homogenous and often vague. The distributed villa pattern of the center has caused there to be no continuous built front on the borders (Fig. 3).

Although it is located on the hill, the physical barrier between the center and surroundings comes to the fore only on the south side where it is enclosed by the sharp slope of the terrain (elevation difference 30m) and urban green belt along the highway (Fig. 4). This contrast by nature protects the CCS and makes great panoramic effect looking from distance. From that side only pedestrian access is possible, and it is connected also with the walkway that leads across the highway. The center also seems hidden with exception of the central tower that dominates the landscape with its height and one of the clinics that is positioned near the slope. Moving to the south-west the margin enters inside the city block and becomes invisible.

The local level streets Pasterova and Resavska bound the northern part. Here the CCS is penetrating into the densely built urban fabric, which radically changes the visibility and accessibility of the center. This city area is a mix of residential space and different public and commercial functions. Here the built structure of the center creates (in) a visible edge and gets into contact with immediate surroundings. There is no continuous built front but a discrete fence that isolates area from the surroundings as there is no clear psychological boundary. The presence of other public and hospital institutions in proximate vicinity in Pasterova Street, in absence of clear margins and entrances, give the sense of confusion that the CCS is larger than it is. Enabled access to some clinics of CCS directly from the border streets contributes to this general image.

The Boulevard of the Liberation directly borders the eastern side. Across the boulevard is located the big city Green Park, National library and Saint Sava temple in vicinity (the area with great simbology and cultural-historic importance). However, high traffic intensity in the boulevard makes these public spaces less accessible for users of the CCS.

Often there are dead spaces, vacant spaces or spaces with inadequate use that further erode enclosure. There is a phenomenon of a concentration of various related and supporting functions in proximate vicinity, such as the increased concentration of pharmacies, shops, laboratories and service

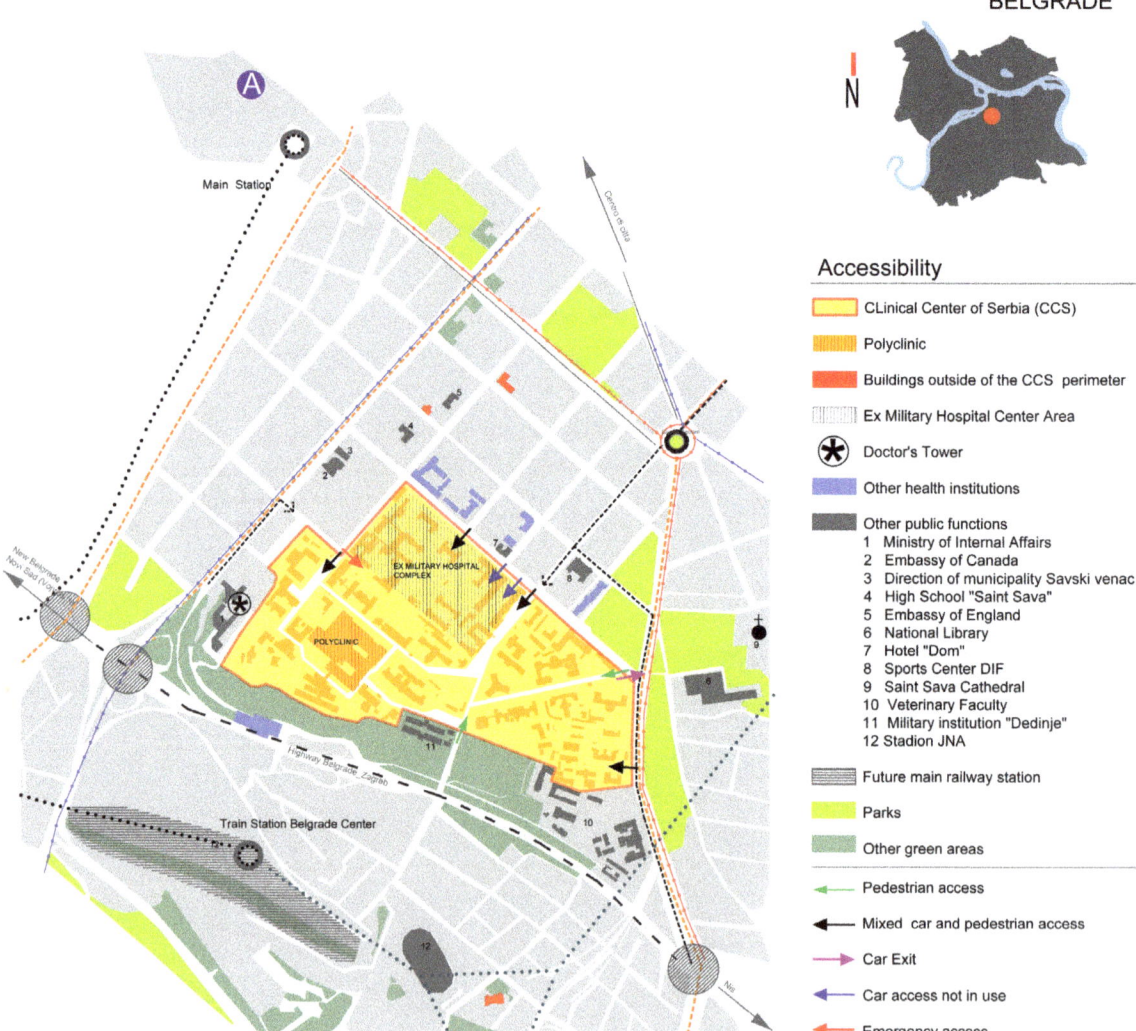

Figure 2: Physical context, accessibility and surroundings

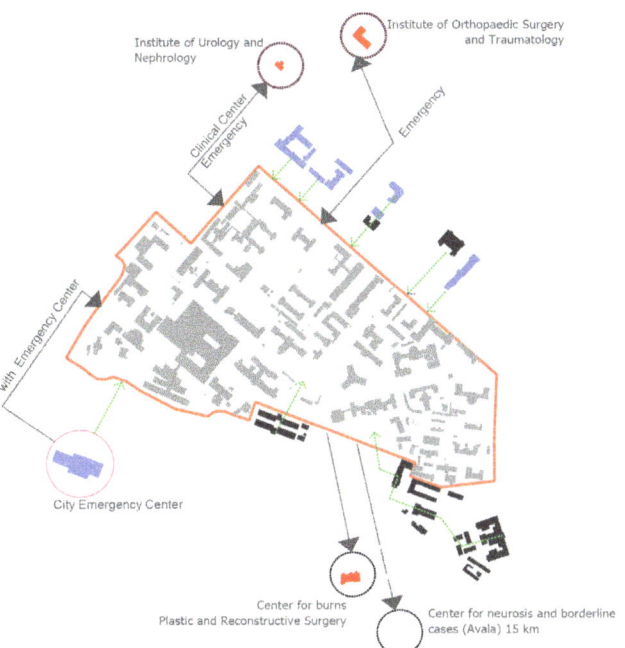
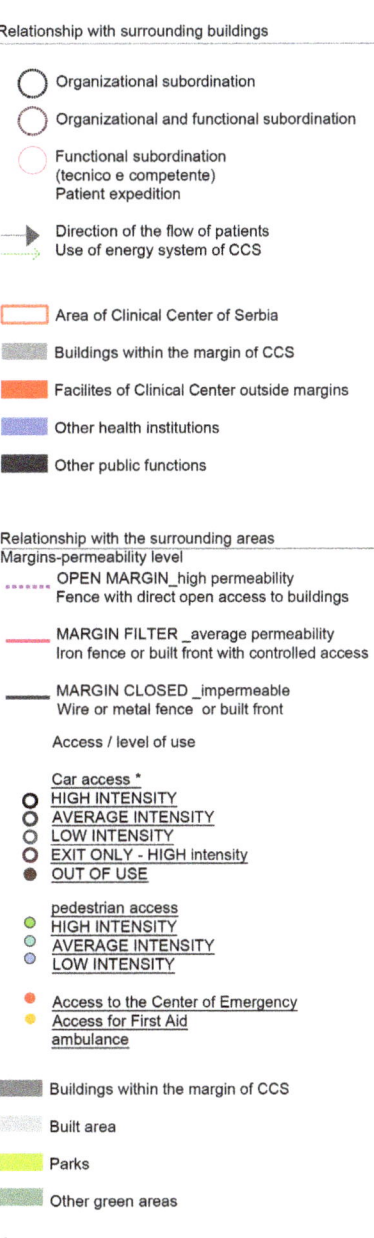
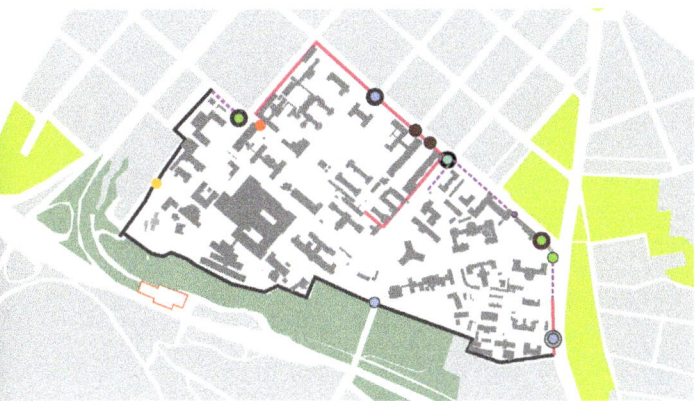

Figure 3: Enclosure and boundaries

facilities. Very frequent is an abusive type of construction, characteristic for countries in transition.

Although more than a half of the CCS perimeter is directly bordering the green areas the only green public area spatially more accessible is Park of Milutin Milankovic (Fig.2) on the corner of Pasterova Street and the Boulevard of the Liberation. The afore mentioned green belt on the southern slope is not adequately equipped and accessible enough to interact more intensively with users.

In proximate vicinity to the CCS are the main bus station, railway station and a fast connection with airport by highway. In addition, surrounding streets are provided with different types of public transport. However, unresolved traffic problems on city level, lack of parking areas and absence of direct accesses from the most important city arteries (that are dedicated exclusively to the CCS), make accessibility of the center very questionable and nullify all the benefits that the location brings.

Accesses are organized through a complicated system of local one-way streets very often poorly marked. There is no clear division of accesses in relation to the type of use. Two principal entrances are on the west side from Višegradska Street where there is also access for emergency and from Deligradska Street that penetrates deeply into the center and divides the area into two parts. These two main accesses present also the most important nodes, anchor points, inside (outside) the Center. The third important point is access (vehicle exit) in Dr Subotica Street (Fig. 2).

It is a characteristic that accesses are not solely points in the space but related more closely to the street or tract, without a clear picture where the Center exactly begins and where it ends.

The Former entrance to the ex-Military Hospital in Pasterova Street (Fig.3), which today serves exclusively for employees and an ambulance is the only entrance built and designed in accordance with the purpose. Its monumentality, carefully shaped gate and the main building that looms from background is one of the rare urban episodes that gives a picture of the seriousness and importance of the institution behind the fence.

The pedestrians use all mentioned points. There are also different minor accesses that are mostly not in use. Non-controlled entrances for pedestrians make the Centre very permeable and very often people cross it to get to the other side of the city.

The long perimeter, the presence of greenery inside and different auxiliary functions as well as permeability even for non visitors make CCs very invisible from the outside in physical terms, which makes a lot of confusion for users. On other side unresolved traffic, functional issues and lack of parking areas generate a lot of crowds both outside and inside the CCS and that makes the center present or visible for its surroundings.

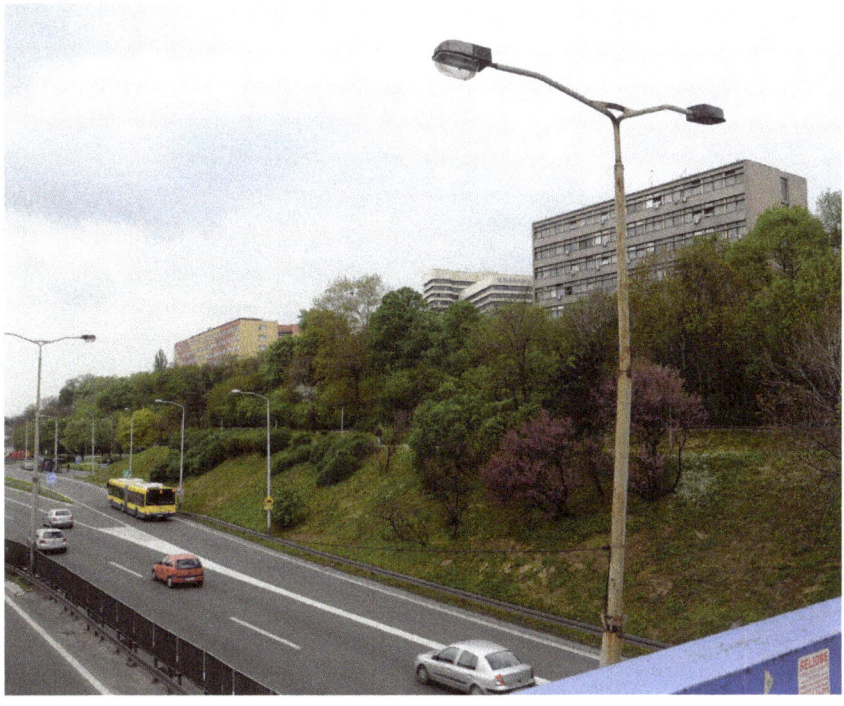

Figure 4: View of the southern border of Clinical center from above the high road, photo by Veljko Koš

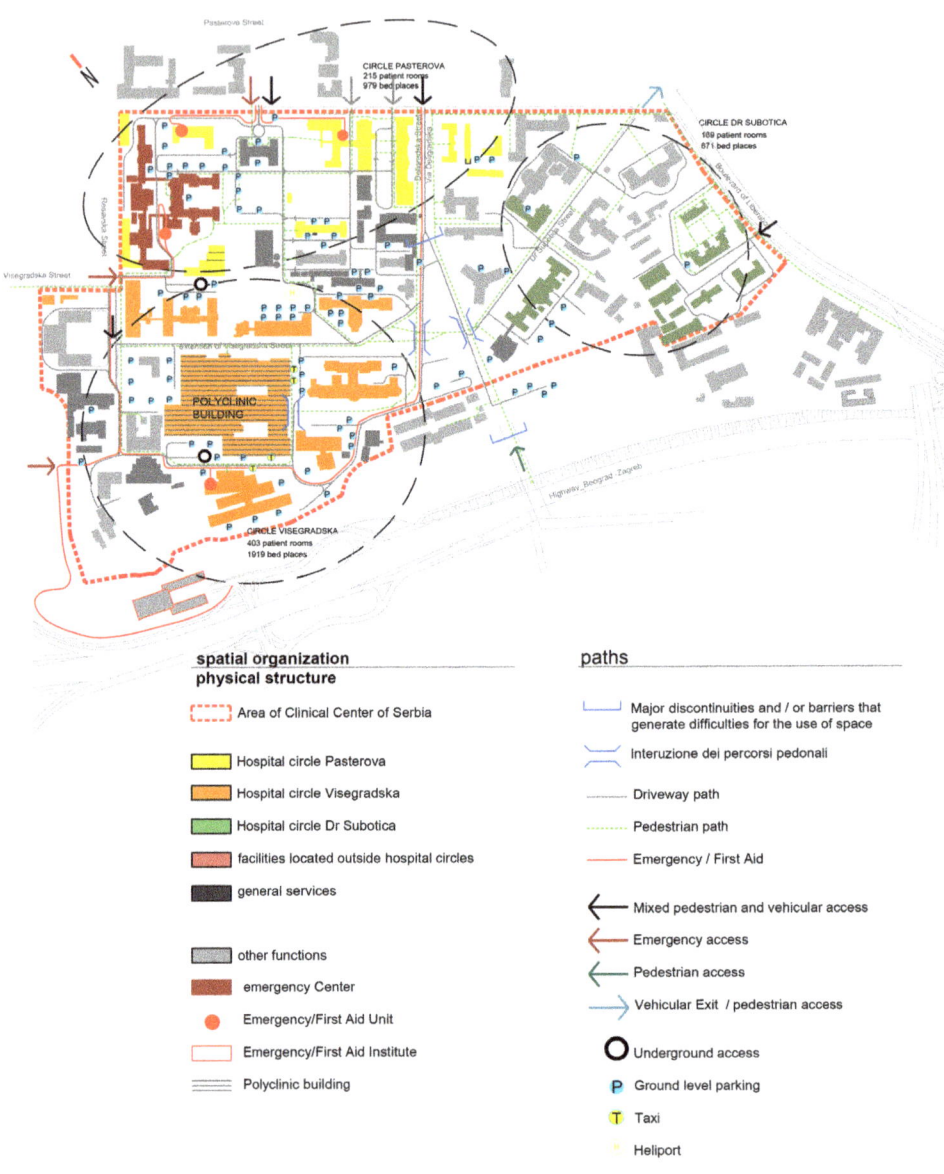

Figure 5: Inner structure of the Clinical Center

Inside the Hospital City: inner structure

Connections and nodes

Presented at the Fig. 5. The main skeleton of this diffused area are the principal traffic routes which act, as explained above, both as main entrances and as distribution corridors: Deligradska, Višegradska (and its extension) and Dr Subotica Streets dividing the subject area in different parts and creating apparent spatial wholes. The basic purpose of the movement to put the space in order and give the visual hierarchy to the environment (Lynch, 1990) here is missing. In the subject area, the central node where the main axes should intersect is actually a point of interruption. There is no physical frame or mark that give the clear image of confluence, of interconnection space between inner wholes (Fig. 6). With its undefined form and broken movement lines, it acts more as a physical barrier in the space. To this impression it contributes also the terrain morphology; the area is sloped in both directions and this comes to the fore in the central area which is on lower altitude comparing to the surroundings: culmination point is in the form of a depression.

Thanks to restrictions of passage and inadequate traffic networks there is no fluidity in moving which is further aggravated by the system of one-way streets. Often users and users with cars have to go out from the center and to enter on other side to reach the destination. The absence of additional nodes that would effectively link spatial areas and inner strategic points with accesses additionally contribute to the mismatch between inner circulation and outer city traffic movement.

The lack of clarity in the movement is amplified by a secondary network of local routes that lead inside the invisible blocks or districts of the CCS. Missing stratification of traffic routes according to the type of users, unresolved parking and unstructured system of entrances, not only to the Center but also to the singular buildings, have created a chaotic network of movements.

Disorganization of the traffic has affected gravely open spaces and their main purpose of connectivity and orientation. The orientation in extensive neighborhoods such as this one largely depends on the spatial relationships and frameworks, especially when adequate signage is absent as in this case.

Pedestrians' flows join vehicular paths and often users through unplanned parking areas access to desired structures. Missing adequate multilevel parking creates serious problems for every day functioning and their expanding at the expense of open space. The present capacities do not satisfy neither the basic stuff need. Other users, such as patients and visitors, mostly park outside the CCS.

Districts and their cores

The principal traffic routes should act as bonds for inner districts. However, In the CCS there is the ambiguous inside-outside sense that derives from undefined enclosure of these inner spatial wholes. The clear physical structuring of the place is missing.

The CCS is spatially organized in three clinical circles (Klinički centar Srbije, 2013) that are a consequence of present physical groupings and the traffic backbones with a visible historical imprint. This subdivision relates to spatial grouping not functional. Clear functional zoning of the hospital city is not possible considering the intertwining and interdependence of the various functions of subjects. The main traffic arteries actually are the spines of these imaginary districts that do not have clear bounds between them. Each of these circles has its visual character that comes to the fore once entered inside of it.

Circle Pasterova includes hospitals that are distributed along the street of the same name and mainly refers to the old military hospital with addition of some dispersed structures. As already mentioned, the Ex Military complex is designed as a separate entity, which in the meantime has become only a quarter within a larger complex. Today it can be assumed according to bounding and disposition of the buildings and entrances. The fenced complex acts as an isolated hospital fortress because of missing both effective visual and physical communication between the core of the circle and surroundings. However, inside reveals a special ambience of interconnected villas and green spaces, with a well-preserved central green park area (Fig. 7). Nevertheless, the core of the circle, once focal point, lost its characteristics of a node and a landmark, once it lost its centrality by integration of the complex into the bigger area of present CCS.

The Circle Dr Subotica is in the form of a street corridor that includes institutes gravitating along the same street and also an isolated entity for infective diseases which for the nature of pathologies treated acts as an independent islands. They were built mostly in the early 20th century in different historic styles but similar typology-pavilions inserted in greenery. The buildings act as separate entities with a special character and notable monumentality of architectural framework. Each of the villas is marked with its own associated open space (lot) with differentiated access zones. Here the well-maintained greenery is the element of connection in the space, which gives a sense of fluidity. The street tract acts as homogeneous spatial setting with multiple roles: as a district, a pathway and as a landmark because of its well-balanced environmental frame.Circle Višegradska includes the facilities that gravitate as satellites around a central tower, and is the core of the complex. It has a completely different character that reflects a functionalist approach in planning as it was a tendency in the second half of the 20th century when the area was remodeled. During socialism it was forced free blocks and international style. The absence of private ownership introduced ambiguities in relation between private and public space. The previous two circles characterize an abundance of greenery and segregation between the hospital open space and public space. In the youngest circle, there is no filter zone between the building and the exterior.

The extension of Višegradska street that connects the main entrance and Deligradska Street is actually the focal open space of this circle. This pendant promenade is one of the main axes of the Center as a whole from where there are accesses to the most known hospital facilities (most of the surgery is concentrated in this circle as well as centralized Polyclinic). The mix of contrasting hospital facilities present in the circle is coherent with the architectural frame. This district of CCS hosts very different architectures and hospital typologies. It is already noted the central tower distinguishes from its surroundings with its dimensions, position on the highest point of the area and its architecture. It is spatially dominant and acts as one of the accents even in the landscape of the whole city. The adjacent Neurosurgery Clinic is one of the reference points because of its characteristic modernist architecture in evident contrast with prevailing present villas.

Green spaces

Green spaces present about 40% of the area. The general impression is an abundance of greenery that offers a diversity of plant species and trees. The CCS

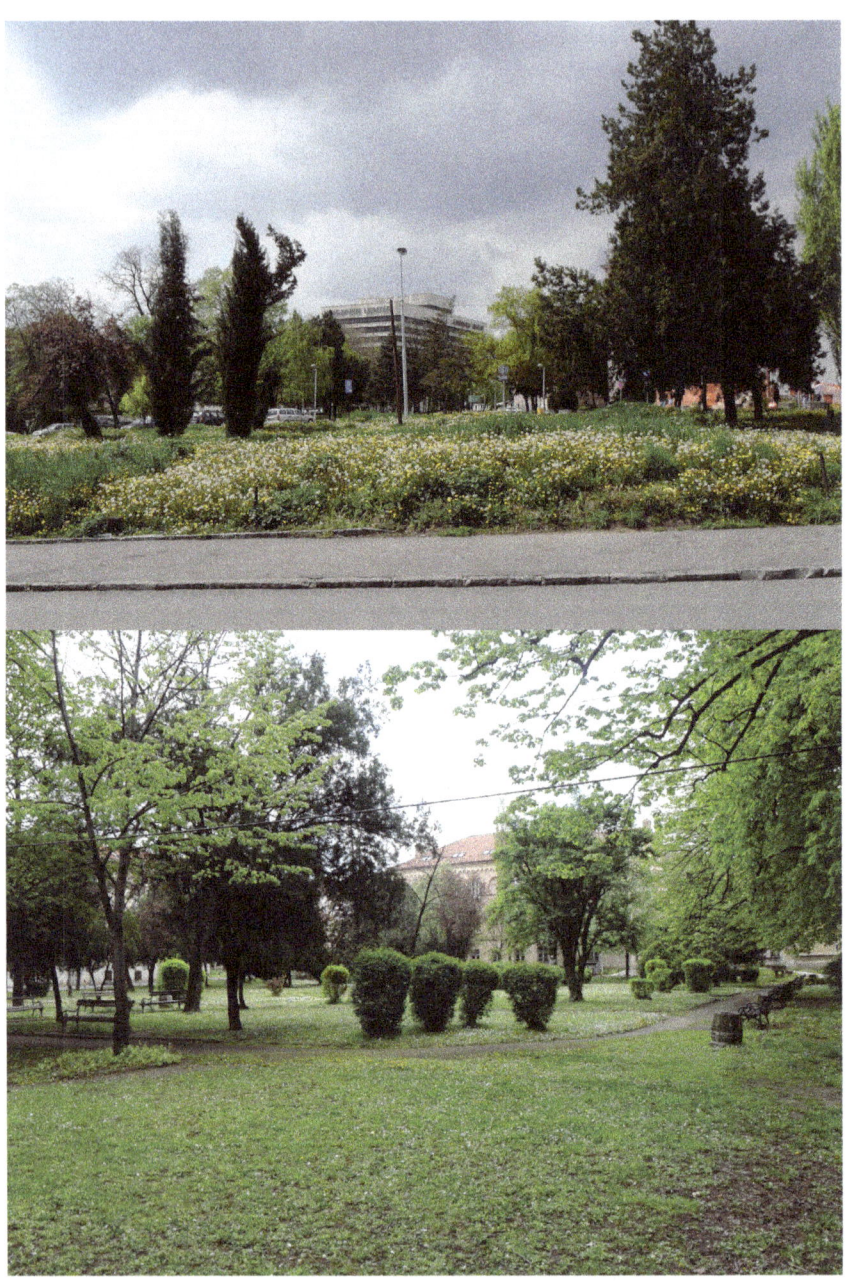

Figure 6-7: The green central node of the CCS with a view to the Polyclinic tower (above) and the central park of Ex Military Hospital Complex (below), photo by Veljko Koš

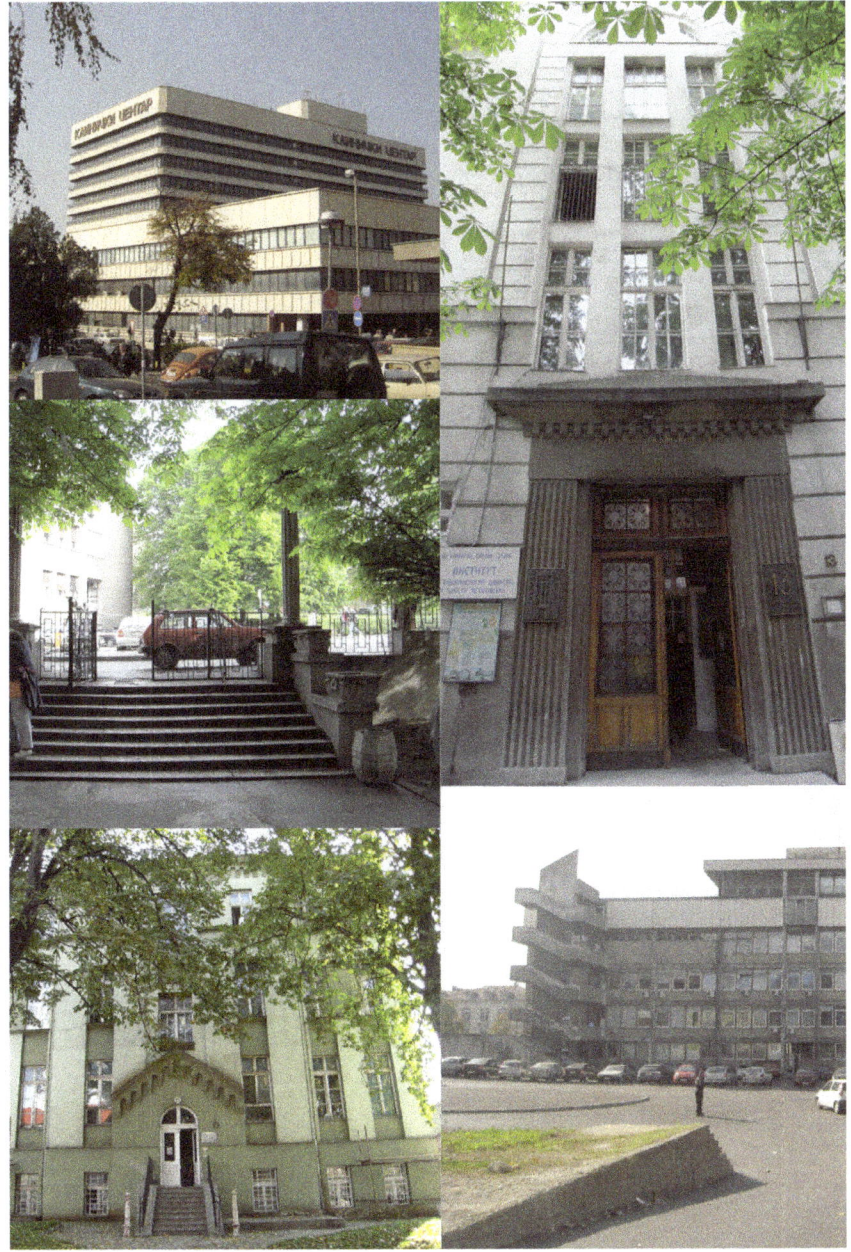

Figure 8: 'Multiple character' of the Clinical center – various urban episodes, personal archive

can is proud of an extremely valuable tree collection more than half of century old, with some more than 80 years old, such as chestnuts, plane trees and linden. There are also pines more than 25 meters tall, not so frequent in central city areas (Popović, 2013).

Although green areas prevail, landscaped parks are only a few that are concentrated in the core of the former Military Hospital. Some spaces as the entrance plateau to the Polyclinic were planed built and planted in accordance with an unrealized Master plan from 1970', but today they are rarely used because of different traffic systems and accesses (Fig. 9).

Other areas, especially grassland, are under the daily threat of extinction due to the uncontrolled and illegal spread of parking spaces.

In preserving and maintaining green areas and open spaces in general, the main problems are difficulties to control accesses in the extensive areas like CCS, which facilitates inadequate behavior and use of space, frequently even being destroyed.

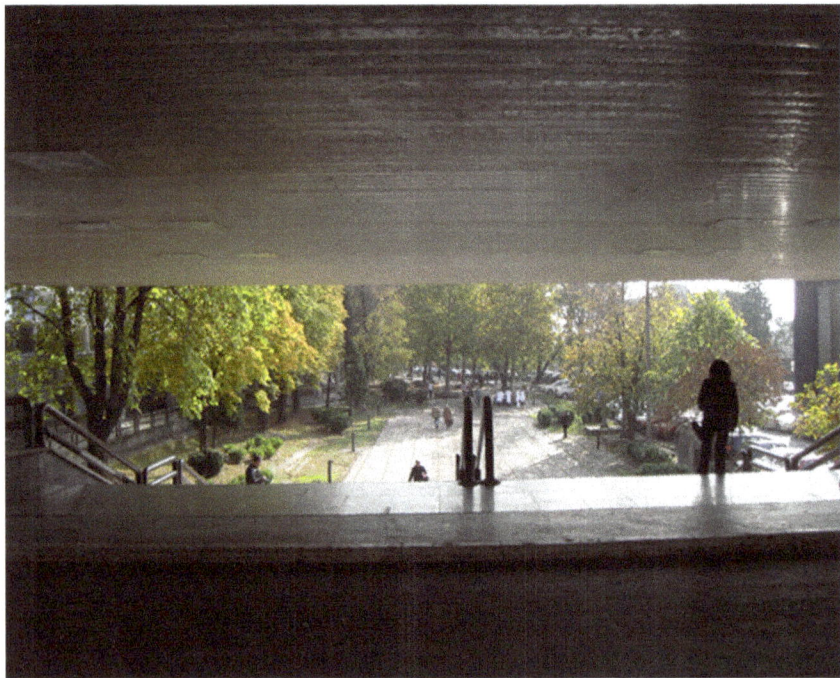

Figure 9: View of the pedestrian access to the central Polyclinic building, personal archive

Conclusion: the sense of whole?

The open space in the Clinical center of Serbia covers over 75% of the area. Nevertheless its physical dominance, the lack in functional organization and inadequate urban setting for the modern hospital, drastically devaluated the role of outdoor space in this healthcare environment.

The fact that the Center is not created from the start as a whole but eventually spread to the surrounding objects and areas produced ambivalent relationships with the environment and the numerous difficulties in constructing its own interior that are unresolved to this day.

Nowadays urban structures are according to the Master plan that was never completed. Consequently, there is no coherence between the functional and physical wholes inside the city, which produce inadequate use of outdoor space. The result is the unfinished Center from the socialist period as with many other unrealized elusive projects from that time.

The conflicts and confusions in open space appear largely as a consequence of ambiguous relations between private and public spaces in post-socialist countries. In addition there are unresolved issues of authorities in managing and planning over the urban land as well as tensions between centralized governing in health care versus increasing autonomy that obtained the Center in a new system. This provoked both misuse and neglect of the open space inside the Clinical Center.

The final image is an amalgam of different urban episodes from different historical periods poorly incorporated into an overall pattern.

Notes

* Inspired by Lynch, K. (1960) *Image of the city.*

(1) Serbia is one of the upper middle-income countries, with population in 2013 (Census) is 7,164,132 which is a decline of 4.4% since the census in 2002. Overall life expectancy in the Republic of Serbia shows a slight increasing trend - in 2013 was 75.05 years. The basic characteristics of the Republic of Serbia population are the changes that have brought the population to the brink of demographic ageing (Institute for Public Health, 2013). The health status of the population is consistent with other Central and Eastern European countries, but below that of Western Europe. 24.6% of the population is on the national poverty line. The major causes of death are cardiovascular diseases (ca. 55%) and neoplasms (ca.22%) The health expenditure in Serbia as a proportion of GDP was 10.4% in 2012 (World Bank, 2014), which is relatively high against regional comparisons with averages of in the EU and in other East and Central European countries.

(2) Health care services in Serbia are organised on three levels and provided through 275 institutions. The Primary healthcare is carried out in primary care centres ("Dom Zdravlja") and include general practice, mother and childcare, dental services, laboratory, home care, patronage, emergency services, etc. The secondary and tertiary level services of the health care network include hospitals, clinical centres, and specialized institutes giving general and specialized inpatient care. Tertiary health care is provided by clinical centres, clinical hospital centres and institutes and for local population offer secondary level services. One of the problems in Serbia is work overload of tertiary structures that often undertake some primary health care tasks to cover perceived weaknesses in the primary health care system (Euro Health Group Denmark, 2004).

(3) The Second Serbian Uprising (1815-1817) was the second phase of the Serbian Revolution against the Ottoman Empire, which ultimately resulted in Serbian semi-independence from the Ottoman Empire. The Principality of Serbia was established, governed by its own parliament, constitution and royal dynasty. Final independence followed during the second half of the 19th century (Wikipedia, 2015).

(4) After political turnovers and civil war in ex-Yugoslavia, in 2006 Republic of Serbia regained is independency. Once referent institution for the state of 25 millions of inhabitants today covers 7 million.

(5) In socialist Yugoslavia, predominant form of property was a public property. The form of private property has survived in a minor amount but never included the property over the urban land. Nevertheless the privatization was carried out since 1990 only in 2009 was introduced legal possibility that different private subjects can become actually owners of a urban land. Additionally, in 1990, the State government appropriated the urban land from the cities transferring all authority to the state level. Therefore, for the long period the cities did not have possibility to dispose with its own territory. This fact made great impact in managing

and transforming the open and public space in period of transition. In general, it blocked urban development.

(6) The healthcare system remained public, but health care providers (among them CCS), started to gain more autonomy nevertheless the healthcare system is still centralized; the Ministry of Health is still the major influencer being the regulator, purchaser/financer and provider of health care services (Euro Health Group Denmark, 2004).

References

Cultural Properties in Belgrade (2010) *Cultural monument Military Hospital at Vračar* (online), available at http://beogradskonasledje.rs/kd/zavod/savski_venac/vojna_bolnica.html (Accessed 12 November 2014).

Euro Health Group Denmark (2004) *Technical Assistance for Assessment of the Clinical Centres In Serbia*. Report to the European Agency for Reconstruction and the Ministry of Health of the Republic of Serbia.

Harvey, D. (1996) Justice, Nature & the Geography of difference. Oxford: Blackwell Institute of Public Health of Serbia (2014) Health Statistical Yearbook of Republic of Serbia 2013, (online), available at http://www.batut.org.rs/download/publikacije/pub2013.pdf.

Klinički centar Srbije (2013) *Osnovne informacije* (online), available at http://www.kcs.ac.rs/ (Accessed 11 November 2014).

RTS (2011) *Kod dva bela goluba* (radio program) Radio Beograd, 21. December 2011, 20:00, available at http://www.rts.rs/ (Accessed 22 October 2014).

Lefebvre, H. (1991) *The production of space*. Trad. Donald Nicholson-Smith . Oxford: Blackwell.

Lynch, K. (1990) *The Image of the City*. Cambridge MA: MIT Pres.

Maki, F. (2008) *Nurturing dreams*. Collected essays on architecture and the city. Cambridge, Massachusetts London: The Mit Press.

Miletić, I. (2009) Clinical Center of Serbia: functional reorganization of Policlinic – Belgrade. Master of II level in Architecture for Health, Faculty of Architecture, Sapienza University of Rome, unpublished.

Popovic, O. (2013), Botanička bašta u krugu bolnica. Politika, (online), available at http://www.politika.rs/rubrike/Drustvo/Botanicka-basta-u-krugu-bolnica.lt.html (Accessed 3 September 2014).

Schaefer, M.: "*Building Hospitals – Hospital Buildings*" in: Wagenaar C. ed. (2006): The Architecture of Hospitals. Rotterdam: NAI.

World Bank (2014) *Serbia data*. (online), available at http://data.worldbank.org/country/serbia (Accessed 15 October 2014).

Wikipedia (2015), Second Serbian Uprising (online), available at http://en.wikipedia.org/wiki/Second_Serbian_Uprising (Accessed 15 October 2014).

11

The role of outdoor public space in a pavilion university hospital. Case study: Policlinico Umberto I of Rome, Italy

Valentina Napoli and Giuseppe Primiceri

Abstract: This paper proposes a reflection on the role of external space in large pavilion university hospital complexes. This type of hospital building was common throughout Europe between the end of the XIX and the first half of the last century. The Policlinico Umberto I of Rome, completed in 1902, was considered one of the best pavilion hospitals of its kind. The hospital has been chosen as a case study to investigate its outdoor space, through the analysis of its phases of evolution from the original project to current day proposals.

Over the course of time the hospital has never been completely renovated, notwithstanding the fact that it was deemed out of date in 1959. There has been ongoing debate in recent years that has produced multiple solutions for its renovation none of which have been implemented. The present situation is the result of different emergency interventions that tried to meet current technological, medical and organizational standards. The relationship between the built and unbuilt space is a measure of the quality of the hospital and its level of humanization, particularly considering the use of outdoor space in the Mediterranean climate.

The analysis of the external space in its current state is based on these considerations and also on the basis of understanding the relationship with its urban surroundings. Along with the study of the evolution of the complex a questionnaire on use and perception of the space was submitted by different categories of users.

Through the process the possibilities that could be linked to the use of outdoor space are highlighted, especially in large university pavilion hospital situations.

Keywords: pavilion university hospital, quality of outdoor space, supportive environment, outdoor activity, users' needs.

Introduction

The open space in hospital complexes is part of the pavilion typology characteristic of the end of XIX century, related to the concept of Garden City and hygienic hospital standards typical of those years. The study of this typology in comparison to a tower hospital, symbolic of the functionalistic culture, give us the opportunity to think about a new scenario for the potential use of outdoor space, finding other possible meanings not only connected to functional aspects: access to the area, parking space, routes and building's entrance.

Studies on outdoor space in hospital campuses started after the seminal article in 1984 in Science by the environmental psychologist Roger Ulrich "View through a Window May Influence Recovery from Surgery". It was the beginning of significant researches on the same topic (Tyson, 1998; Cooper Marcus & Barnes, 1999). The outdoor space assumes specific characteristics, not only important to provide natural light and fresh air into the hospital buildings, but a place to be looked at and physically accessible. Hence, external space in healthcare facilities become truly relevant, giving opportunity to relax, to carry out physical and therapeutic activity and as a place for social interaction. Studies regarding outdoor space linked with environmental and sustainable considerations led the United States in 2002 to create a *Green Guide for Healthcare* (GGHC) (1), the first classification system concerning the sustainable design for healthcare, which through a toolkit gives the opportunity to create a check list on environmental and health issues in a hospital design, from preliminary to maintenance phases. This method gives a specific credit to outdoor space, SS-9.1: "Connection to the Natural World - Outdoor Places of Respite" and SS-9.2: "Exterior Access for Patients". The role of external space becomes consequently of critical importance because it is closely related to the hospital activity and if considerately designed can be a supporting space with therapeutic functions.

The case study of Policlinico Umberto I has become emblematic in an Italian context because it has opened up a debate on the role of outdoor space in hospital complexes in urban areas, analyzing possible new functions to serve both the hospital and the city. The Policlinico of Rome is a University Hospital and the area that it covers is practically a 'city within a city'. The evolution of the surrounding area, from rural to urban area, does not match with the transformation of the hospital, anchored to the old concept of hospital isolated from the city. These considerations open up a new field of investigation concerning open space in healthcare facilities as bothsupporting hospital activity and transitional space between the structure and the city. Beginning with the analysis of the main stages of the historical evolution of the Policlinico, the renewal projects in the last 20 years and of the current situation, we highlight the different role taken on by the outdoor space. Alongside the study of projects and programs, an important aspect of the research concerns direct behavioral observation, layout analysis and questionnaire on use and perception of the space by users (patients, doctors, caregivers, students, visitors, etc.), in order to evaluate the quality of the outdoor space.

Historical evolution of Policlinico Umberto I of Rome

The Polyclinic Umberto I of Rome was built at the end of the XIX century as a result of multiple factors: historical, politic, scientific, cultural, economic and social. The historical context from 1870 (Capture of Rome) to 1888 (ground breaking ceremony) is a complex period from both a national and local point of view. The newly born Italian State named Rome as Capital in 1871 and this gave an impulse to planning development with the first Development Plan implemented in 1873 with an Extraordinary Plan in order to realize public services in the capital (Messinetti and Pedrocchi, 2012). The progresses all over Europe in physics and chemistry brought medicine to a new physiopathology and clinic approach. The University reform legislation in 1870 was published with the aim to educate students of medicine through clinical practice in the hospital, in fact an agreement was signed between the Ministry of Public Education and the Hospital Administrations. To better define the context of the origin of the Policlinico we should mention the Heath Reform of 1888, which tried to overtake the differences and decrease the discomfort, in a country that was still in a miserable position of inferiority in relation to other developed European counties and where is rooted a diffuse sense of health malaise (Boccia, 2006).

The main objective of the reform was to stop the spread of infective illness and to decrease the level of mortality in maternal-infantile sector. This was the start of a Public Health reorganization and a radical change of the hospital layout to meet the new needs in accordance with medical, scientific, hygiene and engineering evolutions. Guido Baccelli, a doctor in the University of La Sapienza and Minister of Health (1881), took into account all of these aspects in the study of the project for the new University hospital of Rome. The main aim was to achieve the concept of unity in the specificity, a single campus to concentrate all the different scientific and professional specialties to support a good medical education (Guarini, 2006). The debate of the commission for the Polyclinic was wide and took into consideration different features such as the typology of the hospital, the departments to include, the right location and the internal layout.

The choices were based on the most current knowledge at that time, the priorities were hygiene, infection control and the availability of diagnostic instruments. A great amount of attention was given to the definition of a new functional model to meet specific needs where the main goals to be achieved have to guarantee the complete independence of each section, the choices of the architects have to be subordinate to the decisionsof the each clinical doctor in order to meet the requirement of hygiene that has to be the priority objective of the project before the aesthetical needs (Pasquali, 1881).

The organization and the numbers of bed places had to be in accordance with the educational and research activity, guaranteeing a significant number of clinical case studies, without forgetting the charitable function of the hospital. The area of the hospital is 160.000 sqm, not centrally located in relation to the urban center at the time and in a salubrious part of the city. The international design competition was won by the Italian architect GiulioPodesti, which designed a 'pavilion hospital', with individual buildings of two or three floors connected with each other by indoor and outdoor bridges. The project of the complex is symmetric, the gross floor area is 40.000 sqm. The main buildings, located on the viale del Policlinico, are the administration building in a central position, the medical clinics on the right and the surgery clinics on the left. In the center of the middle sector there are service zones and on each side different pavilions connected with bridges. On viale Regina Elena in separate buildings the obstetric-gynecologist clinics, infective departments and anatomy-pathology edifice are situated. All the buildings are also connected with a system of underground routes.

The debate on the choice of the area for the campus took into account the possibility of less critical patients' use of the outdoor space. In accordance with these indications and with the idea of 'garden city' typical during those years, the external space was characterized by green boulevards, covered walks and geometrical classical gardens with flower beds between each pavilion and the clinics. The construction works were completed in 1902 and in 1904 the hospital began functioning. Over the next decades different refurbishment works were carried out, for example in 1931 the emergency department and the ambulatory area was extended and located in the basement of the central building. Over the years other interventions were undertaken in order to improve the surgery sections or add buildings to meet new needs. In 1959 when the building was thought to be out of date, the first renovation project was presented. It proposed a radical changes to existing buildings: the demolition of the majority of the pavilions and of the clinics and the transfer of their uses into a large new single block. This was never carried out but was the beginning of the ongoing debate. A Urology Clinic was added in 1980. Changes in recent years relate to mechanical adjustments and extensions, which more than other interventions disfigured the look of the original buildings and have invaded the external space, compromising the usefulness and functionality of this space. The open space in the Polyclinic is not born out of its intention for use as a therapeutic space nor as an extension of the indoor space,but with an idea of 'pavilions in the park'to meet hygienic needs of fresh air and natural light of each pavilion as prescribed by the old legislation. The original project was harmonic, a characteristic that today has been lost, the reason being new buildings were separate in their internal organization avoiding any possible connection with the context. Mechanical additions take over the outdoor space, by blocking pedestrian paths and pulverizing the external space, the original design is compromised, because it is not in accordance with the old organization and therefore of poor quality. Similar considerations on the location of the hospital and on its boundaries, resultant of the thinking at the time of the building construction, hospitals were considered as a risk for the diffusion of illness, therefore located away from the city center and surrounded with high walls, without any relationship to the surrounding environment. Currently the urban growth has enclosed this big 'Island' (around 10 blocks). Planning decisions, since the 1931 development plan, have surrounded the hospital with other State services such as University City, Ministry of Aeronautics and National Library, creating a 'Service District'. The infrastructure system runs all the way around the hospital campus, and road width on viale Regina Elena's is 25 meters emphasizing its isolation, severely disrupting any possible relationship with the neighboring areas.

Analysis of the outdoor space of Policlinico Umberto I through a critical review of planning and building renovation projects from 2000 up to the current date

The conceptual international developments of the use of outdoor space discussed above do not find the same resonance in Italy, where in the same years the focus was on increasing the legislation on the diagnostic and therapeutic aspects (DPR 14th of January 1997) in order to accredit healthcare facilities to the National Healthcare System.

The requalification of the Policlinico started with the intentions of adapting the complex to achieve the 'minimum structural requirements' imposed by the legislation. The state of obsolescence of both building and functional aspects led in 2000 to the first in a series of project proposals for "Planning and Building renovation project of Policlinico Umberto I". Beginning with these considerations a critical review of all the different renovation project hypothesis between 2000 to date are presented, in order to understand the role of outdoor space in each proposal.

2000	January	Preliminary Design Document (Department ITACA Faculty of Architecture University of Rome "La Sapienza")
2003	December	Preliminary Design Document (Department of Architecture and Engineering Eng. Carrara Faculty of Engineering University of Rome "La Sapienza")
2004	November	Preliminary Design Document (Eng. Fecchio Executive Director of Building Project- Hospital Policlinico Umberto I of Rome)
2006	January	Preliminary Design Document (Arch. Bucci Director of Functional Area of Technical and Technological Sanitary Hospital Policlinico Umberto I of Rome)
2008	February	Invited International Design Competition (10 selected competitors)
2009	January	First prized Project (Team Leader - Ove Arup)
2009	June	Decree states that most of the building in the Policlinico are under protection for cultural and historical reasons (Ministry of Cultural Heritage and Activities, Regional Directorate)
2013	September	Preliminary Project for the reorganization of Policlinico Umberto I to realize in three phases between 2013 and 2025 (Hospital Policlinico Umberto I of Rome)

Analyzing all the different hypothesis four keywords stood out in relation to the outdoor space: 'green', 'public space', 'routes' and 'humanization'. The first consideration concerns all of the different proposals and is about the use of the word 'green' to indicate outdoor space. The word takes us back to the Italian planning meaning of 'public green' as it is described by Ministerial Decree 1444/1968 as areas for public space: parks, playgrounds and sports. The term has another significance linked to the 1930 functionalist culture, which used a wide area of 'green' to surround buildings, losing the human dimension of the space. Green as a synonym of outdoor space, this consideration helps a better understanding of the role of this type of space in reference to the hospital complex's functionality. Outdoor space in the Policlinico is residual space between the buildings, beautified and connective space, where only 'secondary activities' or 'necessary activities' take place, as stated by Jan Gehl: "necessary activities include those that are more or less compulsory (...) influenced only slightly by the physical framework. (...) The participant have no choice." (Gehl, 1970 p.9), so they are activities that happen regardless of the quality of the external environment.

The Preliminary Design Document proposed in 2000, besides the restoration of the classical gardens of the architect Podesti relating to the XIX century concept of geometric flower-bed, takes into account the idea of 'connecting areas' furnished with 'waiting, leisure and social areas'. Therefore in the project the outdoor space, alongside the concept of 'green', takes on other important meanings as 'public space' and 'routes', in relation to the surrounding urban context, peoples orientation and internal circulation. The project tries to be not just a hospital renewal but an urban requalification, increasing the value of social relationships but does not achieve the desired effect of a full integration with the healthcare activities. The aim of 'humanizing' the hospital complex appears in the 2004 proposal, it becomes a design requirement, as a result of the importance that this issue carries in the debate about hospital design. The project focuses on humanizing recovery wards, in reference to the internal aspects, as furniture and finishes, without taking into account the possible use of outdoor space. The input of all the different Preliminary Design Projects converged in 2008 on the International Design Competition "Reorganization and Refurbishment Design Plan of Policlinic Umberto I – Masterplan"(2). This step is relevant for the history of the design projects of Policlinic, because give us a good example of design choices taken by different international teams when considering the use of outdoor space. In the competition's brief the aspect of outdoor space is called restoration of interstitial green areas and design of wide areas for studying and meeting. The theme of humanization stays linked to the indoor as waiting and wards areas, and the optimization is intended for the wayfinding and routes system.

Outdoor space is not present in an explicit form, but the design teams, while following indications from the brief, approached the theme in different ways, often giving a precise description of specific function and requirements in relation to the urban context and the hospital activity. All the teams proposed a similar design solution for the position of the wide green area acting as a park or central square. The area is located in middle of the site, in direct connection with the preexisting buildings on the side of via Lancisi, viale Regina Elena and viale dell'Università, this building group is heterogeneous so the space acts as a filter between past and present. The square/park has similar formal characteristics in all the projects for location and scale, but all the different design projects are attentive and sensitive towards the potential contribution of outdoor space in terms of the humanization of the hospital. The external space in the design teams idea is linked with the indoor life of the building, important in improving peoples' interaction, described by the team RTI Ove Arup & Partners International Limited pleasant as a place to pass through and stay, where it is possible to relax during the day, the only functions connected to the hospital activity are the waiting and orientation area, but have a civic value contributing to the urban surrounding. The willingness of the designers is to open the boundaries of the hospital to the city. This idea is the second issue stated in 2001 by the Ministry of Health and the architect Renzo Piano as: Urbanity. Renzo Piano wants to break from the idea of the hospital close into the boundaries, giving a more urban vision, the hospital has not to be detached from the city, but rather become an extension of the city, in other words be an 'open hospital'. The idea of permeability is present in the projects presented for the masterplan of the Policlinico. The connection of two parts of the city by passing through the hospital complex is an important issue, as engine of quality not only for the future asset of the Policlinic but also for that part of the city (RTI Studio Altieri spa), in one of the proposals by RTI Nickl& Partner Architekten Ag became also the elimination of a portion of boundaries' wall. Another common aspect is related to the refurbishment of the classical gardens that are in between the old buildings designed by Podesti along the side of viale del Policlinico. The approach to renew these gardens was to a restore the existing species and the geometrical original design of the flowerbeds in accordance with the oldest buildings that in the masterplan's hypothesis would be converted in to University campus. In relation to the future function of the edifices two design teams tried to give a specific role to the gardens transforming these small spaces, from decorative elements to useful places (RTI Nickl& Partner Architekten Ag), by using specific furniture as benches and places to read and study outside where the University will be part of the outdoor space (RTI Studio Altieri spa). The connection to the 'green' outdoor space with therapeutic, rehabilitation or medical activities, is an important part of some projects. The use of external spaces near each indoor activity, as gardens or furnished places where one can experience the nature and meet people as proposed by RTI Nickl& Partner Architekten Ag, the intent is to give a hierarchy to the outdoor space, from public to progressively more private, where the meaning of green is close to Healing Garden. A 'Children gardens' is one of the examples by ATI Proger spa, in direct relation with the Pediatric Clinic, extension of the indoor activity and respondent to the need to de-medicalize healthcare facilities, in particular for children. The theme of humanization present in the brief was understood as prospective views, spatial quality of ward area, indoor materials and colors (M. Petrangeli, 2009). The humanization issue is associated with the quality of the indoor building space while the outdoor space is treated as a background, not to be used but more to be looked at in an 'internal-external' relation.Observing the concept of humanization from an 'outside-inside' point of view, we can find short comings, as poor quality of transition areas in particular between the urban environment and the building interior. Working on outdoor space is crucially important to take the hospital to human scale, giving a sense of friendliness and support, ensuring protection and openness.

Unfortunately, ten years of design projects ended up in 2009 with the Decree by the Ministry of Cultural Heritage and Activities, which states that most of the buildings in the Policlinic are under protection for cultural and historical reason. The executive phase of the competition stops, and in 2003 the Hospital Administration presents a new preliminary project "Reorganization of Policlinico Umberto I", the design is very conservative in addressing current needs. The external space in the executive project will have a secondary role as beautification and connection, the description of the works reports: "demolition of building alterations and maintenance of connection paths and external areas", excluding a possible new interpretation of the outdoor space in order to add more value to the hospital complex.

In conclusion, a possible way to take action in the process of the renewal of the hospital complex is to find the right balance between two opposing needs: innovation and conservation. Possible design solutions can exist through a deep understanding of technical, medical and economic efficiency systems and of the conservation criteria of the buildings. The project should discover a way to use in its favor structural, typology and formal characteristics in relation to the building and the outdoor space, for a new spatial and functional configuration.

The design proposal should be elaborated beginning with the consciousness of the need of a permissiveness from both the administrations and the designers. The agreement should be defined in advance to evaluate, with the support of interdisciplinary team, the right design project. The aim would be to find a technical, functional, managerial and economic program allowing for the protection of what exists. The Policlinico Umberto I could be a great opportunity to put in place this strategies in order to achieve the current objectives both urban (Healthy City, Salutogenic City) and hospital (de-medicalization, Patient-Centered Design) based on the wellbeing of patients and citizens.

Spatial layout and behavioral analysis

The spatial layout and the behavioral analysis of outdoor space inthe Polyclinic highlightthat the users use only the 30% of the available outdoor space. The observation was undertaken in July (average temperature of 22°), in three different times (morning-afternoon-evening) of a typical hospital day. The study identifies three main areas of major confluence of people underline with the letters A-B-C in the picture (Fig.1).

A: emergency access on Viale del Policlinico;

B: porch and internal courtyard in front of the University Central Pavilion, near the reading room and the medical reservation point (CUP);

C: central area in correspondence with the access on Viale Regina Elena and near the Pediatric, Radiologic and Surgery Clinics.

The highest concentration of people in certain areas depends on: the type of users; the physical conformation of the space; the function of the buildings, in particular the activity on the ground floor in correspondence with the external space. In the case of the latter the main reasons are as follows:
- proximity of ambulatory activities;
- newsagent and bar;
- informal seating areas (low walls, steps);
- trees;
- low vehicular (private and emergency) traffic.

The remaining unused outdoor space needs to be also considered in order to understand the relationship between the behavior of users and the configuration of the space.

The majority of the courtyards in between each pavilion, as previously stated, are not usable anymore, while the ones which are in good condition are linked to the idea of geometric gardens bordered with low walls and not accessible to people with physical impairments. The concept of this kind of garden is more to be looked at and not to be physically experienced, currently, for both reasons location and configuration of the outdoor space, are places without life or only used for necessary activities. The internal routes, which connect each pavilion, represent an other potential usable external space. The boulevards are pleasant because they are denoted with trees, footpaths and furnished with benches, but the high level of transit of private, emergency and supplier's vehicles make it particularly dangerous for vulnerable people. Parking spaces are placed on each side of the lane and the crossing points do not stand out properly, those two aspects increase the isolation of the usable areas making the space only suitable for the circulation of staff both medical and caregivers, precluding an active use by others.

Arising from this analysis the main reasons why the space is not used are listed as follows:
- Accessibility of the space
- Control of the space

- No clear definition between pedestrian and vehicle routes
- Distance from the main activities of the hospital
- Space framework.

Finally, we can state in accordance with Clare Cooper Marcus (2014) that "safety, security and privacy" are the main aims to achieve in outdoor space, in particular when we are in hospital context where the majority of users are vulnerable.

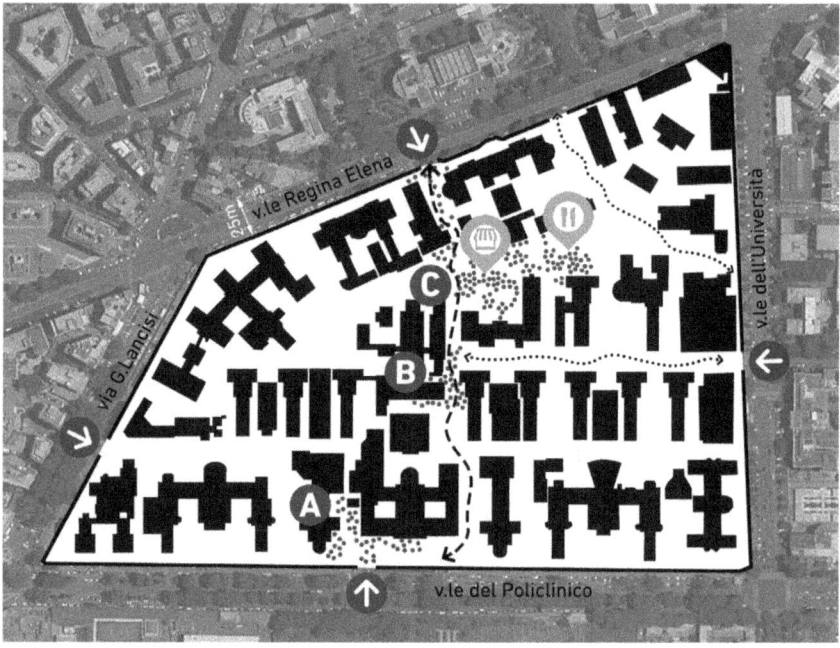

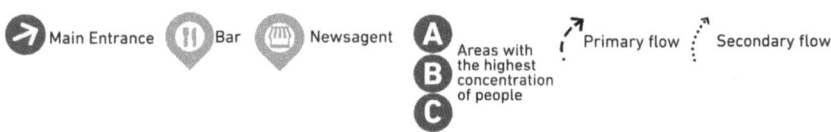

Figure 2: Spatial layout and behavioral analysis, by the author

Evaluation of outdoor space quality: direct observation and questionnaire on use and perception of the space by users

The engagements of all the different categories of users (doctors, caregivers and staff, inpatients and daycare patients, visitors and students) by organized interviews and questionnaires was helpful to understand their behaviors and habits, in order to evaluate the outdoor space of the Policlinico Umberto I of Rome.

Aim of the surveyis to understand the perception of quality of outdoor space of the hospital on the part of users, focusing on functional and emotional aspects related boththe pavilionsystem and the urban tissue.

The questionnaire submitted on site to 100 people of all categories of hospital users, at three different times (morning-afternoon-evening) of a typical day coinciding with the busiest moments of flow due to daycare services and visiting times.

The first lot of questions regards the accessibility, wayfinding, circulation, both to the hospital and to each individual pavilion.

The Policlinic Umberto I is located in a central area, the questionnaire shows that all users admit that is well connected by public transport (metro station, bus and tram line), but most of them, apart from students, reach the hospital by individual transport.

Accessibility to the hospital was also evaluated in relation to the wayfinding system,both from external site boundary entrances and internal access to each distinct pavilion.

High ratings reveals that the signage of the different entrances from the city to the hospital is quite clear, but the internal signs give too many alternatives to arrive at the same place, so most of the users feel disorientated.

All categories, including staff and students that know the campus, recognize that the primary cause of the disorientation is a poor internal wayfinding system. Two main issues were pointed out: difficulties in finding an individual building and the right entrance, because often there are more than one entry in relation to the specific service provided inside.

Almost all users (89%) think that the external paths are not suitable for vulnerable people, in order to improve the current situation the priority is a clear division between pedestrian and vehicular routes, at the moment neglected, and a new wayfinding system. Visitors, students and daycare patients feel this necessity the most, with inpatients and daycare patients asking for more identifiable paths (Fig.2).

Architectural barriers are present along the paths between pavilions but only doctors see the need for their removal, this unexpected result allowed a better understanding of the importance of the other options given (in the following order: clear division between pedestrian and vehicular routes, new wayfinding system and identifiable path) to improve the external paths from the user's point of view. The result also support the direct behavioral observation, that reveal lower capacity by daycare patients and inpatients, especially disabled, of using external paths to walk and in general spend time outdoors. Generally, patients use the outdoor space just at the moment of arrival/admission and leaving/discharge using private or emergency transport, actions that take place directly in front of each building.

The aim of the second part of the questionnaire was to understand the real use and the importance of outdoor space by analyzing the main activities and the frequency of use.

A large majority of respondents, more than 90%, state that the characteristics of external space and above all the existence of green areas are crucially important for the imageand the functionality of the hospital. Most of the people surveyed use the space in the afternoon, apart from daycare patients and visitors, which for practical reason are there in the morning, the space remains completely unused in the evening after 6 p.m., also during the summer time considering the climate could be used for alternative activities (Fig.4). Students, doctors, daycare patients and visitors are the main users of the outdoor space, especially because they can find a moment of privacy and relax far from the stress of indoor environment. Social activities like meeting family, friends and colleagues and socializing are two other important reasonsfor using outdoor space, followed by eating lunch especially by staff. Students, thanks to their ability and willingness, use the space for studying and carry out all the activities proposed apart from therapeutic ones that are almost non present (Fig.4). Conversely, 20-25% of inpatients, visitors and caregivers affirm that they do not use the external space because they think that it is unsuitable to do any of the activities proposed in the questionnaire.

The sample group studied gave priority to the following aspect in order to improve the space: the introduction of a park with seating and sheltered areas. Other elements of high importance is the implementation of the parking space pointed out by all users, and playground areas required in particular by daycare patients and inpatients, visitors (parents) and students. The possibility to have commercial activities in the hospital, apart the ones strictly related with medical activities like pharmacies, do not suit the needs of users. Indeed the results obtained from the final section of the questionnaire relating to the feeling associated with the hospital environment shows that 70% those questioned get a feeling of disorientation (fig.4). It follows that they are afraid that mixing uses and flows, even if well organized, can be a cause of more stress, and can reduce the feeling of safety, perceived today especially by inpatients that represent the most vulnerable part of users.

Two patients out of three have the feeling of being separated from the city, and as they state, a clear distinction between different activities is necessary to make them feel secure. The perception of separation from urban context is present even in other categories of users, only a few doctors and visitors feel part of the surrounding city. The last question submitted tried to understand a possible relationship between Policlinico Umberto I and urban tissue in a future scenario by giving three different choices: a complete permeability of the hospital complex; a clear separation between hospital and city; a partial integration of the structure within the city. The majority of all categories of users excluding patients state that a partial integration of the hospital within the city will be beneficial, as long as privacy levels and respect for those who are in critical condition would be provided. The important issue is linked to "how" to connect the hospital and the city. The survey shows that of those interviewed an approach of differing levels of connection between city-hospital would be ideal, moving from mostly completely open public areas to the city to a private one gradually filtered.

The heart of the future research will be to find the right balance between different needs, which could move forward by testing several ways of possible integration. These issues should concern expertise (hospital administration, architects) and people from different ages, classes, levels of education and cultures, with the aim to establish an innovative evaluation tool able to take into account needs of users and convert them into a design strategy.

DO YOU THINK THAT EXTERNAL PATHS ARE SUITABLE?

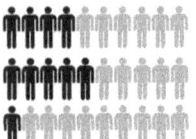

37% Never

52% Sometime

11% Always

89% of users think that external paths are not suitable especially for vulnerable people

WHAT WOULD BE YOUR PRIORITY IN ORDER TO IMPROVE EXTERNAL PATHS?

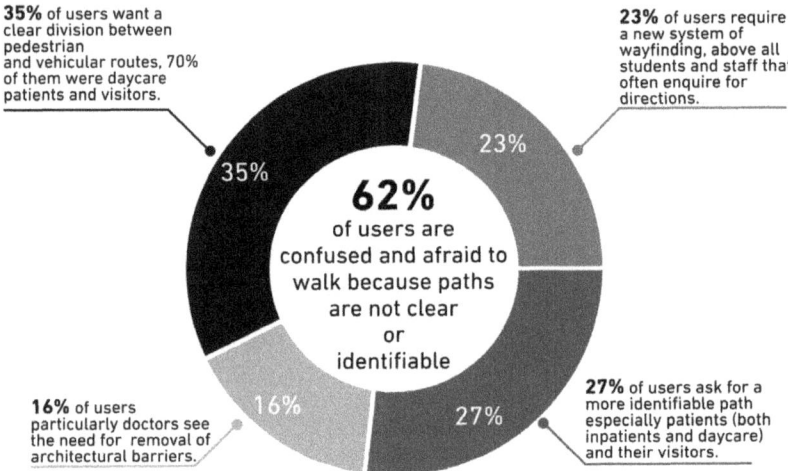

35% of users want a clear division between pedestrian and vehicular routes, 70% of them were daycare patients and visitors.

23% of users require a new system of wayfinding, above all students and staff that often enquire for directions.

62% of users are confused and afraid to walk because paths are not clear or identifiable

16% of users particularly doctors see the need for removal of architectural barriers.

27% of users ask for a more identifiable path especially patients (both inpatients and daycare) and their visitors.

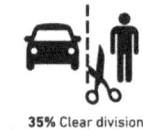
35% Clear division between pedestrian and vehicular routes

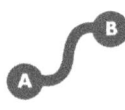
27% Identifiable paths

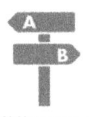
23% New system of wayfinding

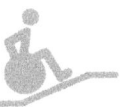
16% Removal of architectural barriers

Figure 3: Graphic of the questions relating to evaluation and improvement of external path, by the author

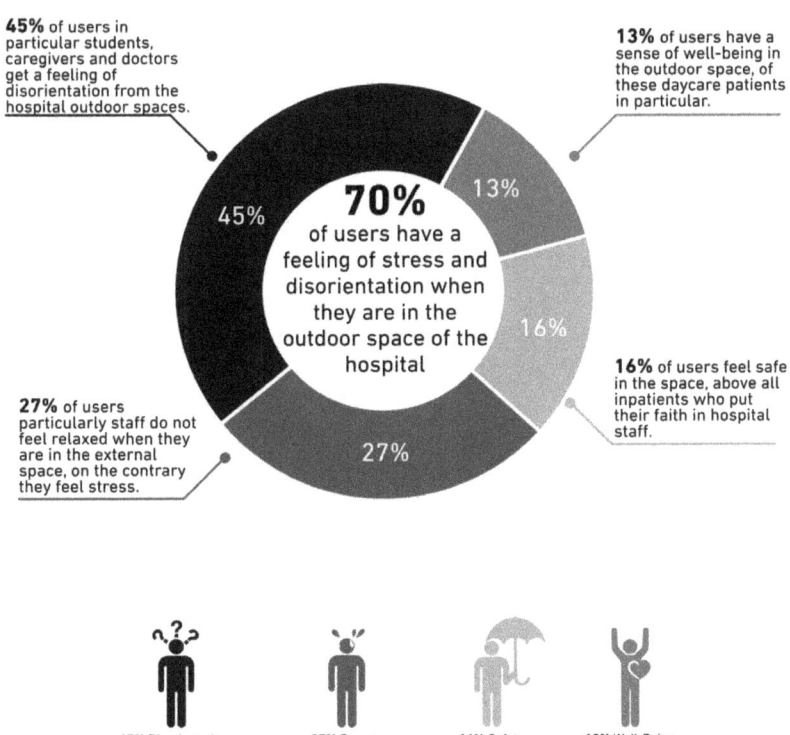

Figure 4: Graphic of the questions about use of outdoor space, by the author

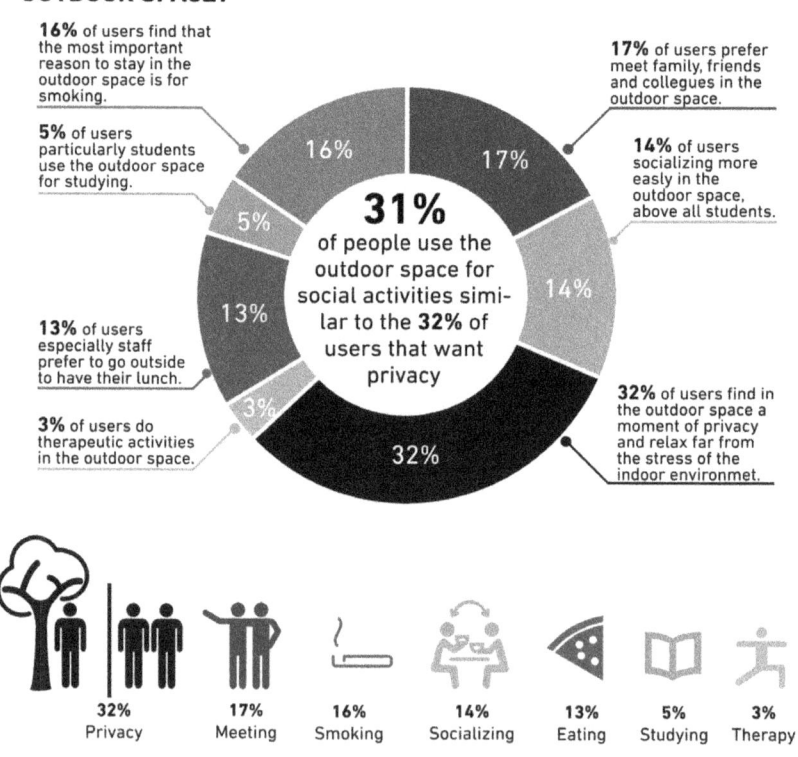

Figure 5: Graphic of the question about feeling in outdoor space, by the author

Conclusions

The analysis of the physical structure of Policlinico Umberto I show the weakness of some issues relating to the ability to provide the right answers to all the needs of current medical innovation. The structure was designed and built on the basis of planning, typology, hygienic, functional, mechanical, administrative and social theories, that we can now consider hospital 'archeology'. The current situation of the hospital shows the difficulty in making radical improvement to the original structure, principally because some of the pavilions are under the protection of the Ministry of Cultural Heritage and Activities. It would therefore be important to highlight the possible strengths of the hospital complex, in order to act as a catalyst for new values, and bring architectural hospital research towards a new future layout, based on different conditions.

Hypothesis on the requalification of Policlinic Umberto I and more general on possible interventions in large Pavilion University Hospitals, which until today were focused on eliminating some impediments concerning functional and mechanical problems, medical innovation and buildings connection. Nowadays for technical, economic and social reasons, already highlighted in other parts of this book, it is necessary to start a process for reallocating specific functional areas like diagnosis and therapeutic activities from the main hospital to the regional para-hospital service (Giofrè and Terranova, 2004). A web of facilities, which do not necessarily coincide with the hospital, can begin to realize the process. House of Health or also the home of the patient can be the place of cure thanks to innovative systems of sanitary services, home care support integrated with teleassistance and telemedicine. This is the basis for a progressive reduction of the characteristically enormous structures that until recently have been the norm in healthcare facilities and in particular in university hospitals.

Current design layouts try to place all the main Functional Areas with high technical-functional complexity (Emergency, Operating Theatres, Intensive Care, Medical Imaging, Hemodynamics, Analysis Laboratories, Sterilization, etc.) in one single new building called 'Technical Unit'. In the existing pavilions, adequately refurbished, all the other Functional Areas with lower and middle complexity (Ordinary Hospitalization, Day Hospital, Ambulatories and Rehabilitation Activities) are often located. The result of this layout arrangement, mostly addressing the optimization of mechanical systems and the proximity of Functional Areas, is building big sealed blocks, often without natural light and far from the outdoor environment, which can be a cause of alienation and stress for both patients and medical staff. The main issue of this model is the connection between the 'Technical Unit' and all the other Functional Areas, above all diagnostic areas, usually located in different pavilions often far from the main block. In order to meet the hospitals functional needs extreme solutions are demanded that are contrary to normal environmental requirements increasing the use of mechanical systems. The schedule of building work often follows an incremental logic. New additions to existing buildings are often oversized and make integration with the original structure difficult.The bigger the hospital the more it attracts patients to it, including those requiring diagnosis and basic medical needs, instead of favoring the process of localization of these basic services in the community. This view demonstrates, particularly in Italy, resistance at various levels to make real changes, and quickly begin the reorganization of healthcare facility infrastructure. The current design solutionsare often invasive, and may be necessary but do not in fact solve definitively the issues of quality of space and life in hospital buildings. In regards to the refurbishment of Pavilion University hospitals we should value the original concept of 'pavilions in the park', instead of upset the balance between open and building space. The complex of Policlinico Umberto I of Rome is an example of 'pavilions in the park', the original project, based on XIX century hygienic and functional reasons, with the characteristic sequences of indoor and outdoor spaces, and relatively low buildings to allow fresh air and light inside. The structure could be rethought without all the recent alterations and minor new buildings, which in accordance with the idea of localization would have no reason to remain, because they are deprived of the original functions. This thought leads to further reflections and new design experimentations in order to give a new function to the outdoor space of old Pavilion University hospital complex. Possible design strategies of the external layout should take into consideration the following issues:

- dialogue with the urban surrounding, in reference to the boundaries that at the moment act like a strong demarcation line between the city and the hospital;
- progressive permeability of the hospital complex to other urban activities to further different levels of hospital-city relationships;
- clear division and regulation of vehicular and pedestrian flows, also at the

urban cross road points, to meet the needs to the most vulnerable users of the hospital;

- organizing the outdoor space by giving it a specific function in order to encourage the use of it;
- increasing the amount of time spent outside, also in the evening, by considering seasonal climate conditions;
- functional integration between outdoor space and indoor activities at ground, first and basement level;
- balance between the protected historical buildings and the flexibility of the new hospital functional and organizational layout;
- location of new highly technologically complex units in small buildings or where possible by using existing ones.

The re-interpretation of the relationship between indoor-outdoor spaces, in all the different cases (hospital complex-city; buildings-surrounding areas; indoor activities-outdoor areas, etc.), show all the potential possible solutions of the innovative refurbishment of the Policlinico Umberto I of Rome and for the most part pavilion type university hospitals. The possibilities given by this kind of hospital complex is the extensive use of the outdoor space, by considering it not only beautification of residual spaces between each building or an area connecting two different points. The functional interdependence of the outdoor space and all the other activities in the hospital could be the key to overcome difficulties of integration between existing and new for the benefit of both the city and all the different type of users.

Notes

* Paragraphs by the author Valentina Napoli: Introduction; Analysis of Policlinic Umberto I outdoor space through a critical review of planning and building renovation projects from 2000 up to the current date; Spatial layout and behavioral analysis; Graphics.

** Paragraphs by the author Giuseppe Primiceri: Historical evolution of Polyclinic Umberto I of Rome; Evaluation of outdoor space quality: direct observation and questionnaire on use and perception of the space by users; Conclusions.

(1) GGHC is a system based on USGBC LEED's (United States Green Building Council Leadership in Energy and Environmental Design) for New Construction but related to health intent. In 2011 was accepted by the USGBC and reformatted as a LEED product. "LEED for Healthcare".

(2) The projects mentioned in the text are in particular by: RTI Ove Arup & Partners International Limited; RTI Studio Altieri spa; RTI Nickl& Partner Architekten Ag; ATI Proger spa.The descriptions of the projects are published in the volume edited by Giovanni Parise:"ConcorsoInternazionale di progettazione per la riorganizzazione e la ristrutturazionedelPoliclinico Umberto I", La Sapienza editions, 2009, where described also are the 10 projects by the selected competitors for the Masterplan.

References

Boccia, A. (2006), "Il Policlinico Umberto I: esigenza della costruzione", in Serarcangeli C. (Ed), *Il Policlinico Umberto I. Un secolo di storia*, Casa Editrice Università degli Studi di Roma "La Sapienza", Rome, IT, pp.22.

Cooper Marcus, C. and Barnes, M. (1999), *Healing Gardens: Therapeutic Benefits and Design Recommendations*, John Wiley & Sons, New York, USA.

Cooper Marcus, C. and Sachs, N. A. (2014), "Design Outdoor Spaces to Fit Specific Patient Population. Healthcare design", available at http://www.healthcaredesignmagazine.com/article/designing-outdoor-spaces-fit-specific-patient-populations(Accessed: 23rd April 2014).

Gehl, J. (2011), *Life between buildings: using public space*,Island Press, Washington, USA.

Giofrè, F. and Terranova, F.(2004), *Hospital and Land*, Alinea, Florence, IT, pp.100-104.

Green Guide for Health Care (2008), "Sustainable Site", available at http://www.gghc.org/tools.2.2.design.php (Accessed: 4th April 2014).

Guarini, R. (2006), "Cento anni di storia del Policlinico Umberto I", in Serarcangeli C. (Ed), *Il Policlinico Umberto I. Un secolo di storia*, Casa Editrice Università degli Studi di Roma "La Sapienza", Rome, IT, p.7.

Messinetti, S. and Pedrocchi, A. M. (2012), "Il Policlinico Umberto I. Progettazione e Realizzazione", in Messinetti, S. and Bartolucci, P. (Ed), *Il Policlinico Umberto I di Roma nella Storia dello Stato Unitario Italiano*, Istituto poligrafico e Zecca dello Stato Spa, Rome, IT, p.6.

Parise, G. (ed.) (2009), *Concorso Internazionale di progettazione per la riorganizzazione e la ristrutturazione del Policlinico Umberto I*, La Sapienza Edizioni, Rome, IT.

Pasquali, E. (1881), *Relazione della commissione incaricata dall'Accademia di studiare il Progetto del Policlinico da erigersi in Roma*, Tipografia dell'Opinione, Rome, IT, p.15.

Tyson, M. (1998), *The Healing Landscape: Therapeutic Outdoor Environments*, McGraw-Hill, New York, USA.

Ulrich, R. S. (1984), "View through a window may influence recovery from surgery", *Science*, Vol. 13, pp.523-556.

12

Hospital open spaces. Healing or threatening environments. Case study: Clinical centre of Niš and Clinical centre of Vojvodina in Novi Sad, Serbia

Vesna Mandić and Tamara Stanisavljević

Abstract: Development of technology, centralization of hospital functions and necessity for optimization of functional connections inside the hospitals result in creating of health mega structures dedicated to efficient treatment and therapy, often neglecting the aspect of external environment. In Serbia, due to the lack of financial resources for reconstruction of the existing or construction of new healthcare facilities, priority is often given to buildings and equipment, rather to open spaces. Focus of this study is the quality of the existing open space in Clinical centre of Niš and Clinical centre of Vojvodina in Novi Sad and possibilities for creating new healing environments. Through analyses of various aspects, current situation in these two clinical centres will be presented, along with aspirations, needs and opinions of users (patients, visitors and staff). Benefits that external environments within the hospital complexes create for all users and positive effects they could make on the visual identity of the hospital will be emphasized through the results of analyses. All aspects of creating positive, pleasant, comfortable and secure ambient, with atmosphere of relief and support will be considered through this case study. Methodology of research process will include desk and internet research, field research, site surveys and interviews with patients, local inhabitants and employees of the Clinical centres. One of the goals of the study is to present the emerging need for developing integrated healthcare systems focused on overall well-being of patients and other users. New approach in planning and designing of open hospital environments could contribute to reduction of costs of treatments and interventions without changing the technology procedures or reducing their quality. Introducing green and colourful, wide and meaningful spaces may help healing process, reduce numbers of hospital days and, in the same time, increase the quality of environment during healing.

Keywords: hospital open spaces, healing process, healing/therapeutic environment, healthcare strategy.

Introduction

The positive effects of open spaces and green areas on the healing process and overall state of patients and other hospitals users is already known not only to hospital planners but also to medical staff and hospital management.

Therapeutic environment which provides physical, emotional and spiritual comfort to the patients, visitors and staff has been neglected due to technological development of hospitals. In the recent years, it was rediscovered as successful way to create users' (mainly patients) oriented hospital, open towards outdoor spaces transmitting a message of acceptance and support.

With rise of the Architectural psychology, humanization of physical space became one of the main tendencies of planning. In case of hospital buildings, the attention was focused primarily on patients, considering both their physical and emotional needs.

This study will explain possibilities for provision of supportive, inviting, secure and non-threatening atmosphere in open hospital spaces, in the two Clinical centres in Serbia, identifying general and specific problems in the process of creating quality therapeutic environments.

Physical potentials of the existing environments within hospital complexes, and their effects on users' perception of space are crucial factors for choice of future intervention model. Overview of user's needs and aspirations will help in definition of possibilities for modification of existing environments in the Clinical centre of Niš and Clinical centre of Vojvodina in Novi Sad.

As patient's perception while staying in a hospital is frequently distorted, limited and influenced by various external factors, it is in constant need of a greater support than in everyday circumstances. Study will recognize and explain possible methods and means of open space planning in order to provide healing environments for different groups of users.

The awareness of positive influences of hospital open spaces on patients healing process has long been present in hospital planning in the world. Focusing on two cities as examples, this study will present actual situation in Serbia, through analyses of various aspects that need to be considered while planning and creating healing environments for the benefit of patients.

Starting Hypothesis

General Hypothesis

1. Permanent progress of technology, leading to centralization of hospital functions and optimization of functional connections, results in lack of necessity for open spaces within healthcare environments.

2. Decision making process is primarily determined by general strategy on healthcare and available budget for investments defined by the Ministry of health of the Republic of Serbia and other relevant institutions.

Specific Hypothesis

3. Pavilion type of hospitals allows focus on both physical structures and open spaces of hospital, i.e. allows contemplation of human approach.

4. Potentials of the existing open spaces are inadequately exploited - Clinical centre of Niš and Clinical centre of Vojvodina in Novi Sad as examples.

5. Lack of financial resources leads to negligence of the existing open spaces and absence of planning of new ones through future interventions.

Clinical centre of Niš and Clinical centre of Vojvodina in Novi Sad

Clinical centre of Niš (1) is a tertiary health care facility (2) constituted of 37 organisational units (Clinics, Centres, Departments, etc.). It is the second largest Clinical centre in Serbia and gravitation area is the territory of the Southeast and South of Serbia with around three million inhabitants. Around half million of patients are treated annually.

It is located in central area of the city with good accessibility potentials. Complex is organized in individual buildings (25 pavilion type buildings and 2 off-site buildings) dedicated to different medical functions (preventive, diagnostic, therapeutic and rehabilitation), non-medical functions and support services. Clinical centre is also a teaching facility of the Medical faculty of the University of Niš.

Clinical centre of Vojvodina (3) provides tertiary level of health care services for the northern province of Serbia. In the same time it represents the main research and education centre of Faculty of medicine of the University of Novi Sad.

It is located in Novi Sad, 1km from the city centre. It consists of 37 buildings organized as pavilions, with 20 specialist clinics, 5 centres, 1 polyclinic and 4 service facilities.

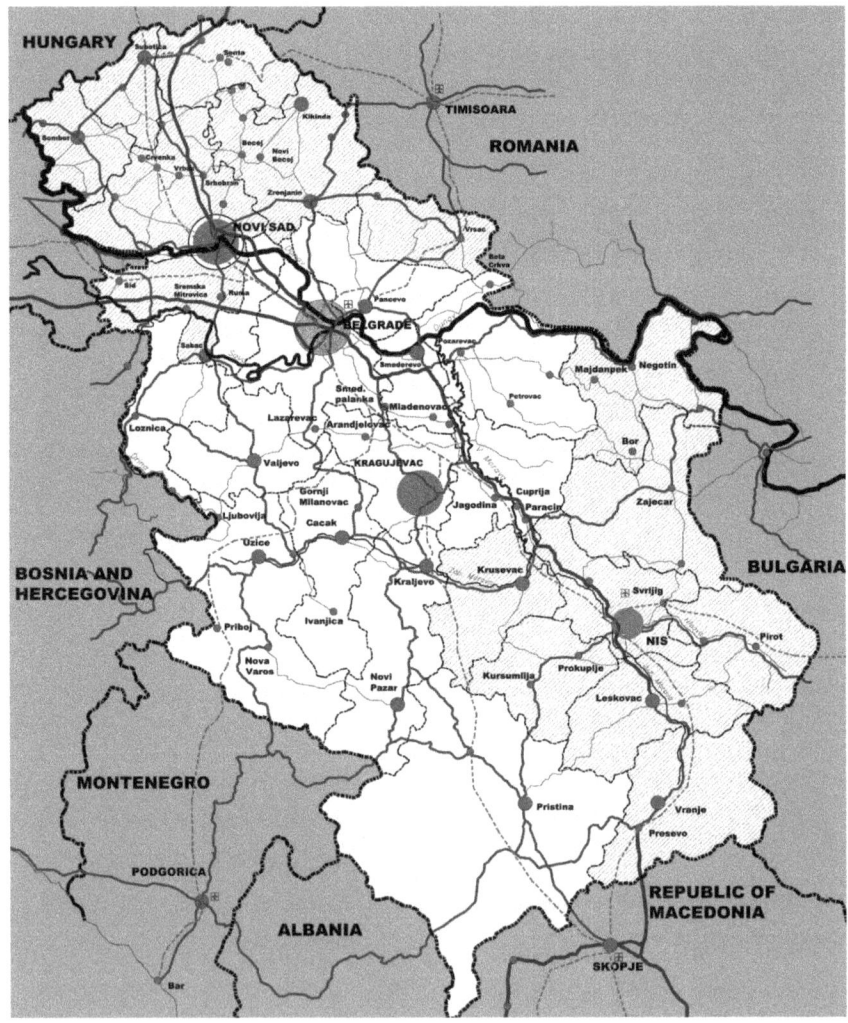

Figure 1: Gravitational areas: Clinical centre of Niš and Clinical centre of Vojvodina in Novi Sad

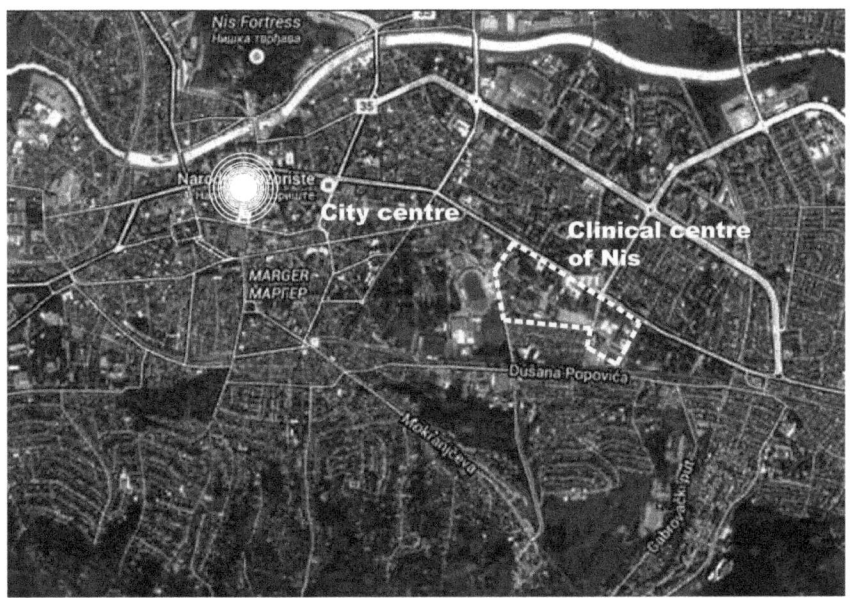

Figure 2-3: Location of Clinical centre of Niš and site borders (above) and location of Clinical centre of Vojvodina in Novi Sad and site borders (below)

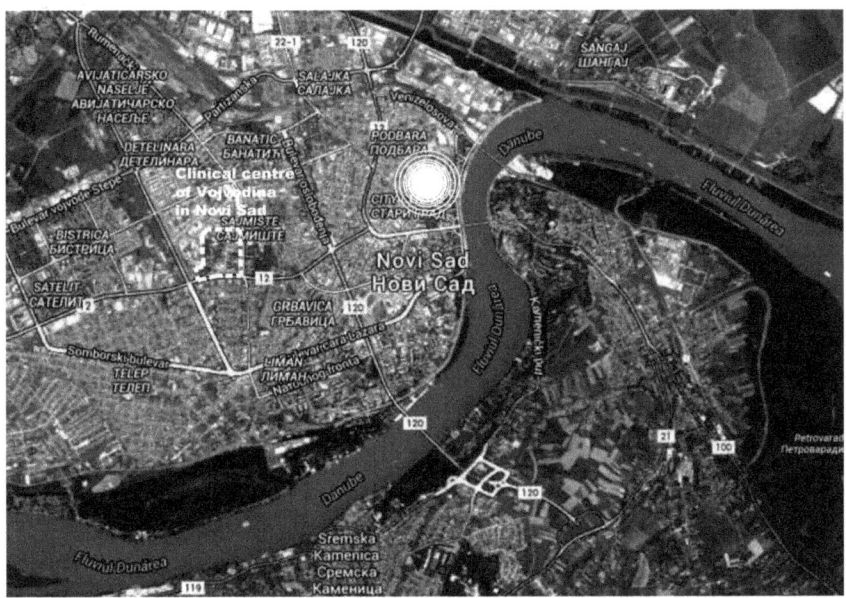

Analyses

Analysis of actual condition of open spaces in Clinical centre of Niš and Clinical centre of Vojvodina in Novi Sad will result in valorisation and possibilities for improvement of the existing open spaces and definition of opportunities for creation of new environments.

Case study will consider the needs of three groups of users:
- patients (outpatients, inpatients) with specific needs based on (dis)abilities, physical or mental state, etc.
- employees (doctors, nurses, administration, technical staff, etc.) who could use open spaces as places for stress relief and energy recovery during the pauses or as an escape in mentally and physically demanding working conditions
- visitors who could use open spaces in company of patients they are visiting as pleasant, balanced and positive environments that encourages the healing.

In conclusion, case study is expected to define models for realization of interventions in both Clinical centres with a goal of creating open spaces that provide feeling of security, relaxation and wellbeing, all in accordance with the needs of all groups of users.

Accessibility: easy way finding/orientation

Users of hospital environment are often stressed, preoccupied and disoriented as they are dealing with potential treat for their own or someone else's health or life. In such mental state, unmarked accesses, unclear circulation routes or confusing ambient without landmarks, info-boards and way finding signs can cause increased sense of insecurity, disorder and anxiety of users.

Moreover, circulation systems in hospital complexes are critical not only to enable clear and intuitive way finding for patients, visitors and staff but also for infection control, i.e. circulation system has to be carefully planned to separate and control public and private, clean and soiled traffic types. In planning the hospital open spaces, a logical and simple circulation system is the essential framework for effective work of the whole system.

Clinical centre of Niš

Clinical centre of Niš is open towards the Zoran Đinđić Boulevard on the northern side and has several accesses for vehicles and for pedestrians. Border between hospital and public area is not defined which could enable connection of the two areas into single environment in planned manner.

Main vehicular access is from Zetska street. This access is controlled by ramp and staff and equipped by information board. From this side also several pedestrian accesses are in function. On the southern side, from Ljube Nenadovića street, high buildings and walls are forming the barrier and preventing access to the clinical centre area. Another vehicular access for patients is from the east, from Vojislava Ilića street.

Main entrance to Clinical centre is marked and can be easily recognized. Other entrances are not clearly marked and seem like accesses to parks or private housing areas. Circulation inside the complex is not distinguished or organized, visitors' and patients' routes are intersecting which results in confusion and causes waste of time.

Outdoor signalisation and way finding signs are not foreseen which creates difficulties in orientation and circulation inside the complex for the first time users that are not familiar with the surroundings. New visitors and out-patients coming for the first time in the Clinical centre will lose time getting oriented. Additionally, insecurity is increased by lack of information boards on buildings specifying either the position of entrance or the functions that are hosted.

Signs and info points are missing also on internal roads, contributing to the disorientation of users. New visually recognizable items with appropriate design and use of light are necessary for functional revival of space.

Clinical centre of Vojvodina in Novi Sad

Main pedestrian access to the hospital area and the vehicular access dedicated for persons with disabilities are from Hajduk Veljkova street, while main vehicular access for visitors, out-patients, staff, logistics and alternative access for ambulance is from the north side, from Novosadski sajam street. Ambulances access the complex from Futoška street on the north border of the Clinical centre area. This access is also dedicated to administrative staff.

Main pedestrian entrance to the Clinical centre is marked, covered by access control and equipped by information board so that users can be informed how to reach the clinic they need. All vehicular accesses are covered by access control.

Situation in Clinical centre of Vojvodina in Novi Sad in relations to outdoor signalisation, way finding signs and info points is similar to the one in Clinical centre in Niš. Patients and visitors often depend on good will and patience of employees to obtain information on desired destinations.

Consideration

Hospital open spaces must be accessible and physically secure for different categories of users with different abilities or age. It is important to create environment visually clear and easy to move through. In the process of remodelling of open hospital spaces accesses to hospital buildings and flows of material, patients and staff have to be planned and marked.

In order to reduce confusion and achieve functional circulation in the hospital complex it is necessary for both Clinical centres to visually highlight entrances to the complex, to clearly mark every building in the complex and to place the way-finding signs in order to enable easy orientation. Signalisation could also have artistic value in order to present visual landmarks in space. Existing visual marks in space are info boards on the entrances of the complexes that are unrepresentative and old. These signs and boards have only informative purpose without any visual value. Validity of the information they are providing is questionable, having in mind that they haven't been replaced or updated for decades.

Information boards should be placed on each entrance and on characteristic places within the complexes (parking areas, internal cross-roads, large parks, etc.). Visually recognizable landmarks will help orientation in space. Besides info boards and signs, sculptures and decorative plants could be used for this purpose. Clear directions, guidance through the hospital environment and existence of landmarks will ensure the feeling of organization and order, security and protection.

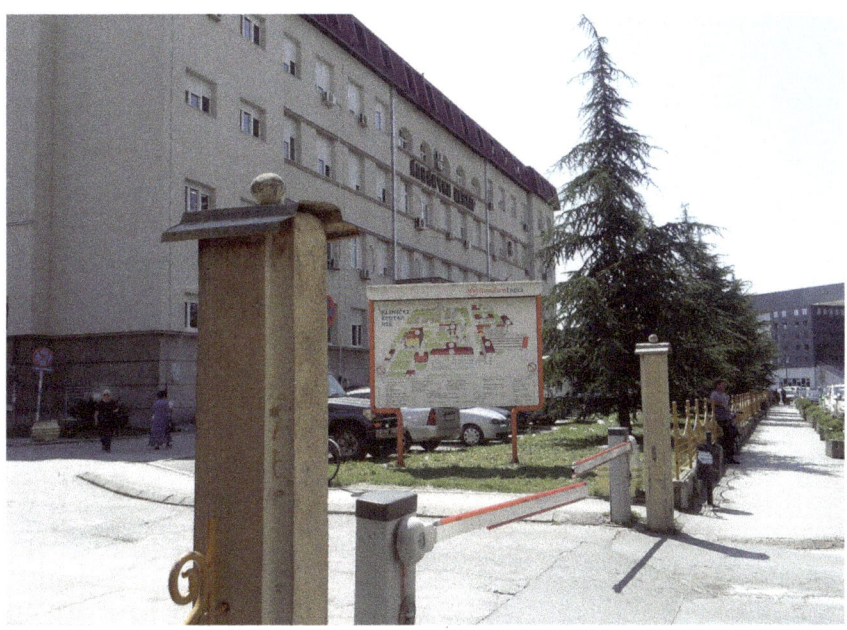

Figure 4-5: Clinical centre of Niš – Main entrance to the Clinical centre (above) and Clinical centre of Vojvodina in Novi Sad - Main pedestrian entrance to the Clinical centre (below) photo by Vesna Mandić and Tamara Stanisavljević

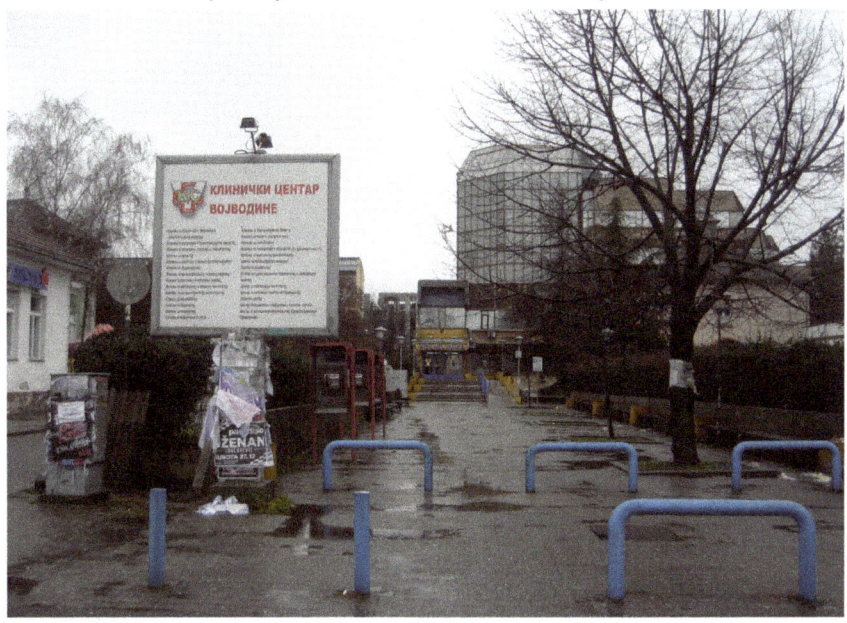

Traffic and circulation

Issue of traffic and circulation is commonly declared as one of the most important issues to be resolved in hospital planning. The very first things that designer and planners think of is to separate different types of traffic/circulation, keep the traffic routes as simple and as short as possible, keep the entrances and public areas well exposed and easily recognizable while keeping the areas with limited and controlled access out of reach of non-authorised users. Even if these principles are essential primarily for internal traffic and circulation, they are fully applicable also to the external areas of hospitals.

As already explained in paragraph "Accessibility – easy way finding/orientation", hospital users, most commonly in a personal distress or in distress for another person, need to feel secure and comfortable in using the space, need to be doubts-free and in position to quickly achieve the goal of their presence in hospital complex. Speaking in practical terms in relation to traffic and circulation, these are some of the principles that would have to be respected to allow comfort for users:

- traffic and circulation must be guided and controlled, i.e. must be planned, not defined freely by individual users
- definition of entrances, depending on the respective users and activities, must be applied
- parking areas must be easily found, logically positioned and connected to the users destinations functions
- drop-of points must be foreseen for individual functions where significant number of patients with inability to move without assistance is expected
- walking distances must be optimized according to the specific characteristics of users
- sidewalks must be provided with sufficient width to comfortably host the circulation of users at its highest frequency.

Even if the users rarely recognize it as direct source of impression and personal feeling, respecting or disrespecting of these elementary principles leads to feeling of comfort or discomfort in using the space.

Clinical centre of Niš

Internal traffic and circulation inside the complex of Clinical centre of Niš does not seem to be severely controlled by the Clinical centre. For start, even if the access control exists in all vehicular entrances to the complex, entrance criteria does not seem strict as access is allowed to majority of interested users. Entrance fee is foreseen (payable directly at the access points), but without real results in reducing the number of vehicles that enter the complex.

Main parking area is located in the zone between the existing part of the complex and zone dedicated to future expansions of the complex, in front of controlled vehicular entrance from Vojislava Ilića street. Smaller parking areas are located in the immediate surroundings of buildings hosting the functions that the parking areas are dedicated to. All parking areas seem to be with insufficient capacity for current organization of activities in the Clinical centres, as they are often blocked and without free spaces.

Excessive number of vehicles and lack of free parking spaces lead to increase of anxiety of users, as either in stress, discomfort, pain or simply in hurry, they fail to find a solution for easy vehicular access to the desired destination.

In addition, either as the result of an objective necessity or due to simple indolence, some of users tend to insist on vehicular access to the points closest to their destination, even without availability of designated parking areas, finding the place for their vehicles on the internal roads, on the internal sidewalks or even in green areas. These actions may provide a solution for objective or subjective needs of individual users. However, they result in inability for other users to comfortably use or sometimes even access the roads, sidewalks and areas that they lead to, resulting in increased discontent, discomfort and anxiety.

Vehicular access to main entrances of other buildings is possible, but these areas are not organized as drop-off points.

Clinical centre of Vojvodina in Novi Sad

Internal traffic and circulation inside the complex of Clinical centre of Vojvodina in Novi Sad seem to be functioning well in accordance to the conditions on site. Separation of entrances is clearly distinguished and access control is functioning in all the entrances.

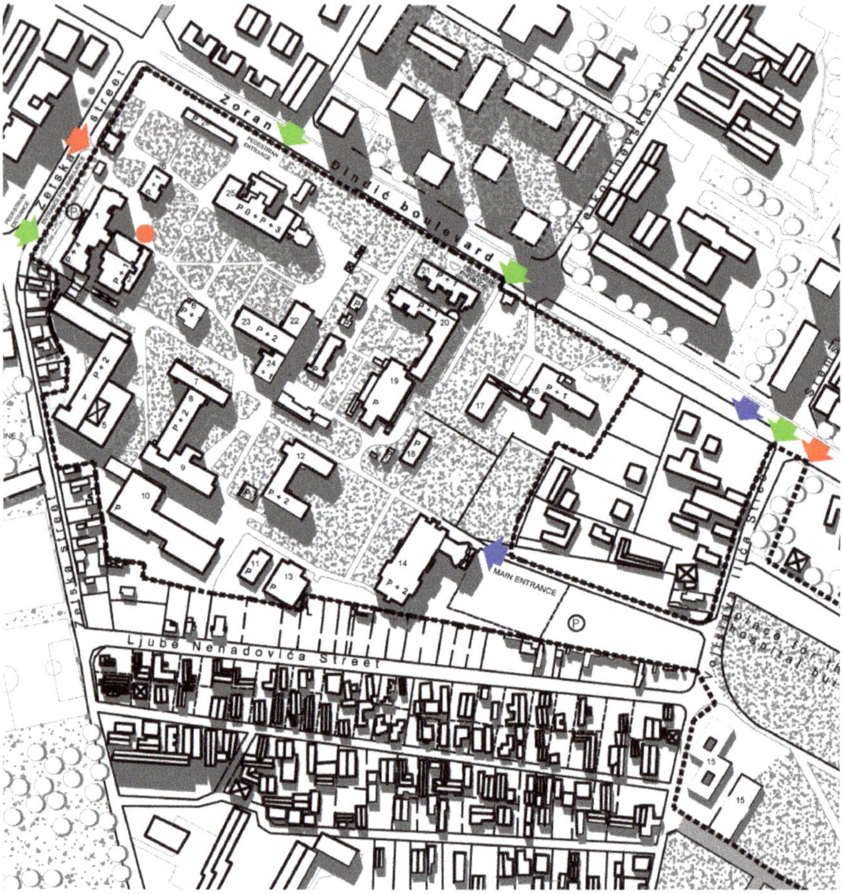

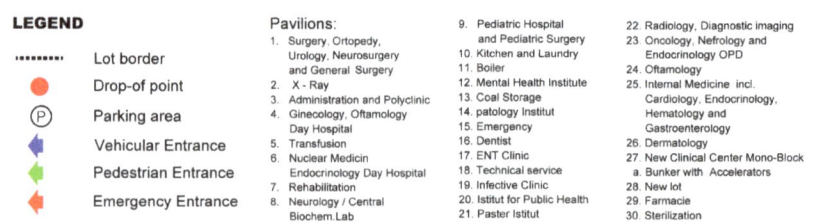

LEGEND

·········· Lot border
● Drop-of point
Ⓟ Parking area
◀ Vehicular Entrance
◀ Pedestrian Entrance
◀ Emergency Entrance

Pavilions:
1. Surgery, Ortopedy, Urology, Neurosurgery and General Surgery
2. X - Ray
3. Administration and Polyclinic
4. Ginecology, Oftamology Day Hospital
5. Transfusion
6. Nuclear Medicin Endocrinology Day Hospital
7. Rehabilitation
8. Neurology / Central Biochem.Lab
9. Pediatric Hospital and Pediatric Surgery
10. Kitchen and Laundry
11. Boiler
12. Mental Health Institute
13. Coal Storage
14. patology Institut
15. Emergency
16. Dentist
17. ENT Clinic
18. Technical service
19. Infective Clinic
20. Istitut for Public Health
21. Paster Istitut
22. Radiology, Diagnostic imaging
23. Oncology, Nefrology and Endocrinology OPD
24. Oftamology
25. Internal Medicine incl. Cardiology, Endocrinology, Hematology and Gastroenterology
26. Dermatology
27. New Clinical Center Mono-Block
    a. Bunker with Accelerators
28. New lot
29. Farmacie
30. Sterilization

Figure 6: Clinical centre of Niš, internal traffic and circulation routes

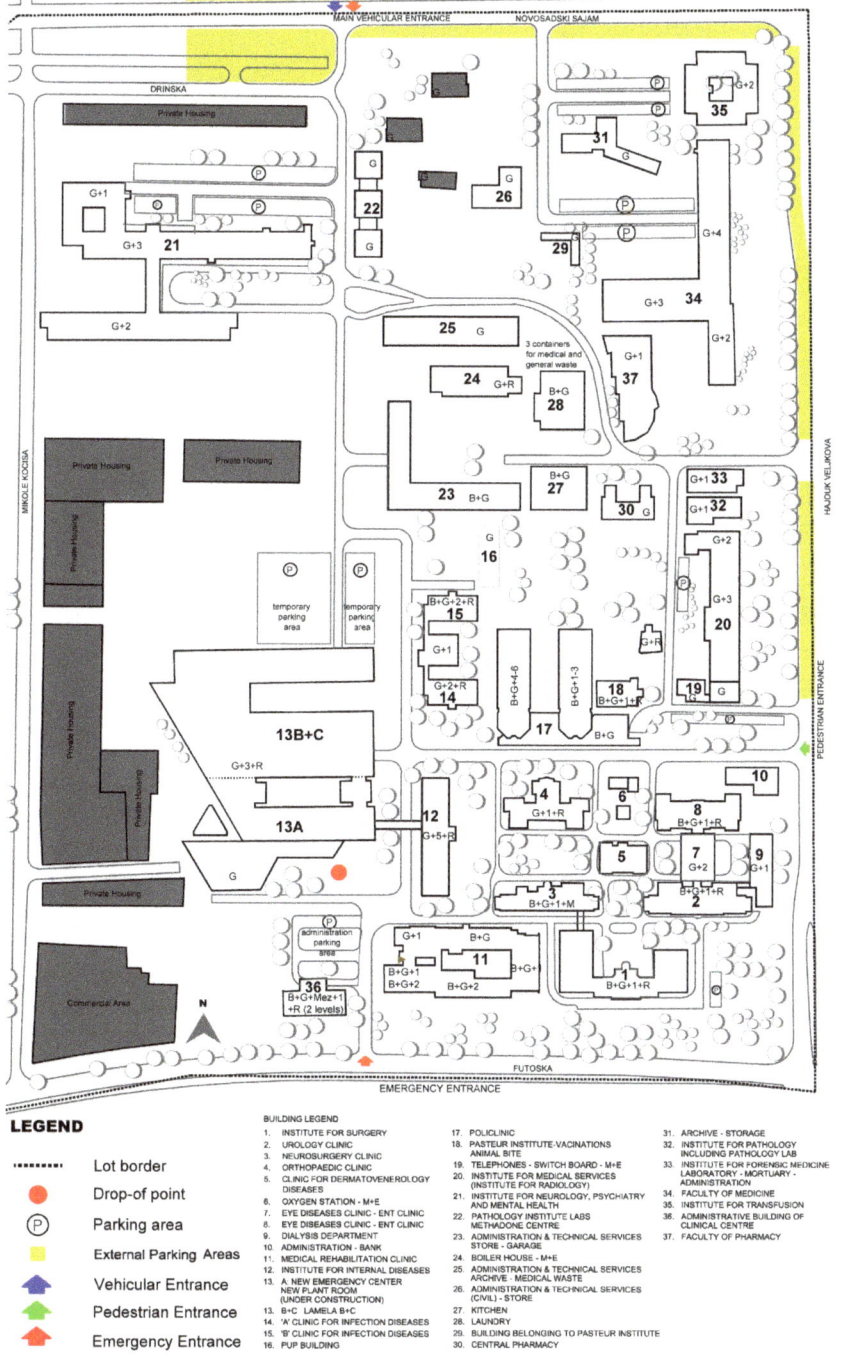

Figure 7: Clinical centre of Vojvodina in Novi Sad: Internal traffic and circulation routes

Small parking areas in the immediate surroundings of function that they are dedicated to are the only parking areas inside the complex, i.e. there is no central parking of the complex. Small capacity of existing parking areas does not seem to cause problems in everyday functioning of the hospital, as vehicles can be found only in parking areas or, alternatively, in the abandoned areas surrounding the unfinished Lamellas B and C. Roads and sidewalks are normally accessible and passable, as the result of control by hospital and/or affirmative attitude of users. Discontent, discomfort and anxiety in circulation through the Clinical centre are reduced.

Adequate drop-off point is foreseen where mostly needed – at the main entrance of lamella A – Emergency centre. Vehicular access to main entrances of other buildings is possible, but these areas are not organized as drop-off points.

Alternative mean of transportation, despite the general function of the complex and related groups of users that are often in uncomfortable situation, is bicycle, one of the typical means of transport in Vojvodina and one of specific characteristics of the local culture.

Walking distances seem to be adequate, both for users accessing the Clinical centre by vehicles (cars and bicycles), as the parking areas are located close to the buildings, and for users accessing the Clinical centre by foot, as main pedestrian access is favourably positioned in relation to entrances to the buildings.

Consideration

Optimal organization of traffic and circulation must be one of the priorities for planning and functioning of hospitals. Valid technical regulations, recommendations in the field and specific characteristics and habits of users must be analysed in order to define the right approach for each single hospital.

Number of vehicles entering the complex must be limited and in line with available spatial capacities. This can be achieved by adequate access control system and later control of movement/parking of vehicles inside the complex. All circulation can be controlled either by dedicated staff or by planned physical barriers in space.

On the other hand, possibility of easy access to the desired destination should be provided, if not by personal vehicles of users then by alternative ways of transport, e.g. mini buses from dislocated parking areas to individual entrances to buildings.

This approach could allow not only the increase of parking capacities in multi-storey parking areas and/or garages in peripheral parts of the complex but also provide more free space for green areas, little squares and other open areas inside the complex dedicated to mental relief of users.

Drop-off points should be established where possible to allow both easy access to the building and uninterrupted flow of traffic.

Sidewalks should be adequately planned and passability should be guaranteed to allow free and uninterrupted movement of pedestrians. Walking distances should correspond to the actual needs of users, e.g. possibilities for reduction of these distances should be analysed to encourage the users in respecting the traffic and circulation plan established by the hospital.

Generally speaking, traffic and circulation should be organized effectively, merely as support service to the primary function of the complex. Accordingly, they must be treated with full consideration of all the aspects through planning phase. Only in this way, rational individual solutions can be found achieving not only the comfort for users, but also other benefits for the hospital (running costs, maintenance cost, etc.).

Persons with disabilities

According to the UN terminology, term "Person with disability" identifies a person with a physical or mental impairment that significantly restricts his or her ability to perform daily living activities. Due to the restriction(s), person with disability faces specific challenges in everyday living activities and often requires assistance and support.

This term refers predominantly to permanent disability. However, person can experience temporary disability due to specific life time events (in case of accidents, after interventions or surgeries, etc.), leading to the increase of number of people requiring special conditions and/or assistance and support in using the space in hospitals.

The most commonly noticed 'obstacles' are physical barriers in space and lack of accessibility conditions. However, also lack of possibility to communicate, i.e. obtain information, is a significant 'obstacle' for persons with disabilities.

Clinical centre of Niš

Current condition on site of Clinical centre of Niš shows low recognition of special requirements of persons with disabilities. Sidewalks are not dimensioned nor equipped for safe and comfortable usage, e.g. ramps on sidewalks in contact with roads, tactile paving surface, off-road and on-road platform edges are missing, etc., dedicated parking areas are not provided, there are no special assistance services and systems applied, etc. Additional barriers are vehicles of individual users that are often parked outside the parking areas, on sidewalks along the internal roads of Clinical centre.

The principle of inclusion is being applied through the on-going project or reconstruction of one of the existing buildings into "Examination & Treatment Block" and construction of new "Ward Units Block" and corresponding external area.

Clinical centre of Vojvodina in Novi Sad

Current condition on site of Clinical centre of Vojvodina in Novi Sad is similar to the one of Clinical centre of Niš. However, recent interventions realized in this Clinical centre show the orientation of hospital management towards the principles of inclusion. In particular, during the most recent intervention in Clinical centre, reconstruction of Lamella A of Emergency-diagnostic centre into contemporary Emergency centre (finalized in 2010), principles of inclusion were applied both to internal space and external area. This tendency is being continued through the on-going project or reconstruction of Lamellas B and C of Emergency-diagnostic centre and corresponding external area.

Consideration

In order to allow equal possibilities in interaction with hospital space for all hospitals users, regardless to their (dis)abilities, it is necessary to plan and apply available technologies, services and assistance methods towards the goal of friendly, communicative surrounding without barriers where the users will feel welcomed and not threatened. Application of the mentioned tools and planning of supportive physical elements, as per principles of inclusion, is the only adequate method of planning and organization of open spaces in contemporary hospitals.

Physical aspects of space

Contemporary approach to organization of hospitals is generally driven by principle of optimization in terms of functionality, reduction of distances and, of course, rational financial plan. In addition, continuous advancement of technology leads to increased possibilities of diagnostics and treatment, widely applicable to all medical disciplines and resulting in the tendency of centralization of hospital functions to provide full availability to all departments. In these conditions, volumes of buildings tend to increase, distances between the buildings tend to reduce, all this to the level where the entire hospital complex becomes a single mega structure hosting all necessary medical functions and support systems.

Even if such structures do correspond to the elementary tasks that they are built for, effect on the users, especially patients, can be understood also as negative. Under the explained conditions, users become simple, tiny parts of huge machinery, where the predominant and single important fact is that they are, e.g., patients, neglecting that they are, before all, humans. Users become, in some sense, irrelevant as individual, relevant simply as a group or element of the system, or, in other words, they become and begin to feel trifling.

The explained negative effect of modern tendencies is being noticed by the professionals and, as the result, concept of humanization in designing of hospitals is being promoted. General principle of humanization is to provide and environment corresponding both to the human's objective and subjective needs, allowing the people to feel important as individuals. Consequently, the tendency becomes to consider the needs of the patients a starting point of spatial organization and planning interventions.

Humanization concept in designing gives the possibility to create hospital environment with the sense of acceptance and familiarity, environment that provides respect for privacy, yet allows easy impression of space and sensory comfort, environment that provides possibilities to fight against or even prevent some of the stress factors.

The possibilities of implementation of humanization concept are numerous. Some of the basic tools can be recognized in different distribution and composition of spaces, use of different shapes and sizes of buildings, use of build structures as a tool for creating adequate external ambient, etc., or simply finding solutions for internal and external spaces to mutually work for the benefit of users. For example, long distances between the buildings contribute to understanding of buildings as separate units, not elements of the same system. Conversely, distances that are too short do not allow creating of external ambient and space is understood as communication only, not as a potential ambient. Buildings that are too high, too wide or simply dominant in space can have threatening impact on users, as they may feel claustrophobic, vulnerable or unimportant.

Clinical centre of Niš

Complex of Clinical centre of Niš is organized in pavilion system, with independent buildings dedicated to individual medical specialization and support services. Buildings are positioned mainly along the streets surrounding the complex, with particularity that the buildings positioned around main entrance, are the highest buildings of the complex.

Each building can be considered a micro unit with corresponding external area, while the distances between the buildings are sufficient to allow creating relief and resting places for all users. Even if there is evidence that open spaces are developed to the certain level and being used to the certain extent, obviously there are still potentials to improvement.

On the other side, organization of hospital complex and promotion of use of open space are sort of legacy from previous periods. In contemporary moments, most recent interventions follow the principle of centralization of functions and reduction of distances, which can be easily noticed on the example of Centre for radiology, constructed in 2005 as a structure directly attached to the existing Clinical for general surgical disciplines. In case this approach in intervention continues, the result would jeopardize the spatial capacities of open spaces and lead to prevail of technology over humanization.

Clinical centre of Vojvodina in Novi Sad

Complex of Clinical centre of Vojvodina in Novi Sad is organized predominantly in pavilion system with several relatively recent buildings organized more following the principles of centralization. Several different approaches in planning can be recognized depending on period of construction:

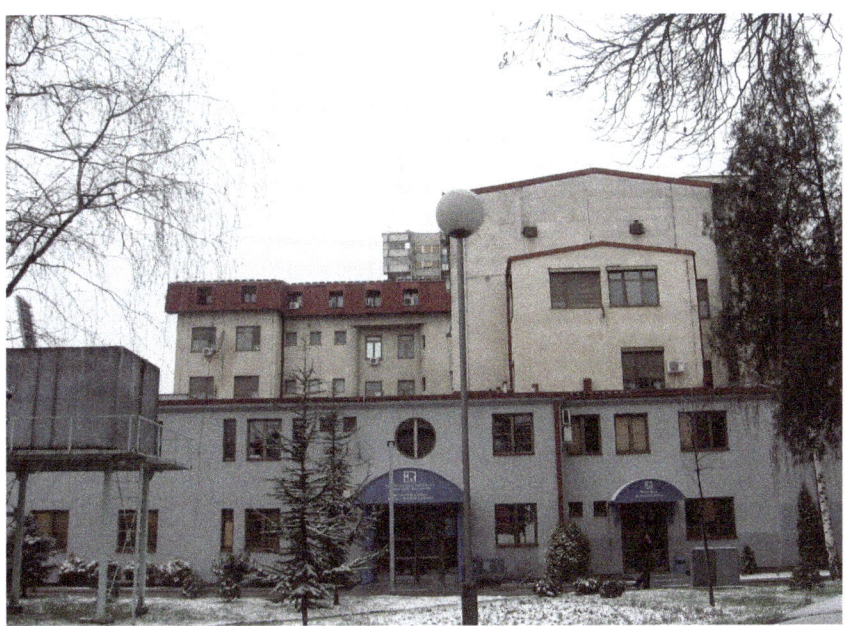

*Figure 8-9: Clinical centre of Niš – Centre for radiology (above) and
Clinical centre of Vojvodina in Novi Sad - Physical aspects of different types of buildings (below)
photo by Vesna Mandić and Tamara Stanisavljević*

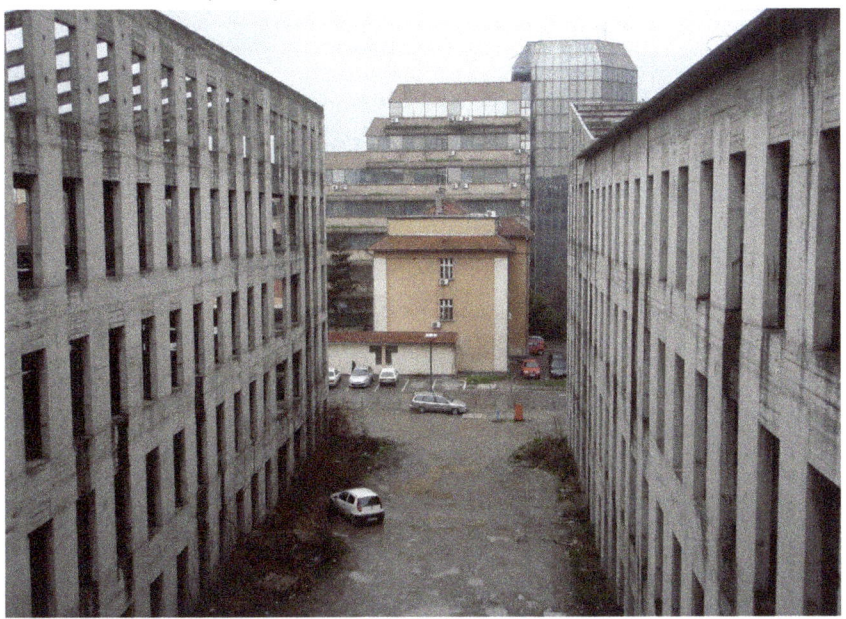

- zone of oldest buildings, constructed in the first half of 20th century, in the southeast corner of the complex, that were positioned on moderate distances and constructed with moderate dimensions, with a clear result of humanized space, generally appealing and non-threatening for the users
- individual buildings (constructed in the second half of 20th century) dominant either in height or in plan surfaces, recognized as independent structures and not particularly oriented towards the users subjective reactions
- mega structure – Emergency diagnostics centre with 3 connected lamellas (structure constructed at the end of 20th century, partly reconstructed at the very beginning of 21st century), oriented directly towards the efficiency of healthcare service denying the subjective factors and emotional states of users.

Appreciation of link with nature and possibilities for use of open spaces as element of healing process is easily recognisable in the zone of the oldest buildings, while this link fades rapidly with increase of dimensions of buildings and reduction of distances between them. Focus on reduction of distances and increasing efficiency of healthcare service is recognizable also through the latest interventions in the complex and the initiative for establishing hot, covered connections between the existing buildings.

Consideration

Architectural forms, concept and typology of hospital buildings evolve over time due to the development of technology. Even if current tendencies are oriented mostly toward the curing and treatment, some of them promote also the values of healing buildings (environments) that are clearly structured with access to fresh air and greenery, exemplifying the belief in the healing powers of rationality and nature.

The relation of technology oriented principles and nature oriented principles in designing might seem simple. However, not only that it is complex to establish theoretical model of the right approach that would combine the most favourable aspects of both principles, but the situation becomes even more intricate when it comes to specific hospitals. Accordingly, individual solutions must be found based on serious, detailed analyses oriented towards the goal of providing a safe, comfortable environment, and reduction of stress and anxiety for users, without jeopardizing the necessary efficiency of the healing and treatment processes. Successful will be only those solutions that recognize both the dimensions of human approach and the needs of efficient operations, i.e. those designs that will succeed in finding the right relation between the technology and nature.

Stress relief

Anxiety is a general term for several disorders that cause nervousness, fear, apprehension, and worry. These disorders affect how we feel and behave, and they can manifest real physical symptoms. Space where people spend time, especially when feeling vulnerable and when their health is jeopardized can affect their behaviour, increase their fears and worry. Open spaces without organization will cause disorder, feeling of abandonment and threat.

Touch of nature: green areas and trees

Green areas provide balance, calm and self-control, and have a positive effect on people's emotional state. The fact that green areas and trees have the most important role in shaping open hospital environments can't be surprising as physical and visual connection with natural environment produces benefits on multiple levels for the patient.

Spending time in nature brings a sense of peace and tranquillity, while social interaction possible in green areas enhances immune functions and produces better reactions on treatments. In hospital environments where everything is controlled (what and when you can eat, what you will wear, when you sleep, time for therapy and medicines, etc.), life routine of each patient is changed and it is normal to feel stress, fear and anxiety. Green areas can offer an "escape" from the hospital environment, giving the patient the sense of control to choose between variety of spaces, from some private and some open, some sunny, some shady, some with background sounds, some without.

Experience of connection with nature for the lying patients can be obtained by indirect contact with outdoors through the windows. For this purpose environments visible from the patient's room have to be planned carefully.

Green roofs are the most effective way of connection between urban structures and nature and could present stress relief points both for patients and for staff. These areas positioned within the building provide possibility of contact with nature for all users, as they are easily accessible even for the patients with limited ability to move.

All flat roofs on the existing buildings could be potential gardens in the future, which is considered positive and recommendable solution from the ecological and energy saving point of view.

Creating open space ambient which promote and encourage different activities dedicated to all users could even reduce the number of hospital days, reduce cost of medical treatments and improve the process of healing.

Choice of plants is important, in order to provide visual effects and natural environment during the whole year and also because of the possible influence of specific plants on the health of the patients. It is not recommendable to provoke allergic reactions by choosing the plants with high pollen production. Some other choices could bring benefits to the patients, especially conifers with the influence of such ecosystems on pulmonary patients.

Clinical centre of Niš

Clinical centre of Niš is rich in green areas but the impression of these areas is not adequately created. Potentials of these green areas and trees should be acknowledged and used for better treatment outcomes. With different levels of interventions, green areas could be organized as places for physical and mental recuperation.

Clinical centre in Niš has great number of buildings with different ward units. Rooms are oriented on different sides of the lot, which is in a great percentage covered with green areas and could be organized in a way to provide pleasant sights and sense of connection with nature for in-patients.

Clinical centre of Vojvodina in Novi Sad

Clinical centre of Vojvodina has enough green areas and trees but they are not predicted to be used by patients or they are not positioned near the buildings hosting medical functions. Patients and visitors are guided directly into hospitals, without any contact with the open space. Buildings within the Clinical centre are oriented in a way to neglect green areas. Poorly designed environments are visible from patient's rooms. Spatial obstacles do not allow creation of anything other than small green micro ambient.

Planned interventions on lamellas B and C include creation of atrium and green roof on the level +1.

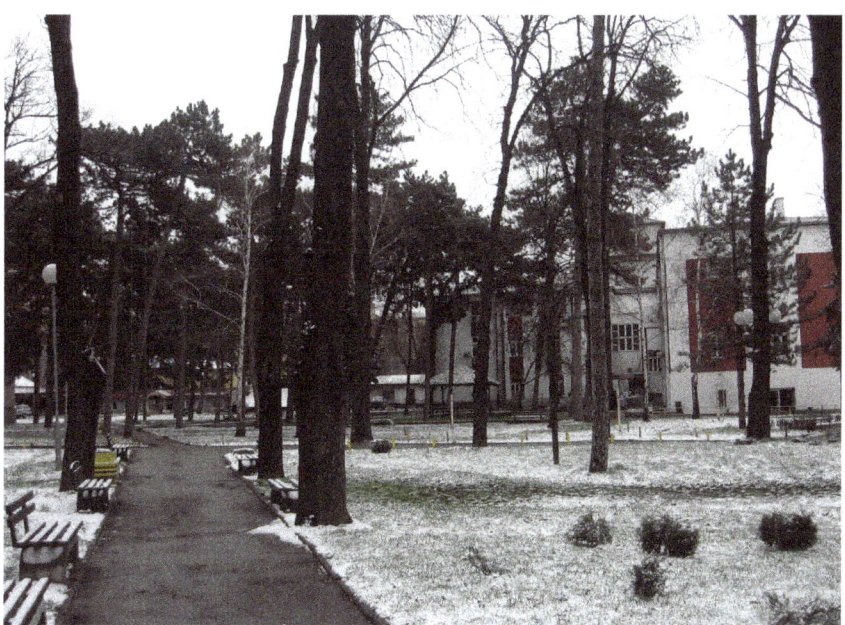

*Figure 10-11: Clinical centre of Niš – Central green area (above) and Clinical centre of Vojvodina in Novi Sad - Emergency, Space dedicated to future green ambient (below)
photo by Vesna Mandić and Tamara Stanisavljević*

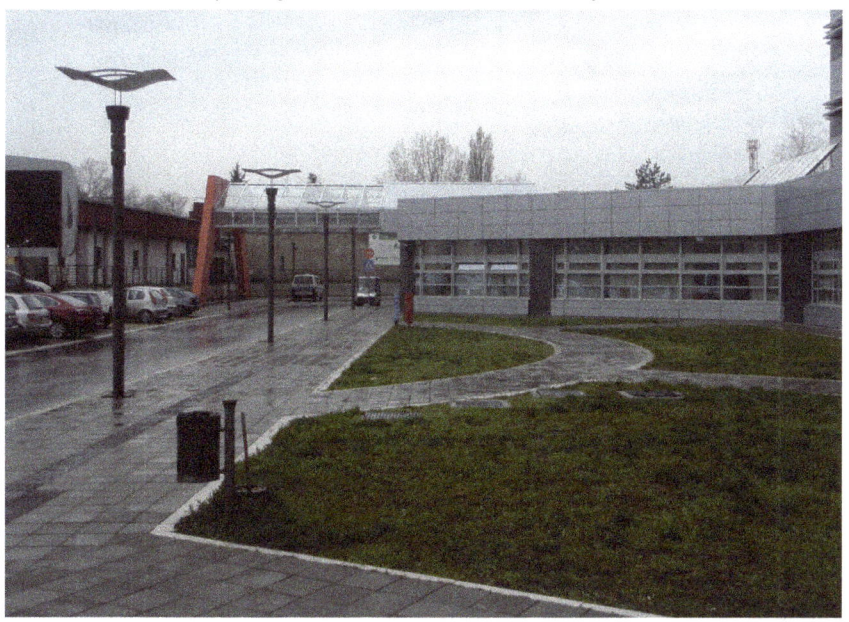

Facades as frame for open space environment

Facades of the hospital buildings present scenery for the open environments. If facades have relation with the open space and they are visually embedded with the furniture, greenery and concept of the space than the environment will be balanced, positive and useful in the process of healing and treatment.

Clinical centre of Niš

Most of the facades in the Clinical centre of Niš are old and were subjects to reconstruction several times. These reconstructions were often done in order to enable expansion of medical functions, but due to insufficient financial resources, the buildings were just enlarged with inadequate annexes. Some facades are under protection of the Government as cultural heritage, but neglected. Shaping of meaningful external areas could make connection between different styles of buildings and help diminishing the effect of eclectic and unplanned construction. Facades in Clinical centre of Niš do not create pleasant scenery as they are old, expended, poorly maintained and colourless.

Clinical centre of Vojvodina in Novi Sad

Scenery created from facades of existing buildings in Clinical Vojvodina in Novi Sad centre is heavy and depressed. Big contrast in façade treatment of the unfinished structure of lamellas B and C and new modern façade of lamella A is creating unpleasant atmosphere. With planned interventions on lamellas B and C, facades of all lamellas will be harmonized. Façade of Policlinic building on the other side of the complex with strong, dominant volume and dark colours gives an impression of aversion, conflict and fear.

Exterior elements: urban furniture, decorative and drinking water fountains

Urban furniture has the purpose not only to satisfy the conformity needs but also to produce beauty. When planning interventions in external areas it is important to choose proper furniture and other elements - comfortable, functional, simple and visually recognizable. The importance of these elements is often neglected, while the lack of simple, affordable elements such as benches, trashcans, lights, points with drinking water, etc. can cause significant discomfort of users and cause irritation.

Clinical centre of Niš

All existing outdoor furniture and exterior elements in open space environment of Clinical centre of Niš, were mounted decades ago, they are worn-out, and their state is not adequate to their purpose due to low maintenance during the years.

For example, place where the fountain was planned to be placed is ruined and neglected. Drinking fountain at the entrance of the complex is functional, but its position and visual impression testify about absence of any artistic criteria.

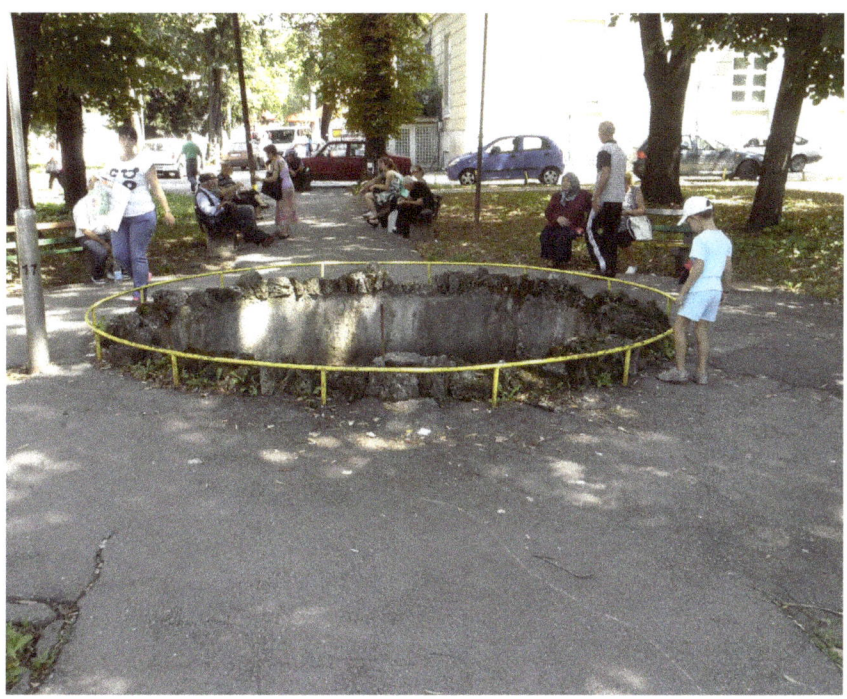

Figure 12: Clinical centre of Niš – Fountain in the central green area, photo by Vesna Mandić and Tamara Stanisavljević

Clinical centre of Vojvodina in Novi Sad

Clinical centre of Vojvodina in Novi Sad demonstrates serious lack of exterior elements. These elements can be found just in the zone of recently reconstructed lamella A and in the zone of pedestrian entrance to the complex, where outdoor furniture is used combined with trees, for creation of pleasant and comfortable surrounding.

Importance of Colours

Colour is a powerful communication tool and can be used to signal action, influence mood, and cause physiological reactions. (5) Colours influence our emotions, our actions and how we respond to various situations and environments. However, perception of colours is individual, personal and often rooted in experience or culture. For this reason and in order to use colours adequately in creating hospital open spaces, local customs, behaviour and needs have to be recognized.

Due to time and weather effects, financial scarcity and common negligence of users, conditions of open spaces inside the complex of Clinical centre of Niš and Clinical centre of Vojvodina in Novi Sad are inadequate for their purposes. Colours are not used as tools in healing processes nor in creation of visual identity of open spaces. The solitary example of creation of visually recognizable place is the façade of the new Emergency centre - lamella A in Clinical centre of Vojvodina in Novi Sad, where big red signs on the entrance façade of the building are indicative and symbolic. Red is recognized as a stimulant and is inherently exciting, known to provide power, protection and good luck.

Consideration

Interventions in external areas of clinical centres should be planned to create opportunities for physical therapy, movement and exercise in the open natural environment. Individual potential for creating various outdoor micro and macro spaces, organized to satisfy the needs of different group of users must be recognized and exploited. For example, capacity of open space in Clinical centre of Niš allows organization of areas dedicated to different activities such as walking and jogging, outdoor exercises, yoga and meditation and other group activities. On the other hand, Clinical centre of Vojvodina in Novi Sad has less capacity for open environments development resulting in possibilities of organization of micro ambient only. These cosy environments with different content can create familiar, pleasant atmosphere for patients, staff and visitors. Increased quality of space can be achieved by careful planning of use of furniture, sculptures, water and other exterior elements.

Sounds are very welcomed in the open hospital areas, helping creation of harmonized ambient, satisfying for all the senses. In some environments, the use of light music can be pleasant bringing great benefits to the patients. Introducing sounds in future planning for development of open spaces within Clinical centres in Serbia seams unreachable aim, from this point of view.

Use of natural light in space is desirable in creating micro spaces and is based on exposure to sunlight and introducing shades. This provides the choice to users to select the space according to their personal preferences – space with open or closed view, isolated, almost hidden ambient or communicative, exposed environment. Shadows can be created by buildings or by artificial elements, in form of e.g. canopies, contributing also to artistic value of space. However, shadows originated from trees are usually more pleasant for users relaxing time, socializing and recovering.

Conclusions and proposals for future actions

This study has shown that present state of buildings and open spaces in public hospitals in Serbia is at unsatisfying level for decades, due to negligence and poor maintenance. Situation can be explained by economic situation in the country, i.e. absence of available financial resources. In such conditions, interventions are done mainly on parts of individual buildings or exceptionally whole buildings, planning just the indispensable works. Available financial resources cannot ensure even reconstruction of hospitals and modernization of equipment, so consequently interventions in open spaces are barely considered. Analyses of potentials of development and improvement on the level of the entire complex are being overlooked, even if this generic approach could lead to reduction of running cost of hospitals. As the result, open spaces in Serbian hospitals never met their reconstruction time.

The solution might seem simple and obvious, as lack of financial resources is identified as the main obstacle. However, the situation is more complex as it should not be resolved at the level of individual hospitals, but based on analyses on state level with a goal of modification of general national strategy of healthcare development and producing new general national strategy in healthcare design. Current lack of this national strategy, but also lack of local regulations, standards and guidelines is already recognized as disadvantage in the on-going project of reconstruction of 4 Clinical centres in Serbia.

For start, assessment of current state in all 3 levels of healthcare system, either of all individual institutions or of selected representative samples, would have to be performed. The approach to the assessment must be interdisciplinary and include different aspects relevant for different disciplines (medical, urban planning, designing, sociology, psychology, financing etc.). Conclusions of the assessment should serve as a starting point for creating relevant set of documents defining the future imperatives of healthcare institutions development. This development should be supported through new legislation framework, interdisciplinary strategy and guidelines relevant to the specific field and supporting disciplines.

Regulations would have to be defined on the national level in cooperation with professional associations specialized in planning process and hospital development, in cooperation of different sectors and engagement of numerous stakeholders. General national strategy in healthcare design and actual plan for future development of hospitals should be produced in line with new general national strategy of healthcare development. Partnerships on all levels (national, regional and local) are necessary to create adequate conditions for realisation of planned actions and to ensure that the actions are executed respecting the needs of actual users.

Goal of these activities would be to allow and promote consideration of multiple criteria and broad perspective for interventions in space. Possible approach is explained in this study. However, the study offers just those solutions that correspond to current state of mind of users and overall awareness of public property in Serbia. Proposed interventions would bring progress in the healing process, but they present merely a starting point for comprehensive consideration.

In time, the orientation and focus towards the improvement can lead also to changes impossible in current moment, e.g. modern tendencies of integration of hospital open spaces into city public spaces that promote abolishing barriers allowing uninterrupted circulation of users. Under the right conditions, application of these tendencies would result in change of group of users and lead to change of perception of hospital open spaces – from places of distress, discomfort and concern to city public spaces that are positive, inviting and companionable.

Having in mind all facts presented in this study, we consider current approach to hospital environments development insufficiently considered and outdated, therefore inadequate for contemporary moment. Change of philosophy in this field is necessary to prevent hospital open spaces from being perceived as threatening and allow creation of healing environment for the benefits of users.

Notes

(1) City of Niš is administrative centre of Niš region, in southern part of Serbia, located on the river Nišava. City covers the area of approximately 600 km², including Niš, Niška Banja and 68 suburbs.

(2) Healthcare system of the Republic of Serbia is organized in three levels depending on the complexity of medical care to be provided to the patients:
- Primary healthcare level (health centres, pharmacies, and bureaus).
- Secondary healthcare level (general and specialized hospitals).
- Tertiary healthcare level (clinics, institutes, clinical-hospital centres and clinical centres).

Serbia has four clinical centres situated in the way to satisfy the needs of patients of the whole country: Clinical centre of Serbia in Belgrade, Clinical centre of Niš in Niš, Clinical centre of Vojvodina in Novi Sad and Clinical centre of Kragujevac in Kragujevac.

(3) City of Novi Sad is administrative centre of Autonomous province of Vojvodina, in northern part of Serbia, located on the river Danube. City covers the area of approximately 700 km², including the 15 suburban settlements at the territory of the city.

City of of Niš and City of Novi Sad are both positioned centrally in their regions providing easy accessibility to Clinical centre for all users from respective gravitating areas. Travelling time to Niš and Novi Sad from other cities from the gravitation areas is less than 2 hours by car. Access to the cities is possible by road, railway and waterway.

References

Nedučin, D., Krklješ, M. and Kurtović-Folić, N. (2010) "Hospital outdoor spaces-therapeutic benefits and design considerations", *Architecture and civil engineering*, Vol. 8, No. 3, pp.293-305.

Ulrich, RS. (1999), "Effects of gardens on health outcomes: Theory and research", In: Marcus, CC., Barnes, M., (Ed.) *Healing Gardens: Therapeutic Benefits and Design Recommendations*, John Wiley & Sons, New York: pp.27-86.

Ulrich, RS. (2000), "Evidence based environmental design for improving medical outcomes", *Proceedings of the Healing by Design: Buildings for Health Care in the 21st Century Conference*, Montreal, Quebec, Canada, March 1-10, 2000.

Ulrich, RS. (1984), "Benefits of nature: View from a hospital bed". *American Association for the Advancement of Science*; Vol. 224, p.420 (2).

Gimbel, T. (1994), *Healing With Color and Light*, A Fireside Book, Simon & Schulster, Inc. New York.

Reuben, A. (1983), *Color Therapy*, Aurora Press.

Kunders, GD. (2004), Hospitals: *Facility planning and management*, Tata MCGraw-Hill Publishing Company Limited.

Royal colleague of physicians of London (1998), *Disabled people using hospitals*, Lavenham Press Ltd, Lavenham, Sudbury, Suffolk.

Schweitzer, M., Gilpin, L. and Frampton, S. (1998), "Healing Spaces: Elements of Environmental Design That Make an Impact on Health", Mary Ann Liebert, Inc., *The journal of alternative and complementary medicine*, Vol. 10, Supplement 1, pp.S-71-S-83.

Topf, M. and Dillon, E. (1988) *Noise-induced stress as a predictor of burnout in critical care nurses*, Heart Lung, 17:567–574, PMID: 3417467.

Morrison, WE., Haas, EC. and Shaffner, DH. (2003) "Noise, stress, and annoyance in a paediatric intensive care unit", *Crit Care Med*, 31:113–119, PMID: 12545003.

Bayo, MV., Garcia, AM. and Garcia, A. (1995) "Noise levels in an urban hospital and workers' subjective responses", *Arch Environ Health*, 50:247–251, PMID: 7618959.

Aldridge D. (2003), "The therapeutic effects of music" in: Jonas W., Crawford C. (Ed.) *Healing Intentions and Energy Medicine*, Churchill Livingstone, Edinburgh, Vol. I/12, pp 151-174.

Ulrich, RS. (2004), "The role of the physical environment in the hospital of the 21st century: A once-in-a-lifetime opportunity", available at https://www.healthdesign.org/sites/default/files/Role%20Physical%20Environ%20in%20the%2021st%20Century%20Hospital_0.pdf (accessed 18 June 2014).

Clay RA. (2001) "Green is good for you", available at http://www.apa.org/monitor/apr01/greengood.aspx (accessed 20 June 2014).

Forbes, I. (2005) "Using Landscapes as Wellness Factor for Patient Therapy", available at http://www.designandhealth.com/uploaded/documents/Publications/Papers/Ian-Forbes-WCDH-2005.pdf (accessed 05 August 2014).

Cooper-Marcus C. (2000), "Gardens and health", available at http://www.designandhealth.com/uploaded/documents/Publications/Papers/Clare-Cooper-Marcus-WCDH2000.pdf (accessed 28 July 2014).

Astorino LD, (2003), "Enhancing the design process through visual metaphor", available at http://www.healthcaredesignmagazine.com/article/enhancing-design-process-through-visual-metaphor (accessed 15 June 2014).

University of Minnesota, Center for Spirituality and Healing and Charison Meadows, Kreitzer, MJ, "Healing environment", available at http://www.takingcharge.csh.umn.edu/explore-healing-practices/healing-environment (accessed 31 May 2014).

http://www.un.org/disabilities

www.GGHC.org

Republic of Serbia (2012), *Law on health protection*, Official gazette of the Republic of Serbia from 03.08.2012.

13

Analysis of some renovation projects indoor and outdoor.
Case study: Policlinico Umberto I of Rome, Italy

Rosalba Belibani and Martina Cardi

Abstract: This paper introducesthe Policlinico Umberto I, historical hospital of Rome, briefly illustrating its constructive history. The description mainly focuses on the original project analyzing, therefore, the pavilion type and the relation between indoor and outdoor spaces, deeply modified over the years. The growth of the hospital highlights its own critical issues and in this assay we propose some sustainable intervention strategies, justifying the theoretical and practical methodologies. In this paper are also analyzed some of the several renovation projects of the hospital, particularly focusing on the one regarding the re-functionalization of Pediatrics and Obstetrics Clinics, in which, actually, the architectural and planning problems are interfering with the healthcare service. Currently, the efficiency of the hospital is severely compromised by the continuous interaction between the two clinics and by the wrong manages of some units. The departments are, therefore, re-designed in every detail, considering the physical and psychological condition of the patients, the interaction between education and healthcare and the needs of the staff. We investigate also the tools for the design of green spaces pertaining to a hospital, in order to satisfy of an high quality of the hospital landscape. The contribution, overcoming the distinction between open and closed space, enters a broader formulation of the outdoor space, which become a place of social interaction and a design object, complementarily to the building.

Keywords: sustainable design, renovation project, hospital landscape, outdoor spaces.

Brief history of the pavilion hospital

When the pavilion model was designed for hospitals, now-common diseases were a scientific phenomena and so their classification, study and treatment lead to early specialisations, hence the arising of polyclinics and, consequently, the building type. From the experience of medieval xenodochias, in which contagious diseases still spread because of the promiscuity among patients, the arch. Filarete, during is first assignment on hospitals, designed the Ca 'Grande Hospital, which later became Maggiore Hospital, in Milan. It is one of the first geometric campuses and it is characterized by a large central courtyard with, at its side, quadrangles with secondary courtyards, and a church corresponding to the entrance axis. The design is also notable for its innovation in some technological aspects, such as the inclusion of copper canals for the collection of the waste from latrines, leading to an underlying duct, flushed with a constant supply of flowing water, then used for irrigation.

An important step in the typological and technological progress of the hospital type is marked by the reconstruction of the Hotel Dieu Hospital in Paris, destroyed by a fire in 1772. The design group, appointed by the Academy of Sciences in Paris after the event, revised the design criteria for the construction of hospitals and created a first model for hospitals with specific functional requirements, in order to respond to the new healthcare needs with architectural solutions that were scientifically substantiated.

The separation of the patients in independent pavilions had been already advocated in the middle of the eighteenth century by the Englishman John Howard, as a way to overcome the common and now problematic model of the hospital with unsegregated departments. Infact, the work done by that commission will have an unequivocal historical value thanks to the competence and the authority of each member involved and to the conclusions it reached, all for which we can say that the Academy of Sciences of Paris is the mother of the modern hospital.

The coordinator of the Commission's work, Tenon, talking about the motivational charge of the study of the new project said: "... *I think I have to make my remarks to preside over the anatomical and pathological knowledge.*

It is about man and sick man: his own rule, the length of the bed, the width of the stairs; his step less outstretched, less free than an healthy manone, gives the height of the steps, such as the length of the stretchers on which it is transported, determines the width of the hospital stairs..." (Tenon, Memoire sur les hospitaux, Paris 1788).

The design criteria behind the new pavilion model requires quantitative standards for the building complex and for the internal distribution, such as:
- Not more than 1200-1500 beds per hospital complex;
- Minimum distance between halls calculated as twice their height;
- Separate departments for men and women;
- Arrangement of beds in the wards into two rows, with a maximum number of 36 patients for each room;
- Presence in every ward of autonomous services (latrines, kitchens, nuns local and infirmaries);
- Windows extended up to the ceiling;
- Open and ventilated stairs.

The new hospital buildings constructed in Europe, therefore, follow the functional criteria formulated in Paris and, between 1839 and 1854, the first pavilion hospital was built; the Lariboisière Hospital.

The evolution of the hospital type, then, followed with the transition from the pavilion to the hospital block type, and the reason of this switch is rooted in new medical discoveries, as in all the previous typological and functional transformations. In fact the block type is seemingly more flexible than the architectural system made by independent pavilions, suggesting a new solution to the new healthcare demands. Like all the following architectures will answer to the new medical needs, the new type and all the others formal research that will come, will be required to not only meet new internal needs, but also the needs to identify the hospital building for its social relevance. The will also arises from the representation of health research at the social level that will lead, therefore, to the location of the building, often monumental, more closely related to the urban context. The structures, over the years, reached an unheard-of size and majesty, allowing designers to focus their attention on the aesthetics of the building rather than on the disposition of several buildings, and as in

Barcelona Plan Cerdà the hospital type confused in the city mesh.

In Italy the whole development process of the hospital architecture was incorporated after 1861, year of the Unification of the State. Meanwhile, Giordano and Ziino, two Italian hygienists, analysed the European experience in the Giordano's essay "DegliSpedali in Genere e dellaMaternità in particolare" (1876) where they described the 'Hospital City' as an 'aggregate of many buildings, possibly in the green, to be located in a large area adjacent to the city but separate from it', indications that seem to anticipate different realisations of the century, not least the one of the Policlinico Umberto I in Rome.

The large amount of studies on hospitals, widely publicized in the late nineteenth century, undoubtedly influenced the birth of the Policlinico Umberto I.

Guido Baccelli gave the decisive impulse in 1881, when he became Minister of Education, by convening a commission of experts to clarify the rules and the way to build a modern hospital in Rome, analysing the disciplines to include and the number of clinics to predict (Commission report of 1881). During his speech on the 16th of March of the same year, Baccelli describes his idea of the hospital in this way: "*...it is a scientific and practical institute, in which assemble sick men (...) is an institution in which the civil charity, in a happy union with medical-progressive science, works to the advantage of the most miserable people (...) thus harmonising education and care, science and philanthropy: here is the Polyclinic*".(Messinetti, Bartolucci, 2012)

In Rome, the dislocated placement of all the medical clinics throughout the city created considerable inconvenience to patients and students, forced into strenuous and time consuming travel from one side of the town to the opposite and, therefore, the idea was welcomed of joining them together in one unified complex with a single administrative direction, able to efficiently handle the needs of the several departments.

"*...and because of this concentration, the derelicts of fortune, those who with their suffering bodies offer subject to the student, ... will find in the Policlinico healthy shelter ... to their beds, as to princes', will rush the most distinguished scientists of the city; there they will animate a noble competition between them* *for their own and scientific benefit. These unhappy people will no longer, as is now the case, move from one hospital to another, with the danger of missing the street, before being rescued in any way"*.(Messinetti, Bartolucci, 2012)

In conclusion, January 19, 1888 in Rome, King Umberto I, the Queen Margherita and all the highest political and institutional state members attended the groundbreaking ceremony of the Policlinico Umberto I, hailed as "the greatest monument to charity and science."

The Policlinico Umberto I: from the original design to the current status

The area of the hospital was obviously chosen among the healthiest places in Rome, and is located in the center of the city, between San Lorenzo and Porta Pia, just outside the Aurelian walls. Originally the area devoted to the Polyclinic was in a location nearby Via di Porta Maggiore, but itwas later considered unsuitable because of the unfavourable road access already available to the area and for its size, which was much less than the site eventually chosen.

"....the shape is a quadrangle ... the view that can be enjoyed is one of the most enchanting of the Roman countryside; and the horizon is outlined by the picturesque chain of the Colli Albani and Monti della Sabina." (Messinetti, Bartolucci, 2012)

The project of the general hospital, inserted in the works financed by Law n° 209 of 14th of May, 1881, provided 500 beds for medicine, 400 beds for surgery and 350 beds for university hospitals. The general setting of the masterplan presents a large quadrangle divided by a central axis (for requirements such asadministrative spaces, hospitality, retreats of reports, kitchen, chapel, etc...) to the right of which there is an area dedicated to Medicine (medical clinics, preparatory, and pavilions),while on the left there is an area dedicated to Surgery (surgical clinics, ophthalmology and pavilions). The layout design is completed with pavilions arranged radially around the chapel of the hospital and some isolated clinics for those diseases requiring increased ventilation and green spaces. The whole area is surrounded on the main front on Viale del Policlinico by an iron railing leaning over a small concrete base and, on the other fronts, enclosed by retaining walls which, in correspondence with the location of the infectious diseases clinic, rise up to six meters fromstreet level. And it is this fence with the high gate that defines the boundary of the hospital; it contains and constitutes the border of the city. The perimeter of the body becomes a threshold not only conceptual but physical, unsuperable, between the hospital and the urban district that remains separate.(Fig.1)

Under the authoritative direction of the Architect GiulioPodesti, the construction works of the clinics began in September 1889 and ended on December 20th, 1896, because in 1897 both the design and the direction of the works went to Ing. Biglieri, engineer of the GenioCivile office, who was supposed to continue Podesti'sWork. He started work from the current status, by modifying the general distribution of the internal pavilions of the original system, designing a new pavilion type to be constructed on the second row parallel to that of the clinics overlooking Viale del Policlinico. Between 1900 and 1902, in fact, nine pavilions were built, seven on the same line of the first and two in the third line. The inclusion of the two pavilions in the third row altered the face of Viale dell'Università, a concern previously solved by Podesti by maintaining a similar external fascad eto that of Viale del Policlinico.

In 1903, the Ministry of Public Works delivered the constructed buildings of the complex to the Ministry of Education and to the Commission of the United Hospitals of Rome, and it was only in 1904 that the new hospital welcomed. The following building work, made in order to complete the original construction plan, greatly modified the Podesti original design and it was only in 1904 that the new hospital welcomed his first patients. Then, the constructive history of the complex went on through the building of the missing clinics: between 1912 and 1927, according to new projects and at a lower level than the original one, were built the Pediatric Clinic and Pathological Anatomy Clinic, which appear therefore more autonomous and detached from the complex; between 1927 and 1930, finally, were completed the buildings of Tropical Diseases, Medical Clinic V, Radiology, Technical Offices and Paediatric Pavilion.

The several modify made to the original plant designed by the Arch. Podesti lied to a distorted image of the hospital and after the numerous enlargement the volume rose from 300.000 to 800.000 cubic meters, including about 3000 beds. In fact the original coverage ratio, which was about 1/4 of the surface, increases considerably, distorting in some ways the design of open spaces, which automatically switched to the second level.

The Pavilion Type of the Policlinico Umberto I, unique in its kind, has two floors and the wards are built over an open porch, at an elevation of 7,80mtswhere air can circulate freely. The pavilion contains 18 beds, each one 3 meters away from the other, and has, in the back, an isolation room with 4 beds plus three individual isolation rooms for patients for which is equipped a medical center and separate services. The project incorporates the kind of historical hall, which has a floor plan, T in shape, the type of clinics designed by Podesti on the main front, with the tripartite division in a central area, with general services and classroom for lessons, and two side wings symmetrical intended to hospitalization.

"To experience the reasons that reflect the soil of Rome hygienists do not feel convenient to lay the infirmaries at the level of the natural terrain. Since then build a new hospital was to study a type of craft pavilion that matched those reasons."(Messinetti, Bartolucci, 2012).

To make easier the services of all the buildings that need to rely on the administration building, he conceived the idea to connect them through a tunnel, and precisely to connect with underground sections of masonry, and the infirmaries of the first floor through tunnels covered shelters in iron and crystal. The ground floor of each building remains so naturally connected from the area of tunnel that is established on the vault of the underlying traits masonry, with distance between buildings not exceeding mts. 30. It plans to build between a building and the other a simple iron footbridge consists of two strong girders, which are used to stop the parapet of the gallery itself at the first floor, supported by four cast iron columns. These are empty inside and they do pass, in winter and summer, the ventilation air from the basement below, so that will be placed on the first floor and then expelled from special fans located in the top of the cover.

The plant continues to undergo significant changes and the amount of works executed around 1945 is due, as a result of the war, the onset of problems of space and technological upgrading of facilities and services. The various changes on the historical artifacts are to be considered as autonomous responses, given in the absence of planning and coordination of the initiatives, also because of a lack of alternative proposals for localization of universities and health. They build volumes ex novo green spaces of the project, which are increasingly reduced, and when the useful surface is missing, one resorts to a rising phase with vertical elevations and replacement of coverages. This completes the distortion of logic composition with the proliferation of bodies added, accretions, employment and degradation of green spaces, particularly of the domestic courts to the halls.

Over time it becomes necessary to the program of building renovation of part of the buildings of the hospital, through a Plan Framework, launched and funded by Law 843 of 12.21.1978, emerged from the analysis of the status quo and by the criteria concreteness and organic. The program, which sees an agreement for the concession of the restructuring program does not exhaust the problem of functional restructuring of the hospital as a whole even if filled with dignity the most glaring deficiencies.

The many problems encountered in the centralization of services and revise the system to adapt to the current needs are still waiting for a solution, if it can not be total, can definitely start with the re-functionalization also part of some buildings, with their recovery functional and technological adaptation.

Contemporary research in the design of hospitals beyond the traditional sense typological skillfully combining the acquisitions of scientific research with the functionality, the devices bioclimatic with the intentions of the architectural language and communication.

Critical issues and possible strategies

Although, at the end of 19th century, the Policlinico Umberto I represented one of the most advanced medical facilities in the European scene, today the largest Roman hospital is inadequate to meet both theinternational standards imposed upon the hospitals and the space requirements of contemporary medicine. On one hand this is due to the huge scientific progress in the medical field during the 20th century, and on the other, is justified by the constructive history of the complex, which, since the end of World War II could barely continue with unified planning. The result was a distortion of the compositional logic already partly compromised, and the alteration of the original structure and layout of the site, proliferation of added bodies, raising of floors, filling, especially of the courtyards between the pavilions, and degradation of green spaces. Consequently some critical issues are today related to the complex and they belong mainly to two categories:
    1. Accessibility and relations with the urban context;
    2. Internal functionality and resulting efficiency of the healthcare service.

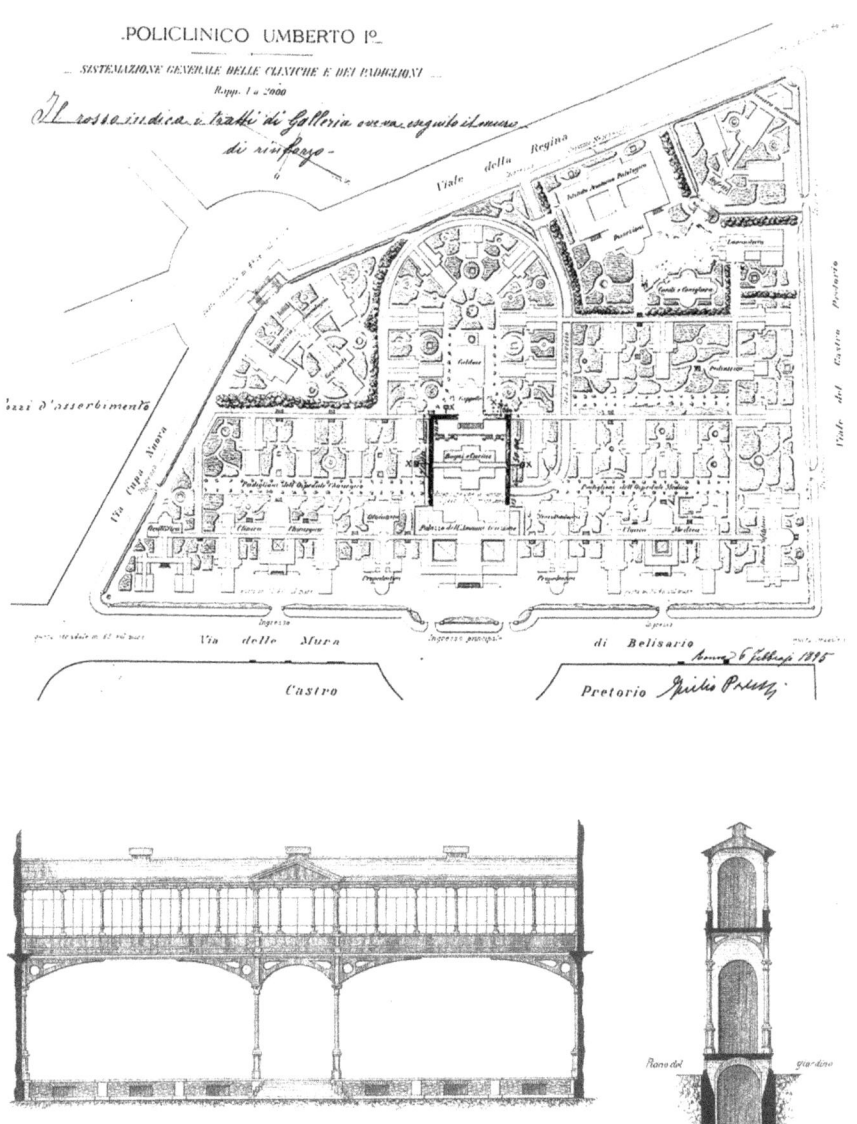

Figure 1: Policlinico Umberto I, original plant and section detail, by G. Podesti

Within the first, certainly falls the problem of the current segregation from the city. The hospital, since the beginning, has been an "introverted" place, enclosed in a boundary wall that restricts permeability with the surrounding urban context, in the same manner as with the adjacent Castro Pretorio and Sapienza University. The lack of navigational clarity when accessing and the absence of internal spaces of urban interest make the complex isolated and cut off from the urban texture, inhibiting integration with the city (despite the large amount of people that spend time in the complex every day, between staff, patients and visitors). Disorientation and a sense of bewilderment are common feelings in patients and visitors who are about to enter the hospital, increasing the feeling of distance between the hospital and the citizens. Another problem to be mentioned is the numerous enlargements and additions, which have altered the original facades and have contributed to clouding the monumental aspect, typical of nineteenth-century buildings, characteristic of the original design. Among the most representative facades is one on Viale del Policlinico, marked by a series of pavilions immersed in the green spaces of the grounds, now marred not only by mismanagement of the site but also by the presence of numerous parking areas at street level added over the years to make up for the lack of parking dedicated uniquely to the hospital. The parking lots, obviously subtracted accessibility and reduced the space dedicated to original green areas.

Within the second category, however, fallall issues related to programmatic, functional and architectural aspects that interfere with the health service, thus decreasing efficiency. The most significant of these issues is the lack of an overall project that provides the programming steps for interventions, restoration or demolition and new construction, which is the main cause of the continuous waste of resources, both economical and of the energy of the Polyclinic. Moreover, the red tape associated with this kind of operation in Italy, further burdened by the presence of constraints imposed by the *Superintendence of Cultural Heritage of Rome* to the entire complex, is one of the main causes of the current condition of the healthcare service. By addressing the design of a unified project for the renewal of the hospital, we have unavoidably to deal with the pavilion template, which is a widely utilized model of healthcare architecture, and that, in this particular case, can only be improved and never entirely overturned. As it is based on the old principle of hospitalisation differentiated by pathology, the design causes dispersion between the numerous pavilions of all the highly technological functions, which in contemporary hospitals are generally enclosed in one area named "technology block", featuring operating rooms, intensive care units, diagnostics and services related to the hospitalisation. Currently they are still distributed throughout the different specialist clinics, despite numerous attempts towards centralisation made over the last few years, with a great deal of strain on space and energy demands.

The great challenge for the Policlinico Umberto I, for which the possibility of relocation to urban level was never officially considered thanks to the privileged position it enjoys in infrastructure and the large catchment area that it currently covers, is to succeed, despite the unfavorable typology, to meet the needs of healthcare today. The intervention strategies that can be expected to achieve this ambitious goal concern both critical areas abovementioned.

Among the first steps needed, is the improvement of accessibility, meaning the ability of the hospital to be easily navigated and enjoyed by patients and visitors, thus facilitating the identification of the main entrances, both emergency and pedestrian, and positioning of signage to decrease the sense of bewilderment linked with the approach to the structure. Following this is the planning of a parking lot in an exclusive domain of the complex, in order to improve the architectural and urban quality of Viale del Policlinico, facilitate parking for health staff to allow easy access to their workplace, and help visitors or patients who need to park temporarily. Moreover, to give back identity to such a historical hospital, it will be necessary to eliminate all measures deemed inadequate on four fronts in order to restore the original monumental character, especially to the one on Viale del Policlinico. Among the strategies that are indicated to improve the internal functionality and efficiency of the health service, is certainly the design of a centralsquare, open to the public, within the perimeter. It must be seen as an area that gives recognition to the complex, which aids with orientation inside the pavilions, thus increasing the usability of the hospital for staff, visitors and patients and, in turn, opening the Policlinico Umberto I 'citadel' to the city of Rome through the insertion of commercial functions including a library, temporary exhibition hall, restaurant and bar. It will also be necessary to review the whole functional distribution of the hospital, by providing the "technology block", possibly in a central location, and with links to the current wards, with constant attention to the flexibility that today must be a core principle to a hospital building. Consequently it will be necessary to assign a new function to the areas that will be left unused, as a result of the centralisation of functions in the technology block, for which it is inconceivable not to provide a unified project of restoration. Finally, the elimination of superfluous additions and a return to the original layout, and therefore the redevelopment of green spaces, which return livability and quality to the outdoor spaces. In parallel to the whole process described, will always be consideration for the aspects relating to the improvement of the spaces dedicated to teaching and their integration with the care services; the economical feasibility studies; and the inclusion of devices for the reduction of energy requirements.

Some redevelopment projects

The hospital, thanks to its importance in both healthcare and the historical-artistic Roman landscape, hasover the last few years been the subject of a great number of projects, not always realised, for the redevelopment of the whole complex or of some of its pavilions. Among them, in the year 2000, the "Plan of the renovation of the architectural and urban plant of the Policlinico Umberto I in Rome" commissioned by the hospital to the ITACA Department (Innovazione Tecnologica nell'Architettura e Cultura dell'Ambiente) of the Architectural Faculty of the Sapienza University of Rome, aimed to entirely renew the structure of the hospital complex with the main intention to open the hospital to the city, outlining several main elements of the proposal. These are: the system of the original buildings, the Agora, the system of the inpatient pavilions, the system of the great technologies, the system of isolated buildings in the park. The main idea is to create a central square, the Agora, as the heart of a continuous architectural element that joins the front facades of all the impatient halls of the hospital, connecting the empty spaces existing between them. This new wall, starting from the entrance on Via Lancisi, covers the whole area up untilVialedell'Università, at the site of the Urological Clinic. This element on one hand faces the courts restored between the back of the inpatient halls, and on the other hand overlooks the central area of the complex which will host the new "system of great technologies," following two hypotheses, which have in common the idea of opening up to the front of Viale Regina Elena. In the first case the technology block is placed in the basement (corresponding to the current ground level) and glass elements emerge to give light to the underlying operating rooms and diagnostic spaces. The second hypothesis can be considered an extension of the first one, as the only block of operating rooms is based on the previous system and connected by walkways to the new connecting front of the pavilions. The systems of the entrances, of the parking lots and of the green a reorganised accordingly, with specific attention to the study of tree species to be included within the complex. The project has never been realised.

In 2008 the company of Policlinico Umberto I announced an international design competition for the renovation and expansion of the hospital compound. The winner of the competition was *RTI Ove Arup & Partners International Limited*, in collaboration with other companies. The project proposal essentially calls for the demolition of pavilions 1, 2, 3, 4, 5 and 6, and of the Finance Building, replacing them with modern pavilions linked together, creating a strong spatial relation with the opposite clinics of Viale Regina Elena. The row of new halls is designed behind the clinics overlooking the Viale del Policlinico, which remains unchanged due to being bound by Superintendence of Cultural Heritage of Rome. The new building includes, at ground level, all the functions of admissions, outpatients and emergencies; on the first floor, services and department facilities; and from the second up to the fifth floor, the centralised surgical block, intensive and sub-intensive care units, and all the inpatient wards. Vertical connections are planned in each of the new pavilions and there is a differentiation of the paths and entrances decided by type of user in order to rationalise the flow of movement. For this master-plan for all 15 hectares of the general hospital, there are five stages of demolition over two and a half years, in order to allow the health service to continue its activities in the health facility. The project involves a decrease in the existing volume, from 270 to 240 thousand square meters, and the freed spaces will be converted in new green areas and will be used by both the university and hospital. This project, which had been scheduled to start in 2009 and finish in 2012, was never built. (Fig.2)

A further feasibility study on the Policlinico Umberto I was conducted in agreement with the hospital by the Department of Architecture and Urban Planning for Engineering of the University of Study of Rome, specifically by a research team headed by prof. ing. Gianfranco Carrara, full professor at the Faculty of Technical Architecture. The aim of the research was the development of a proposal for a Preliminary Design Document, which, rather than aspire to a configuration design of the new building to plan, wants to provide a methodological information basis as a start point for the redesign of the hospital. It therefore analyses more deeply some legal, economic and technicalaspects, identifying possible demolition within the complex in relation to the historical and artistic value of each pavilion and the possibility to maintain thefoundations of some pavilions for the construction of a new block, thus avoiding unexpected, delay-causing discoveries of archaeological finds, so probable in the Roman underground. The proposal of this research group, after a long preliminary analysis phase, consists of the creation of a new building of 31,000 square meters (according to the financial resources of the hospital) on the foundations of the current Tropical Diseases and Medical V Clinics. Their demolition is allowed, in fact, by the low level of historical and conservation quality of existing architecture and the opportunity to transfer somewhere else the few functions left in them after centralisation of the services. The new technology block, square in shape, includes within it the services for the upgrading of the DEA (Department of Emergency and Admittance) as well as radiology, endoscopy, a surgical unit with twenty operating theatres, an intensive care area with thirty-five beds, and an area designed to accommodate units of short-term and ordinary inpatients. This project was also never realised, but it is certainly a thorough starting point for anyone who wants to try their hand in the redevelopment of the hospital complex.

Some other projects, at a smaller scale, have been made over the recent years to improve the condition of some individual clinics and to reactivate inoperative or partlyunusable departments. Among the various noteworthyproposals stands out the project for the new Department of Paediatric Nephrology and Gastroenterology, carried out byStudio Schiattarella& Associates, which was inaugurated in May 2009. The project represents a landmark in the search for new forms of expression, alternative to the established image of the therapeutic space, and new ways of interaction between hospitals and patients, and has as its main objective the achievement of the highest quality of humanisationand psychophysical comfort for children and their families. Young patients are the main actors of the new space and they leave the hospital after an experience characterized by the discovery of howlights and colourscan positively affect the humor duringhospitalization.In the original department patient rooms, small and without bathrooms, onefollowed the next connected by glass corridors that prevented privacy and resulted in a jumble of people forced to promiscuity, whereas the new plan provides rooms equipped with large windows letting in natural light, but where privacy is guaranteed by a systemof curtains and films that protect from internal introspection. There is attention by the designers focusing mainly on the lighting design issues,which are totally integrated with architectural ones, to create a colourful environment that stimulates the imagination and fantasy of the children, and in which the light works as a therapeutic support.

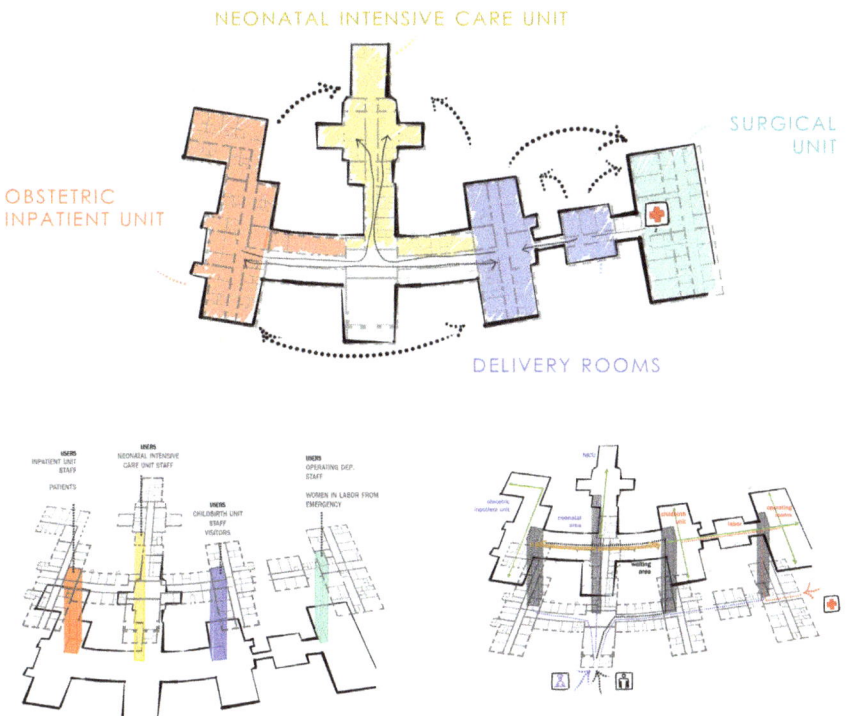

Figure 2: Policlinico Umberto I competition, render, by RTI Ove Arup & Partners International Limited

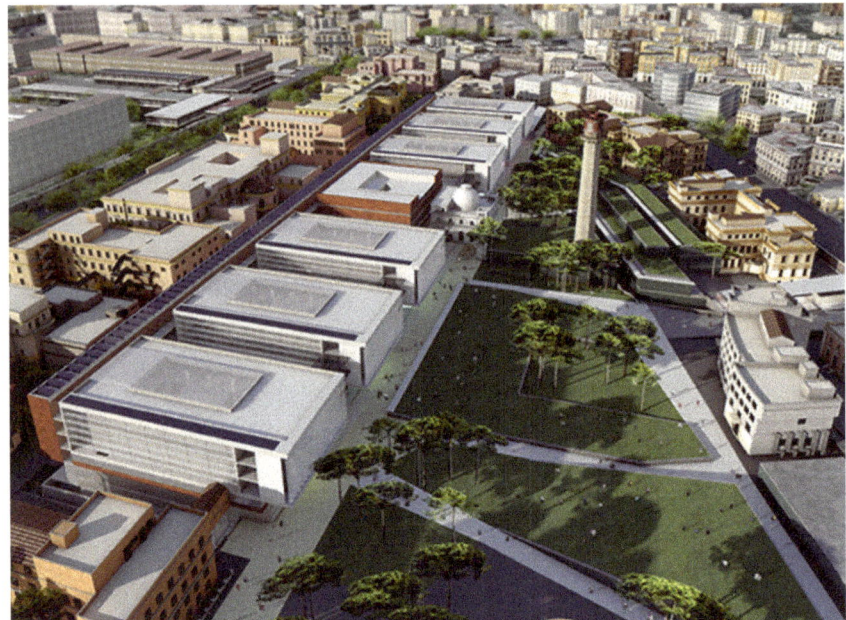

Figure 3: Gynaecologic-Obstetric Clinics, functional schemes and routes, by Martina Cardi

The new functional design of the Paediatric and Gynaecologic-Obstetric Clinics

Among the architectural projects concerning the PoliclinicoUmberto I, we suggestthe master's degree design made by Martina Cardi, supervised byprof. arch. RosalbaBelibani, both authors of this paper. The design only addressesthe renovation of two clinics, namelyPaediatrics and Gynecology-Obstetrics. It was assumed to bemore sustainable and economically affordable to re-functionalise these two buildings alone, as single units, self-consistent and related to each other, than providing a global project for the whole complex.The two clinics, since the time of the original project, represent a nearly independent pole of the hospital, which contains within it all the services pertaining to this medical area such as operating rooms, intensive care units and related services, making hardly any reference to centralised systems. Over the years, lots of departments inside the clinics stopped operating due to uninhabitability or for lack of staff owing to the economic crisis and this left huge, empty spaces within the pavilions. But, while in paediatrics this process was followed by an extension of some units in these spaces, in the gynecological-obstetric clinic the percentage of currently unused spaces is actually equal to 30% of the area of the entire clinic. The basic premise of the thesis design is therefore for the redistribution of internal functions for the two clinics, which currently share some units without adequate connective accessibility between them. Currently, the functionality of this wing of the hospital complex is severely compromised by the continuous need for interaction between them and clearly this represents an issue, most of all in the case of emergencies. An example of this matter is the path of Paediatric Emergency: This path is interrupted in the event of an imminent need of operating rooms as the department of paediatric surgery inside the Paediatric Pavilion is currently inactive due to the facilities having been deemedinadequate and so operating rooms are 'borrowed' in the Urology Clinic, located over 300 meters away. This discontinuity greatly decreases the efficiency of the structure and increases the risk of infant mortality in emergencies. In fact, increasing this risk further,are both the pathleading to the operating rooms, and the route of return, in which the post-operative child is in a delicate state of health and is not ready to face the environmental conditions of open air or of the underground pathways. The status of the project will therefore inevitably reactivate the Department of Paediatric Surgery, resulting in restoring safety to the Emergency path. Similar to the case above is the obstetric emergency route which, in this case, is interrupted by the splitting of the Neonatal Intensive Care Unit into two separate units, one inside paediatrics and the other one in Gynecology-Obstetrics. The two clinics, however, are on split levels andbarely connected via underground paths, even in this case of about 300m. The problem therefore lies in the need to take such a long route in the event of the birth of an infant with immediate need of care in the NICU. In such unstable conditions, the newborn is currentlyforced to be taken through underground paths, or over-ground by Ambulance (removing the vehicle fromEmergency urban service in the city of Rome) to finally reach the NICU inside paediatrics. In this case, the project will therefore restore the safety of the maternity unit through the placement of the Neonatal Intensive Care Unit entirely within the Gynecology-Obstetrics clinic, expanding it enough to include the number of beds currently located in Paediatrics.

The decision to deepen the internal design of the maternity unitinside this clinic is the result of the process of analysis described above. Between the two clinics, it was considered more necessary to intervene in Gynaecological-Obstetrics because the current condition of this structure is significantly more disadvantaged than paediatrics, which in recent years has been the subject of a series of projects of redevelopment, including the new Emergency Department and the Department of Paediatric Nephrology and Gastroenterology aforementioned.The clinicwas built between 1893-1897with few changes compared to the Podesti's original project. The elaboration of the project of this clinic has been the subject of particular attention to the need to place new mothers, pregnant women and infants in an environment as safe and healthy as possible.The original three buildings

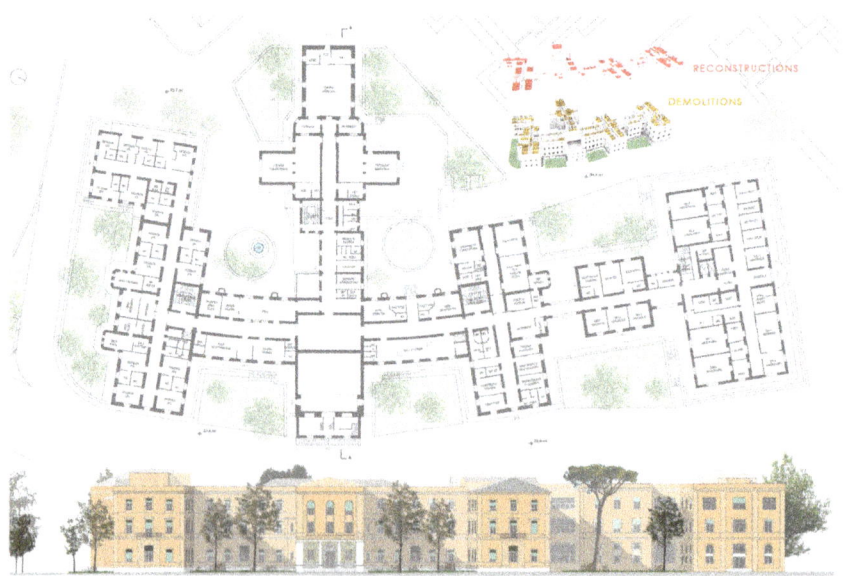

Figure 4: Gynaecologic-Obstetric Clinics, second floor plan and façade by Martina Cardi

presented in the main atrium porch with columns and pilasters of the Tuscan order, originally crowned by a pediment decorated with stucco later removed. In the post-war years, the site has lost the central symmetry due to the addition of two appendices, and a fourth building.(Fig.4)

During the redistribution of functions, the maternity unit was placed entirely on the second floor of the clinic, and it is on this level that the planning section of the thesis focuses on. On this level is a spatial discontinuity characterised by an open terrace at the lower levels of the atria. The first operation to restore the functionality of the whole plan is to remove the gap and close the terrace, using the lower floor of the mezzanine as decking and building a new ceiling closure of the atrium. Subsequently, we proceeded to the location of the four departments making up the maternity unit: the surgery department, delivery rooms, the NICU and the obstetrics inpatient ward. The path was chosento be horizontal, across the 2nd floor, a plan particularly suited to the shape of the clinic, leveraging secondarily a vertical plan, which would necessitate the use of elevators and stretchers. With this principle as the basis of the design, next came the arrangement between the four wards that make up the maternity unit,paying special attention to the relationship between them, and between the spatial configuration of the wings of the structure, without neglecting the position of Emergency Obstetrics, crucial to ensure efficiency at that location. Indeed the emergency path leads to an intermediate zone, located between the delivery rooms and operating theatre, ensuring that there is quick access in case of emergencies both with natural births and those requiring surgery. Next to the delivery room is the Neonatal Intensive Care Unit, extended, compared to the original one, to allow safe transfer of premature infants or those in unstable conditions. Adjacent to this is the obstetrics in-patient unit, which shares with the NICU the newborn observation area.The in-patients department has a rooming-in service, recommended by experts to foster a good relationship between the new mother and baby and prolong the period of lactation, as well as some single rooms reserved for more complex or unsuccessful cases, and a room dedicated to sharing the stage of lactation, with other mothers and relatives. Also included is a waiting room, in a central position between the delivery rooms, the NICU and the ward, which enjoys an independent lift to ensure that the central corridors are free to facilitate travel in cases of emergency. The vertical path is differentiated by type of user, and the study of flows from the floors below allows for increased efficiency of travel within the plan, increasing the feeling for medical staff and patients of being in a controlled and structured environment (Fig.4).

After defining the structure of the maternity unit, the last phase was a more in-depth study of each of the four units following the same process methodology. In fact, each of them has been designed primarily taking into account regulatory standards related to the specificity of each department, and then the criteria of technological innovation, humanisation and choice of colour. To have the elements to be able to design a therapeutic environment appropriate for the activities of each department, the study has thoroughly examined the physical and psychological status linked to any type of user, from pregnant women, new mothers, infants, to members of the hospital staff, and occasional visitors. The operating department features a relaxation room for surgeons and anesthesiologists, a telecommunications system allowing students to follow the action from a neighbouring room, external to the department, and a communication system whereby relatives in the waiting room are able to be updated on the surgical proceedings. These measures are intended to minimize any contamination due to the continuous entry and exit from the ward, often without passing through the appropriate washing steps (Fig.5). The delivery unit design includes a therapeutic environment that supports the woman during the acute pain related to childbirth. This area is painted and decorated predominantly with the colour blue, in addition to the use of natural imagery, which is thought to help the woman to relax and encourage the dilation phase during labour and childbirth. The labour rooms are private, so that the mother feels free to express pain without inhibition, and are equipped with all the necessary facilities to allow her to deal with said pain, such as a pilates ball and mat. In addition, one delivery room will contain a birth pool should any expecting mothers wish to choose this method. For obvious reasons a specific system of acoustic insulation is to be expected, to help staff to reduce work-related stress, as well as patients and visitors (Fig.6). In the case

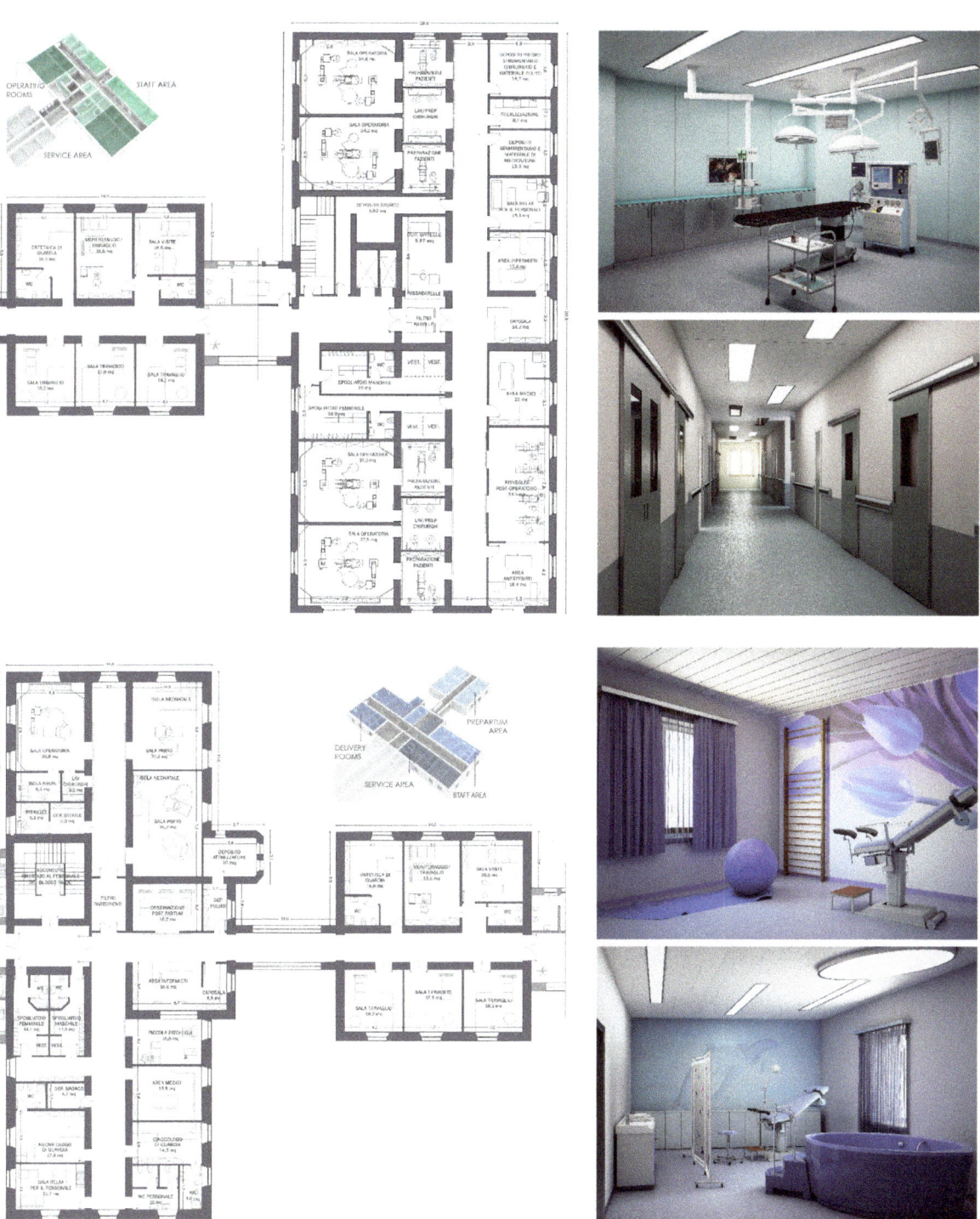

Figure 5-6: Surgery Unit and Birth Unit, plan and renders, by Martina Cardi

of the NICU, the main objective of the design is to encourage and assist the staff of the department with the arduous task of observing and caring for newborns 24 hours a day. This is achieved by placing workstations in a central position within the halls of the ICU. The choice of the colour beige was made, taking into account the high reflectivity of the skin of a newborn child, which, surrounded by any more vibrant a pigmentation, would alter his appearance and,therefore, the diagnosis resulting from a visual examination. Furthermore, the high sensitivity of the retina of newborns has necessitated the inclusion of a system of low overall lighting, with additional lamps for examining a child in its cot without disturbing surrounding newborns.

The design aspects of the redevelopment of the relationship between the exteriors and interiors

The space in front of an hospital always conveys the feeling of belonging to the hospital itself, regardless of the type and of the specific building. It is an area of absolute pertinence, defined in this way by the design, as a form of respect - or fear - toward the institution which is providing it. It frequently appears as a not designed space which, therefore, is not easily perceived as a place of mediation with the features and the sense of semi-private space, as it should be. It is a private hospital area that belongs to its users only when they enter it, and this matter would not be regrettable if, in fact, the user could enjoy it for personal use or if the patient could have the possibility to use it also for therapeutic purposes. The design of outer space is often conceived as a natural consequence of the building type and it has no ambitions: it does not reflect a careful study of the landscaping and functional intentions.

The dialogue between the city, with its urban fabric, and the complex of the Policlinico Umberto I, with its typological features, is interrupted. Even thought the original design contemplate this relation, even only in a formal way, actually the complex no longer communicates with the urban context because of the distortion, widely described above, of the original setting. The undifferentiated growth of both the city and the hospital, misrepresented their relation and the complex actually belong to the city only by perceptive custom. Neither the hospital and consequently nor its green spaces seems to belong to the city, so it happens to be an exclusive, bad quality pertinence of the hospital. Unfortunately, the current green spaces status have no longer the grace of the parterre represented in some original drawings with an institutional finality. It lost, over the years, its function as comforting and pleasant place where to rest, and actually the few free spaces are wild vacant spaces between the parked cars and the buildings.

It is necessary, therefore, to provide some tools and methods for the design of hospital green spaces. The aim is to define the main quality criteria for an hospital facility, selecting indications and methods to satisfy the objectives. The contribution must be centered on the study of the full and empty spaces connections, overcoming the customary distinction between open and enclosed spaces, entering into a broader and more heterogeneous interpretation of the outer space as a place of social interaction at different levels, to be designed along with the building. The methodological difference is in the transition from the objective and environmental parameters and to phenomenological interpretation, the individual perception of the formal aspects and well-being state. An important aspect in the design of the hospital landscape, bounded to the perception, and also on the design of new complex, is the role of the natural elements, especially in the mediation with the surroundings.

The whole body of the hospital, currently, needs more "green" and even the accessibility provided by the green spaces. In a project of re-functionalization, as well as the internal restructuring matters, the aspects of the green design play a crucial role. They mostly concern:

- The edge of the area of relevance of the hospital, that is the threshold with the urban context;
- The areas dedicated to the entraces;
- The open spaces adjacent to the halls and clinics;
- The inner courtyards;
- The small pertaining areas;
- The green walls;
- The green roofs.

As an unavoidable aspect of the renovation project is the definition of new areas, with their duties and delineate boundaries, interactions. The design of outdoor spaces, both in the case of new construction and recovery, as in the case of the Policlinico Umberto I, therefore, has to be defined in its intentions about highlights, communicability and, why not, therapeutic function. Each space, although segmented, through the use of special plants and flowers, specifically chosen, may have a dedicated function to entertain and comfort (if it provides comfortable seating in the free spaces), and even have a therapeutic function, because, such is known, the use of the color of the flowers - and sometimes their scent - in as a treatment for certain diseases. The color, moreover, is scientifically used in the interior spaces as treatment of the floors and walls, so it can be used as well in the outdoor spaces to increase great perceptions and the sense of well-being (Fig.7).

The use of a grassy meadow may facilitate the perception of the entrances, cancel the thresholds; a great design of flowerbeds and hedges will let the possibility to enjoy the facing from the upper floors; some deciduous essences will favor shade and oxygenation in the summer, and solar radiation in winter; green walls will improve the microclimate and adorn walls without architectural quality allowing the construction of backdrops; green roofs could provide additional walking areas and entertainment as well as mitigate temperatures and noise in the spaces below.

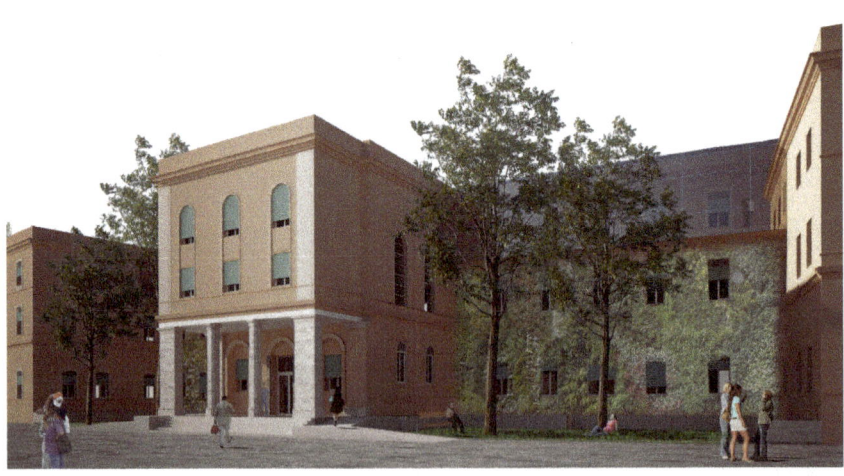

Figure 7: Gynaecologic-Obstetric Clinics entrance, façade and green wall, by Martina Cardi

References

Carrara, G. (2006), *Metodi e tecniche di approccio per la riqualificazione di un policlinico universitario. Il caso del Policlinico Umberto I di Roma*, Palombi & Partner srl, Roma.

Del Nord, R. (2006), *Lo stress ambientale nel progetto dell'ospedale pediatrico. Indirizzi tecnici e suggestioni architettoniche*, Motta Editore, Milano.

Dincer, I., Midilli A., Kucuk, H. (2014), *Progress in Sustainable Energy Technologies Vol II CreatingSustainable Development*, Springer International Publishing, Switzerland.

Dipartimento ITACA, Innovazione Tecnologica nell'Architettura e Cultura dell'Ambiente, (2000), *Piano di ristrutturazione del sistema urbanistico e edilizio del Policlinico Umberto I*, Gangemi Editore, Roma.

Felli, P., Laurìa, A. (2006), *La casa di maternità: una struttura sociale per il parto fisiologico. Linee guida per la progettazione*, Edizioni ETS, Pisa.

Fondi, D. (2002), *Architettura per la sanità. Forma, funzione e tecnologia*, Edizioni Kappa, Roma.

La Franca, G. (2010), "Luce e colore. Ristrutturazione all'Umberto I", *Progettare per la sanità*, Vol. Luglio 2010, pp.30-35.

Messinetti, S., Bartolucci, P. (2012), *Il Policlinico Umberto I di Roma nella storia dello stato unitario italiano*, Istituto Poligrafico e Zecca dello Stato, Roma.

Serarcangeli, C. (a cura di), (2006), *Il Policlinico Umberto I. Un secolo di storia*, Casa Editrice Università La Sapienza, Roma.

AA. VV. (2009), *Concorso internazionale di progettazione per la riorganizzazione e la ristrutturazione del Policlinico Umberto I*, Casa Editrice Università La Sapienza, Roma.

Editors

Francesca Giofrè (1968). Architect, PhD in Technology of Architecture, full time Associate Professor at the Faculty of Architecture of Sapienza University of Rome, Department Planning, Design, Technology of Architecture. She teaches Technology of Architecture since 2004. Since 1995 she has carried research and consultancy work through the University and other institutions national and international. Her research areas are mainly: innovation in design process, regarding planning, the focus is placed on studying and crafting new tools helping the operators of the building process in the decision-making; innovation in construction process; design for all, the research activities within this area build on the analysis of the needs of people in order to find architectural and technological solutions in different context which can provide all with equal opportunities. She has published various papers, articles and books and she made many feasibility design studies in the field of architecture for health. She has been Member of Teachers College PhD in "Regeneration and recovery of the settlements" (2004-10); since 2013 she is member of the Teachers College PhD "Engineering-based Architecture and Urban Planning". Teaching co-ordinator, member of scientific board and teacher of the II level Master in Architecture for Health for architects and engineers comes from Developing and emerging countries (since 2004). From 2014 she is director of the Master in Architecture for Health. Since 2004, she is member of Interuniversity Research Centre TESIS, Systems and technologies for health care buildings. She has different responsibilities inside the Faculty and the Department. Since 2015 vice – dean at the Faculty of Architecture, Sapienza University of Rome and delegate for Extra UE International cooperation. She has the scientific responsibility of executive agreements with foreign Faculties of Architecture (Belgrade, Sarajevo, Ethiopia, Guatemala, Mozambique, Paraguay, etc.).

Zoran Đukanović (1962). Architect, Assistant Professor at the University of Belgrade, Faculty of Architecture, Department of Urbanism, since 1992. He teaches at several courses of urban spaces, town and spatial planning. He was a leader of several national and international workshops. He is the founder of the international, interdisciplinary, scientific, research and educational Program "Public Art and Public Space" at Faculty of Architecture, University of Belgrade. Also, he teaches at the University of Belgrade, Faculty of Forestry, Department of Landscape Architecture and Horticulture. He has been mentoring at the interdisciplinary master postgraduate studies for "Stage Design" at the University of Arts in Belgrade. In the course of several past years, his field of interest has been gradually shifted to the domain of planning and designing of public urban space, art in public urban space, urban management, and participative work with the local community. He realized and managed several significant projects, implemented with the support of many national and local institutions. He took part in the realization of several spatial plans, master plans and regulation plans for many cities in Serbia. He was member of consulting and advisory bodies as well as planning committees, in many Serbian citie's territories; cooperates with several academic institutions from the EU, SAD and far East. He took part in several research projects of town planning, architecture, urban design and public art and numerous scientific/expert conferences, as well. His recent research books include Urbophilia (2007, University of Belgrade, with Radović); Placemaking (2008, University of Belgrade, with Živković); Belgrade Fortress – Dream Book of White Town's Continuity (2009, P.E. Belgrade Fortress, with Andrić); Art in Public Space (2011, Academica, with Živković, Bobić, Vuković, Đerić); VinoGrad / The Art of Wine (2015, University of Belgrade, with Živković) and other.

Authors

Rosalba Belibani. Architect, PhD in Architectural Composition and Theory of Architecture, is a researcher and professor of Architectural Design at the Faculty of Architecture, Sapienza University of Rome, with skills on sustainable design and environmental education.

Nađa Beretić. Msc of Landscape architecture and Urbanism and Regional Development Planning. PhD student at the Department of Architecture, Design and Urbanism in Alghero, University of Sassari. She is program and production coordinator of Public Art & Public Space program.

Ružica Božović Stamenović. Architect. Phd, Associate professor of design, University of Belgrade and National University of Singapore. Her main research interests deal with human ecology and relations of design and health in contemporary urban spaces.

Martina Cardi. Architect, has been interested in the renovation of the Policlinico Umberto I in Rome since her thesis project, for which she received some recognitions. Actually she lives and works in London, where she deals with healthcare architecture.

Rosalba D'Onofrio. PhD, researcher in Urban Planning at the School of Architecture and Design "E. Vittoria", University of Camerino. She conducts researches in the field of Regional Planning and Landscape and Urban Sustainability.

Anna Maria Giovenale. Architect, PhD, full professor at Sapienza University of Rome, Department Planning, Design, Technology of Architecture. Dean of the Faculty of Architecture. Her main research interests deal with planning and architecture of healthcare services.

Vesna Mandić. Architect from Belgrade, Serbia. She has a Master in Architecture for Health, Sapienza University of Rome. Employed in Mace d.o.o. as Health Facility Specialist of Ministry of Health of the Republic of Serbia for the Project of Reconstruction of four Clinical centers in Serbia.

Ivana Miletić. Architect, graduated at Faculty of Architecture, University of Belgrade. Msc of Architecture for Health and the PhD in Technology of architecture, Sapienza University of Rome, Faculty of Architecture; she discussed a thesis on Re-development and Recovery in Situ. She works in Italy as an architect specialist in social housing and healthcare design.

Valentina Napoli. Architect, PhD student in Environmental Design, Department Planning Design Technology of Architecture, Sapienza University of Rome. She is carrying out a research on "Transitional space between healthcare facilities and city".

Giuseppe Primiceri. Architect, PhD in Technology of Architecture. He has collaborated to many researches with the Department Planning Design Technology of Architecture, Sapienza University of Rome. Expert in healthcare design.

Fabio Quici. Architect, PhD Research Professor in the Department of History, Drawing and Restoration of Architecture, Faculty of Architecture of Sapienza University of Rome. His research fields: Architectural Drawing, Visual Studies, Urban Regeneration, Contemporary Architecture.

Tamara Stanisavljević. Architect from Belgrade, Serbia. Master in Healthcare Design, Sapienza University of Rome. Employed in Belgrade office of Steam S.r.l., as Project coordinator for the Project of Reconstruction of four Clinical centers in Serbia, financed by the Ministry of Health of the Republic of Serbia.

Ferdianando Terranova. Full professor, Sapienza University of Rome, Faculty of Architecture (retired from 2010). Him main research interests deal with the planning of healthcare system and the effect of technological innovation on the healthcare design.

Elio Trusiani. Architect, PhD associate professor of Urban Planning. His activity regards urban renewal for historical/contemporary/informal city, landscape planning and cultural heritage/landscape.

www.ingramcontent.com/pod-product-compliance
Lightning Source LLC
Chambersburg PA
CBHW061934290426
44113CB00025B/2911